Cardiac Mechanical Assistance Beyond Balloon Pumping

Susan J. Quaal, PhD, RN, CVS, CCRN

Fellow, Council on Cardiovascular Nursing
Associate Clinical Professor
University of Utah Health Sciences
Cardiovascular Clinical Specialist
Department of Veterans Affairs Medical Center
Salt Lake City, Utah

with 125 illustrations

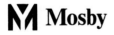 Mosby

St. Louis Baltimore Boston Chicago London Philadelphia Sydney Toronto

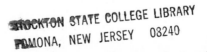

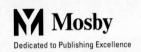

Dedicated to Publishing Excellence

Editor: Robin Carter
Editorial Assistant: Chris Kuehne
Project Manager: John Rogers
Production Editor: Chuck Furgason
Designer: Susan Lane

Printed in the United States of America

Mosby–Year Book, Inc.
11830 Westline Industrial Drive
St. Louis, Missouri 63146

Library of Congress Cataloging in Publication Data

Cardiac mechanical assistance beyond balloon pumping / [edited by]
    Susan J. Quaal.–1st ed.
        p.   cm.
    Includes bibliographical references and index.
    ISBN 0-8016-6442-X
    1. Heart, Mechanical.   I. Quaal, Susan J.
    [DNLM: 1. Heart-Assist Devices.   WG 168 C2663]
    RD598.35.M42C37   1992
    617.4'120592–dc20
    DNLM/DLC
    for Library of Congress   92-25096
                                                                CIP

93 94 95 96 97   UG/MV   9 8 7 6 5 4 3 2 1

Contributors

Nancy Abou-Awdi, RN, MS, CCRN
Clinical Research Coordinator
Cullen Cardiovascular Research Laboratory
Texas Heart Institute
Houston, Texas

Abhijit Acharya, PhD
Director, Division of Cardiovascular, Respiratory,
 and Neurological Devices
Office of Device Evaluation
Center for Devices and Radiological Health
Rockville, Maryland

Kazuhiko Atsumi, MD
Professor, Nihon University School of Medicine
Tokyo, Japan

Ronald N. Barbie, MD
Cardiothoracic Surgeon
Humana Heart Institute International
Louisville, Kentucky

Lawrence E. Barker, RN
Perfusionist
Psicor, Inc.
Honolulu, Hawaii

Terry K. Bavin, RN, MN
Cardiovascular Nursing and Critical Care Clinical Instructor
Fresno Community Hospital & Medical Center
Fresno, California

†Jean-Pierre Brugger
Cardiovascular Research Institute (IRCV)
Sion, Switzerland

Ray C.- J. Chiu, MD, PhD
Professor of Surgery
McGill University
Quebec, Canada

†Deceased.

Marilyn Cleavinger, MSBME
Assistant Director, Artificial Heart Lab
University Medical Center
Tucson, Arizona

Sheldon E. Cohen, MD, FACS
Chairman, Cardiothoracic Surgery
Fresno Community Hospital & Medical Center
Fresno, California

Chris L. Coleman, MD
Research Associate Professor
Baylor College of Medicine
Houston, Texas

Marguerite Corda, RN, MSN, CCRN
Clinical Nurse Specialist
Open Heart Unit
Maimonides Medical Center
Brooklyn, New York

J.N. Cunningham Jr., MD
Chairman, Dept of Surgery
Maimonides Medical Center
Brooklyn, New York

Carolyne Desrosiers-Clarke, BSc
Research Assistant
Dept of Surgery
Montreal University
Quebec, Canada

William C. DeVries, MD
Cardiothoracic Surgeon
Louisville, Kentucky

John F. Dixon, RN, MSN, CCRN
Clinical Manager
Cardiothoracic Surgery/Transplant ICU
Baylor University Medical Center
Dallas, Texas

Steve H. Dougherty, MD
Associate Professor of Surgery & Microbiology
Texas Tech University Health Sciences Center
El Paso, Texas

Robert W. Emery, MD
Director, Cardiothoracic Transplantation
Mechanical Devices Division
Minneapolis Heart Institute
Minneapolis, Minnesota

Una Loy Clark Farrer
Des Moines, Washington

Charlotte D. Farris, BSN, RN
Supervisor, Cardiovascular Surgery/Transplant ICU
Baylor University Medical Center
Dallas, Texas

O.H. Frazier, MD
Chief, Transplantation Services &
Surgical Director, Cullen Cardiovascular Research Laboratory
Texas Heart Institute
Houston, Texas

Iwao Fujimasa, MD
Professor, Institute of Medical Electronics
University of Tokyo
Japan

Elizabeth A. Galvin, RN, MS, CPN
Pediatric Critical Care Clinical Nurse Specialist
University of California-Davis Medical Center
Sacramento, California

Elisabeth George, RN, MSN, CCRN
Critical Care Clinical Nurse Specialist
Presbyterian University Hospital
University of Pittsburgh Medical Center
Pittsburgh, Pennsylvania

Marv Gohman, CCP
Perfusionist
Cardiac Systems
Minneapolis, Minnesota

Tom Golden, CCP
Perfusionist
Cardiac Systems
Minneapolis, Minnesota

Charles Hahn, MD
Cardiovascular Research Institute (IRCV)
Sion, Switzerland

Jane B. Hansen, RN, BSN
Nurse Clinician
Minnesota Thoracic Associates
Minneapolis, Minnesota

J. Donald Hill, MD
Chairman, Dept of Cardiovascular Surgery
California Pacific Medical Center
San Francisco, California

Marilyn Hravnak, RN, MSN, CCRN, RRT
Formerly Head Nurse, SICU
Presbyterian University Hospital
University of Pittsburgh Medical Center
Pittsburgh, Pennsylvania

Kou Imachi, MD
Professor, Institute of Medical Electronics
University of Tokyo
Japan

G. Kimble Jett, MD
Director of Mechanical Assistance
Baylor University Medical Center
Dallas, Texas

Keith Johansen, CCP
Perfusionist
Cardiac Systems
Minneapolis, Minnesota

Kristen E. Johnson, RN
Formerly Program Director
Mechanical Devices Division
Minneapolis Heart Institute
Minneapolis, Minnesota

Lyle D. Joyce, MD, PhD
Thoracic & Cardiovascular Surgeon
Minnesota Thoracic Associates
Minneapolis, Minnesota

Jay Katz, MD
Elizabeth K. Dollard Professor of Law, Medicine, and Psychiatry
Yale Law School
New Haven, Connecticut

Willem J. Kolff, MD, PhD
Distinguished Professor of Medicine & Surgery
Research Professor of Bioengineering
University of Utah
Salt Lake City, Utah

Bette Lemperle, BSN, MPH
Chief, Circulatory Support Devices Branch
Division of Cardiovascular, Respiratory, and Neurological Devices
Office of Device Evaluation
Center for Devices and Radiological Health
Rockville, Maryland

S. Jill Ley, RN, MS, CCRN
Clinical Nurse Specialist
Cardiovascular Surgery and Transplantation
California Pacific Medical Center
San Francisco, California

Mary Beth Farley Liska, RN, CCRN
Mechanical Devices Coordinator
Minneapolis Heart Institute
Minneapolis, Minnesota

David H. Loffing, MS, CCE
Senior Clinical Engineer
Dept of Bioengineering
University Medical Center
Tucson, Arizona

Marco Meli, MD
Cardiovascular Research Institute (IRVC)
Sion, Switzerland

Dennis Mills, CCP
Chief Perfusionist
Cardiac Systems
Minneapolis, Minnesota

Jeffrey N. Neichin, RN, MS
Regional Sales Manager
Johnson & Johnson Interventional Systems
Warren, New Jersey

Maura L. Neichin, RN, BSN, MHS
Clinical Research Associate
San Diego Clinical Research Associates
San Diego, California

George P. Noon, MD
Professor of Surgery
Baylor College of Medicine
Houston, Texas

Yukihiko Nosé, MD, PhD
Professor, Dept of Surgery
Baylor College of Medicine
Houston, Texas

Roland Odermatt, PhD
Director
Cardiovascular Research Institute (IRCV)
Sion, Switzerland

George J. Olding, BS, CBET
Senior Clinical Engineer
Dept of Bioengineering
University Medical Center
Tucson, Arizona

Don B. Olsen, DVM
Director of Institute for Biomedical Engineering
& Artifical Heart Research Laboratory
University of Utah
Salt Lake City, Utah

Philip E. Oyer, MD
Professor
Dept of Cardiothoracic Surgery
Stanford University Medical Center
Stanford, California

George M. Pantalos, PhD
Research Assistant Professor
Departments of Surgery and Bioengineering
Total Artificial Heart Program Clinical Coordinator
University of Utah
Salt Lake City, Utah

Janice T. Piasecki
Manager, Clinical Research & Regulatory Affairs
Abiomed, Inc.
Danvers, Massachusetts

Marc R. Pritzker, MD
Cardiologist
Minneapolis Heart Institute
Minneapolis, Minnesota

Daniel M. Rose, MD

Chief, Cardiovascular Surgery
St. Vincent Medical Center
Bridgeport, Connecticut

W. Donald Rountree, RN, MS, CCRN, CS

Critical Care Clinical Nurse Specialist
Humana Hospital Audubon
Louisville, Kentucky

Peter M. Rutan, RN, BSN, CCRN

Clinical Nurse II
University of California-Davis Medical Center
Sacramento, California

Stephanie Sevcik, BS

Manager, Technical Services
Lifespan Clinical Equipment Services
Minneapolis, Minnesota

Yukiyasu Sezai, MD

Professor, Institute of Medical Electronics
University of Tokyo
Japan

John Shafer, CCP

Perfusionist
Cardiac Systems
Minneapolis, Minnesota

Julie A. Shinn, RN, MA, CCRN, FAAN

Cardiovascular Clinical Specialist
Stanford University Medical Center
Stanford, California

Motomi Shiono, MD

Research Assistant Professor
Baylor College of Medicine
Houston, Texas

Bruce J. Shook

Vice President of Clinical Affairs
Abiomed, Inc
Danvers, Massachusetts

H. David Short III, MD

Assistant Professor of Surgery
Baylor College of Medicine
Houston, Texas

V.I. Shumakov, MD
Research Institute of Transplantology
Moscow, Russia

Richard L. Simmons, MD
George V. Foster Professor Surgery & Chair, Dept of Surgery
University of Pittsburgh
Pittsburgh, Pennsylvania

Richard G. Smith, MSEE, CCE
Technical Director
Artificial Heart Lab
University Medical Center
Tucson, Arizona

F.C. Spencer, MD
Chairman, Dept of Surgery
New York University
New York, New York

Timothy A. Thorstenson, MDiv
Dept of Pastoral Care
Abbott-Northwestern Hospital
Minneapolis, Minnesota

Carol Toninato, RN
Surgical and Clinical First Assistant
Minnesota Thoracic Associates
Minneapolis, Minnesota

R. Keith White, MD
Resident in Cardiothoracic Surgery
University of Utah
Salt Lake City, Utah

Roxi Wolfe, CCP
Perfusionist
Cardiac Systems
Minneapolis, Minnesota

To
the physicians, nurses, clinical engineers, perfusionists,
and, most importantly, patients,
whose pioneering efforts have advanced
cardiac mechanical assistance beyond balloon pumping
into a most successful medical science.

Foreword

Many years ago I wrote "a physician who does not listen to his nurse should have his head examined." It is still true. It is also true that many physicians do not quite understand as much about intra-aortic balloon pumping, heart/lung machines, LVADs, and artificial hearts as the technicians and nurses who deal with them daily and actually manage them.

There is the same problem with biomedical engineers. To present a current example: Centrifugal pumps are being used in more than 120,000 cardiopulmonary bypasses per year. The centrifugal pump usually stands on the floor or close to it. When the pump slows down or stalls, because it is nonocclusive, the 1 meter long arterial line acts as a siphon, the blood flows back in the oxygenator, and air is sucked into the aorta. When air is seen in the arterial line, it is already too late because the aorta is already full of air. A simple check valve* will prevent the backflow of blood and eliminate potentially deadly air embolism. If engineers from the centrifugal pump manufacturers would spend 1 day in the operating room, they would understand this; but they do not, and some even deny that the problem exists! It is fortunate that people who have had "hands-on" experience have contributed their expertise to this book.

In 1983 Susan Quaal wrote a book entitled *Comprehensive Intra-Aortic Balloon Pumping.* The last chapters were about VADs and the artificial heart. The book was successful, and it continued to sell well over the next 9 years. In 1985 the publisher asked Susan Quaal to write a second edition. However, she was too busy with other things plus working on her Ph.D. and she did not feel qualified to write about other mechanical assist devices beyond the balloon pump. The publisher has persuaded her to write a second edition about the balloon pump, and to become the editor of this companion volume, which describes LVADs, artificial hearts, etc.

It is noteworthy that the chapters of this book have been written by or with the help of nurses, clinical engineers, and perfusionists. In all but 7 chapters, physicians are co-authors as well; and in some chapters, experienced physicians are the principle authors.

From a practical point of view this book should be very helpful for people who work with all these diverse devices. It also gives a glimpse of VAD technology in the former Soviet Union and in Japan.

---

*Kolff WJ: Letter to the editor, *Ann Thorac Surg,* p 512, Sept 1990. This simple check valve is available through Cardiac Systems, Inc., 1027 Conshohocken Road, Conshohocken, PA 19428, (215) 828-4564.

Susan Quaal is still "running" balloon pumps. Her practical and theoretical knowledge of every subject in this book is amazing. She is well-qualified to be its editor.

I predict that this book will be just as successful as the first edition of *Comprehensive Intra-Aortic Balloon Pumping.*

Willem J. Kolff, MD,   PhD
Distinguished Professor of Medicine & Surgery
Research Professor of Bioengineering
University of Utah
Salt Lake City, Utah

Preface

It is a great privilege for me to serve as Editor of *Cardiac Mechanical Assistance Beyond Balloon Pumping*. In 1983, when I wrote the first edition of *Comprehensive Intra-Aortic Balloon Pumping*, the two chapters covering those devices that go beyond the limits of balloon pumping to support the failing myocardium seemed adequate. Nearly 10 years later there is a wealth of information that deserves to be published. I felt compelled to recruit leading experts in the field, who could provide a compendium of knowledge that reflects the current state of the art in mechanical assistance.

This complete work provides a definitive tome, covering many different aspects of mechanical assistance. Comprehensive chapters are presented on multiple devices, including Japanese and Russian; perfusionist, engineer, and nurse team member roles; process of device development; and FDA and corporate sponsors' involvement in VAD programs. These chapters are essential for readers to understand device function and patient management. I am, however, very pleased that in addition to its technical information, this book holistically addresses ethical and spiritual issues and a family's perspective from first-hand experience with the total artificial heart.

I extend my sincere appreciation to all contributors who kindly extended their trust and confidence in me as Editor for their scholarly and well-developed chapters. This book could not have reached its genesis without the competency of many individuals on staff at Mosby–Year Book; I am especially grateful to Robin Carter, Chris Kuehne, and Chuck Furgason for their expertise, support, and patience.

Susan J. Quaal

Contents

**PART THREE
DEVELOPMENT AND SUPPORT OF
A VENTRICULAR ASSIST DEVICE PROGRAM**

†Deceased.

PART ONE

INTRODUCTION

CHAPTER 1

Adult and pediatric
ventricular heart failure

Peter M. Rutan and Elizabeth A. Galvin

INTRODUCTION

Attempts to treat the failing heart have a long and interesting history. Pien Ch´iao, a fifth century BC, Chinese physician, is reported to have attempted a heart transplant (Fig. 1-1).[1] Ancient Europeans were known to have used dried toad skin to treat dropsy (edema). Later, rural folk medicine practitioners in England used a concoction of herbs that included foxglove. In 1776 William Withering isolated the cardiotonic ingredient in foxglove, digitalis, and investigated its proper use in the treatment of heart disease.[2] A manuscript listing the medicinal use of plants, compiled by a fifteenth century Aztec physician, discusses the use of an extract of the magnolia tree to treat heart problems.[2] It was not until the twentieth century, however, that the treatment of heart failure was based on a more accurate understanding of cardiac anatomy and physiology, rather than by treating symptoms such as dropsy, which were believed to be the primary disease.

Death from heart disease is the leading cause of mortality in the United States. Greater than 35% of the total number of deaths each year are attributed to this cause. The Centers for Disease Control estimate that 11.2 million people suffer from coronary heart disease alone.[2] In addition approximately 2.3 million individuals experience chronic heart failure, with an additional 400,000 people advancing to this stage each year. Of those who develop heart failure, 50% die within the first year.[3] A recent literature review (1989-1990) found that over 75% of reported heart failure patients were male and the average age was greater than 50 years.[4]

PATHOPHYSIOLOGY
Definition

Cardiac failure is a syndrome characterized by an alteration in the heart's pumping ability (pump failure). As it progresses, the heart is increasingly unable to meet the body's metabolic needs. Thus delivery of oxygen and nutrients to the cells becomes inadequate, leading to cellular dysfunction, and a decrease in systemic blood flow and

3

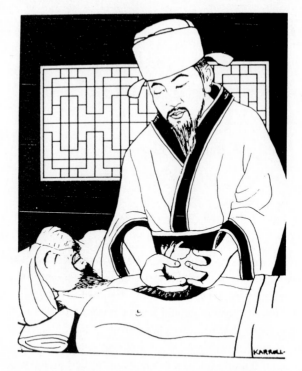

Fig. 1-1. Pien Ch´iao and his legendary exchange of hearts in the fifth century BC. (From Kahan BD: *Transplant Proc* (suppl 2) 20(2):3, 1988.)

cardiac output. This results in further deterioration and impairment of cardiac function. Changes can be rapid or slow (acute or chronic) depending on the factors contributing to the pump failure.[5]

Myocardial physiology

The heart can fail due to an impairment in systolic function (decrease in stroke volume and impedance to forward flow), diastolic function (elevation of ventricular filling pressures leading to congestion), or a combination of both. These changes can be structural and/or biochemical in nature. Changes in systolic function can be related to such things as cardiac cell loss, decreased contractile force generated by the cell, chemical abnormalities in the excitation-contraction phase, inadequate energy stores to sustain contraction, or problems with the regulatory and contractile proteins. Changes in diastolic function may be related to structural changes such as a shift in the intraventricular septum, or to abnormalities in relaxation such as an abnormal calcium uptake into the cardiac cell.[6,7]

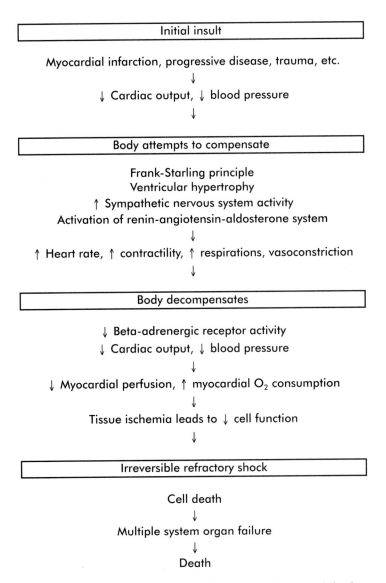

Fig. 1-2. The sequence of events leading to heart failure and shock.

Sequence of events

There are a multitude of causes for heart failure; some cause acute failure and others lead to chronic failure. After an initial insult occurs, a downward trend will take place that will ultimately result in death unless proper therapeutics are instituted (Fig. 1-2). At first the body compensates for a fall in cardiac output by activating several major

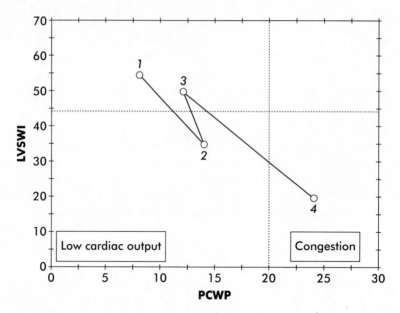

Fig. 1-3. Progression from normal cardiac function to heart failure and cardiogenic shock. *1,* Normal cardiac function; *2,* An initial insult affects the patient's contractility or left ventricular stroke work index (LVSWI). The body attempts to compensate for the cardiac depression and decreased flow. *3,* Initially the contractility improves as the sympathetic nervous system reacts, but eventually the heart decompensates; *4,* This leads to decreased contractility, increased preload or pulmonary capillary wedge pressure (PCWP), and imminent cardiogenic shock. (Normal LVSWI: 44-68 gram•meters/m^2; normal PCWP: 0-12 mm Hg.[11])

compensatory mechanisms: (1) the Frank-Starling principle, (2) ventricular hypertrophy, (3) sympathetic nervous system and renin-angiotensin-aldosterone system responses, and (4) baroreceptor reflexes. As a consequence cardiac output is increased, tissue perfusion is improved, and vital organ function is preserved. These compensatory mechanisms will eventually take a toll, leading to decreased cardiac output, decreased perfusion, and tissue ischemia. This proceeds to an irreversible or terminal stage, resulting in cell death, damage to the major organs, and the eventual death of the patient[8-10,12-14] (Fig. 1-3).

Frank-Starling relationship

The Frank-Starling principle describes the heart's ability to increase cardiac output in response to a variety of stimuli. This is accomplished by its ability to alter the force of contraction when wall stress is impacted by increased ventricular filling. The sarcomere is stretched to a greater length, which results in a more forceful contraction. Thus a failing heart will require higher filling pressures (end-diastolic pressure and volume) to maintain the same cardiac output. This corresponds to the clinical improvement observed when pulmonary capillary wedge pressure (PCWP) is increased to 15 to 20 mm Hg, concomitant with volume loading. As cardiac failure worsens, PCWP increases to greater than 20 mm Hg. The sacromere finally yields to overstretching, and cardiac output is no longer augmented by increases in end-diastolic pressure and volume.[6,13-15]

Hypertrophy

Hypertrophy is stimulated by pressure and volume overload conditions and results in an increase in myocardial muscle mass. Weber further defines this change as remodeling of the ventricle, which involves modifications in myocardial structure or biochemical composition of muscles, vessels, or interstitium. Several factors can contribute to ventricular structural alteration: (1) hypertrophic growth of myocytes, (2) inability to maintain blood flow to the increased muscle mass, and (3) excess collagen formation, which can affect the ability of the myocyte's ability to stretch during ventricular filling.[7]

These changes can be global or regional, depending on the type of heart failure (e.g., regional hypertrophy occurs when noninfarcted parts of the ventricle undergo hypertrophy in response to changes in end-diastolic volume and pressure and take over the function of the infarcted parts, following a myocardial infarction).[7,16,17]

Sympathetic nervous system

As the heart fails, there is reflex myocardial sympathetic stimulation. This results in a release of catecholamines by cardiac adrenergic nerve endings and adrenal glands, leading to increased contractility, heart rate, and systemic vascular resistance. Along with local autoregulatory mechanisms, this response helps preserve circulation to the brain and heart and decreases blood flow to other organs. Along with the effects of angiotensin-II and vasopressin, this increased activity helps maintain arterial pressure, venous return, and ventricular filling.[13-15,17]

Renal system

Renal hypoperfusion, increased sympathetic tone, and changes in plasma sodium levels that result from heart failure activate the release of renin. This release stimulates the production of angiotensin-II, which causes vasoconstriction. Angiotensin-II, in turn, stimulates production of aldosterone, which acts on the renal tubules to decrease sodium and chloride secretion and increase potassium excretion. Angiotensin-II can also stimulate production of arginine vasopressin, which also causes vasoconstriction. The net result is an increase in intravascular volume, preload, and afterload.[5,15,17]

Baroreceptor reflexes

Decreased cerebral perfusion activates carotid baroreceptors. This results in increased sympathetic tone and stimulation of the pituitary gland to release arginine vasopressin.

Atrial baroreceptors react to the increase in filling pressures related to heart failure by increasing the release of atrial natriuretic peptide (ANP). ANP causes arteriodilation and venodilation, promotes sodium excretion, inhibits renin and aldosterone production, and reduces sympathetic vasoconstriction, thereby regulating circulating fluid volume and lowering arterial blood pressure. It is believed that the effects of ANP may be overwhelmed by other compensatory forces at work.[13-15,18]

β-Adrenergic receptors

β-Adrenergic receptors are located in the myocardium (β_1) and in the smooth muscle (β_2). β_1 receptors are responsible for positive chronotropic, inotropic, and dromotropic responses. β_2 receptors primarily mediate vasodilatation. Investigations have demonstrated that the β_1 receptors are "down-regulated" with a decrease in both numbers and function in the presence of heart failure. In addition, the amount of down-regulation seems to be related to the severity of heart failure. β_2 receptors are thought to "uncouple" in heart failure. Receptor sites do not decrease, but their activity diminishes. Research has demonstrated that G proteins (guanine nucleotide–binding proteins) mediate beta receptor activity. G proteins can either stimulate (G_s) or inhibit (G_i) myocardial activity. Research findings suggest that there is an increased level of the G_i protein in heart failure that is capable of inhibiting myocardial contractility.[19,21]

CAUSES OF HEART FAILURE

Patients experiencing heart failure span all age-groups and exhibit different levels of severity and varying degrees of muscle damage. Published results of investigations into heart failure reveal that the predominant causes fall under the ischemic heart disease category. This is a change from earlier studies in which nonischemic heart disease, primarily hypertension, was the primary cause of heart failure.[4] Although it is commonly thought of as a specific disease entity, cardiac failure is related to a large number of different disease causes. Many different schemes are used in the literature to categorize heart failure. Schlant and Sonnenblich present a useful method based on three broad categories: (1) mechanical problems (e.g., stenotic valve), (2) effect on the myocardium (e.g., myocarditis), and (3) electrical problems (e.g., dysrhythmia).[5] (See the box on pp. 9-11.)

Heart failure may affect preload, afterload, contractility, and heart rate, determinants of myocardial performance. Clinically, these are estimated by pulmonary capillary wedge pressure, systemic vascular resistance, and ventricular stroke work. An alteration of one or more of these factors may lead to a change in myocardial function. The box on p. 12 lists some conditions which can adversely affect these factors. The reader is referred to Brozena and/or Schlant for a more detailed discussion of this topic.[5,15]

————————— **SELECTED CAUSES OF HEART FAILURE** —————————

I. Mechanical abnormalities

1. Increased afterload
   a. Aortic stenosis
   b. Systemic arterial hypertension
   c. Coarctation of the aorta
2. Increased preload
   a. Valvular regurgitation
   b. Shunts
   c. Increased venous return
3. Altered contractility and preload
   a. Myocardial infarction
4. Obstruction or impairment to cardiac chamber filling
   a. Mitral stenosis
   b. Tricuspid stenosis
   c. Pericardial constriction
   d. Tamponade
   e. Massive pulmonary embolus
   f. Intrachamber tumor
5. Traumatic injury
   a. Ventricular aneurysm
   b. Myocardial contusion
   c. Penetrating injury of the heart

II. Myocardial abnormalities

1. Idiopathic cardiomyopathies
   a. Dilated cardiomyopathy
   b. Hypertrophic cardiomyopathy
   c. Restrictive cardiomyopathy
2. Cardiomyopathy due to neuromuscular disorders
   a. Friedreich's disease
   b. Myotonica atrophica
   c. Duchenne's muscular dystrophy
3. Myocarditis
   a. Bacterial
   b. Spirochetal
   c. Rickettsial
   d. Viral
   e. Mycotic
   f. Protozoal
   g. Helminthic
4. Metabolic deficiencies
   a. Diabetes mellitus
   b. Beriberi
   c. Protein-calorie malnutrition
   d. Acid/base imbalance
   e. Electrolyte imbalance

Continued

SELECTED CAUSES OF HEART FAILURE—cont'd

5. Cardiotoxic/cardiac depressant effect
   a. Alcohol
   b. Cobalt
   c. Cocaine
   d. Radiation exposure
   e. Electrical shock
   f. Tricyclic antidepressants
   g. Phenothiazine antipsychotics
   h. Certain chemotherapeutic agents
      (e.g., Adriamycin, daunomycin, vincristine)
   i. Theophylline
   j. Poison—plants
      i. Cardiac glycoside effect—foxglove
      ii. Effect similar to cardiac glycoside
         (e.g., oleander, lily of the valley, jerusalem cherry, milkweed, jessamine)
      iii. Other cardiotoxic effects
         (e.g., larkspur, jimson weed, mistletoe, tapioca)
   k. Poison—animal/insect
      i. Snakes
      ii. Scorpions
      iii. Arthropods
         (e.g., bees, yellow jackets, hornets, wasps)
      iv. Spiders
   l. Poison—environmental
      i. Carbon monoxide
      ii. Halogenated hydrocarbons
      iii. Arsine gas
      iv. Lead
6. Effects of aging
7. Impaired performance secondary to a preexisting mechanical abnormality
   (e.g., hypokinesis, akinesis, dyskinesis)
8. Ischemia
   a. Acute
   b. Chronic
9. Infarction

_____ **SELECTED CAUSES OF HEART FAILURE—cont'd** _____

10. Metabolic disorders
    a. Acromegaly
    b. Hypoparathyroidism
    c. Pheochromocytoma
    d. Hyperthyroidism
    e. Cardiac glycogenosis
    f. Hemochromatosis
11. Other disease
    a. Amyloidosis
    b. Carcinoid heart disease
    c. Sacroidoisis
    d. Endocarditis
    e. Progressive systemic sclerosis
    f. Acute cardiac allograft rejection
    g. Crohn's disease
    h. Chronic obstructive pulmonary disease
    i. Connective tissue disease
    j. AIDS-related cardiomyopathy
    k. Cocaine-induced heart disease
    l. Anaphylactic shock
    m. Septic shock

III. **Conduction system abnormalities**
    1. Bradydysrhythmias
       a. Extreme sinus bradycardia
       b. Junctional rhythm
    2. Tachydysrhythmias
       a. Prolonged supraventricular tachycardia
       b. Ventricular tachycardia
    3. Conduction disturbance
       a. High grade heart block
       b. Atrioventricular dissociation
       c. Complete heart block
    4. Fibrillation
       a. Atrial fibrillation
       b. Ventricular fibrillation

EXAMPLES OF CONDITIONS THAT MAY AFFECT
PRELOAD, AFTERLOAD, AND CONTRACTILITY

Increased preload

Valvular regurgitation
Shunting
Increased venous return

Decreased preload

Mitral stenosis
Tricuspid stenosis
Pericardial constriction
Tamponade
Pulmonary embolus
Intrachamber tumor
Atrial fibrillation
Atrial flutter
Ventricular ectopy
Hypovolemia
Venous dilatation
Anaphylaxis
A-V dissociation
Right ventricular failure
Pneumothorax

Increased afterload

Thromboembolism
Increased sympathetic
    nervous system activity
Drug side effects
Systemic arterial hypertension
Aortic stenosis
Coarctation of the aorta

Decreased afterload

Anaphylaxis
Fever
Septic shock
Hypercarbia
Drug toxicity

Decreased contractility

Trauma
Acute myocardial infarction
Myocarditis
Ischemia
Drug toxicity
Dysrhythmias
Coronary artery embolism
Sepsis
Hypoxemia
Acid-base imbalance

PEDIATRIC HEART FAILURE

Although some causes of cardiac failure occur in both the adult and pediatric populations, there are those that are unique to children. In the adult, cardiac failure typically results from ischemic myocardial dysfunction, whereas in children cardiac failure is more often related to congenital cardiac lesions. The pathophysiology of heart failure is the same for patients of all ages. However maturational physiologic differences affect the progression of and responses to cardiac dysfunction. In addition, cardiovascular compromise occurs in some disease processes that are seen primarily in the pediatric patient.

Heart failure in the child, as in the adult, exists when the heart is unable to pump sufficient blood to meet the metabolic needs of the body. Since the causes of heart failure are multiple and can be primary or secondary in nature, various categorization methods have been employed to aid in its discussion. The causes of pediatric heart failure can be classified as resulting from (1) mechanical abnormalities, (2) myocardial abnormalities, or (3) cardiac rhythm or conduction disturbances. It is clear that some causes fall into more than one category. For the purposes of this discussion, however, the major abnormalities will be addressed.[5]

Mechanical abnormalities

Congenital heart disease. The intracardiac pressure and volume load can be altered by congenital cardiac defects. The incidence of congenital heart disease is approximately 8 to 10 of every 1000 newborns.[22,23] Heart failure due to congenital defects typically occurs in the first year of life.[24] Hemodynamic changes, in addition to the size and complexity of the lesion, will determine the degree of increased ventricular work needed to meet the metabolic needs of the body.

The congenital heart defects are classified as acyanotic or cyanotic, depending on the overall hemodynamic alterations and clinical manifestations that occur. The acyanotic lesions are those in which blood is shunted from the left to the right side of the heart. Deoxygenated and oxygenated blood are not mixed in the systemic circulation. In the cyanotic lesions, blood is shunted from the right to the left side of the heart, causing systemic mixing of oxygenated and deoxygenated blood. Because deoxygenated blood is present in the systemic circulation, varying degrees of cyanosis are present.

Examples of acyanotic defects are atrial septal defect (ASD), ventricular septal defect (VSD), patent ductus arteriosus (PDA), aortic stenosis, coarctation of the aorta, endocardial cushion defect, and pulmonary stenosis. The cyanotic defects include transposition of the great vessels (TGA), tetralogy of Fallot (TOF), truncus arteriosus, total anomalous pulmonary venous connection (TAPVC), tricuspid atresia, and hypoplastic left heart syndrome (HLHS). An increase in pulmonary blood flow and ventricular volume load is seen with a PDA, ASD, VSD, endocardial cushion defect, TGA, truncus arteriosus, and TAPVC. Pulmonary blood flow is usually decreased in TOF, tricuspid atresia, and pulmonary stenosis.

In aortic stenosis, coarctation of the aorta, and pulmonary stenosis, heart failure is related primarily to outflow obstruction and the subsequent increased ventricular pressure load. Hypoplastic left heart, the most severe form of left ventricular outflow tract obstruction,[25] is the leading cause of death from cardiovascular disease during the first 2 weeks of life.[23] Death due to hypoplastic left heart failure occurs because the left ventricle is inadequate to maintain systemic perfusion.[23]

It is not uncommon for these defects to coexist as a complex cardiac lesion. Indeed patient survival is often dependent upon shunt patency to provide flow in the presence of valvular or vasculature obstruction.

Systemic arterial hypertension. Children do not typically have essential hypertension. Hypertension may be found in children with renal disease, congenital heart disease (e.g., coarctation of the aorta), central nervous system disorders (e.g., encephalitis, lead poisoning), trauma to the back or abdomen, tumors (e.g., neuroblastoma, Wilm's tumor), and endocrine disorders (e.g., aldosteronism, Cushing's disease).[26] If severe enough, hypertension can cause heart failure because of the increased pressure load on the left ventricle (LV). Sustained resistance to ventricular outflow (increased afterload) can eventually cause LV and septal hypertrophy resulting in a left ventricular outflow obstruction.

Pericardial tamponade. Although an uncommon occurrence in children,[23] pericardial tamponade can result from blunt or penetrating chest trauma or as a complication of cardiac surgery. After injury, blood or fluid accumulates in the pericardium and exerts pressure on the heart. Ventricular filling and pumping action become impaired, causing hypotension, tachycardia, venous congestion, a narrowed pulse pressure, and low cardiac output. Sudden death may occur after a rapid and massive cardiac tamponade.[26]

Myocardial abnormalities

Cardiomyopathy. Cardiomyopathy, a disease involving the heart muscle itself, is distinct from coronary, hypertensive, valvular, pericardial, and congenital heart disease. Cardiomyopathies can be primary disorders in which the cause is unknown, or they may occur secondary to other illnesses or disease processes. The cardiomyopathies are categorized clinically into three types: (1) dilated cardiomyopathy, characterized by ventricular dilation and symptoms of congestive heart failure; (2) hypertrophic cardiomyopathy, characterized by hypertrophy of the ventricle; and (3) restrictive cardiomyopathy, marked by scarring of the ventricle, which interferes with diastolic function.

In the United States, dilated congestive cardiomyopathy is the most common type of cardiomyopathy seen in childhood and is the most common diagnosis of pediatric heart transplant recipients. Although hypertrophic cardiomyopathy may produce symptoms during childhood, it generally does not become apparent until the second or third decade of life. Restrictive cardiomyopathy in children is more prevalent in equatorial countries and is thought to be related to repeated tropical infections.[23] End-stage heart disease due to cardiomyopathy is one of the major indications for pediatric cardiac transplantation.[27]

Inflammatory lesions. Myocarditis, or inflammation of the heart muscle, is caused by a number of infectious agents, but is most typically attributed to a viral cause. It may also occur in several noninfectious diseases, including polyarteritis nodosa, trichinosis, rheumatic fever, and systemic lupus erythematosus.[23] In myocarditis, pathogen invasion and inflammation result in myocardial structural injury, including tissue necrosis, scarring, and fibrosis. Manifestations of cardiac injury include depressed cardiac contractility with ventricular dysfunction, valvular insufficiency, and dysrhythmias. Most often recovery from myocarditis is complete, but some patients succumb to sudden death and others develop a progressive, chronic impairment of cardiac contractility. It is difficult to estimate the incidence of pediatric myocarditis because many mild cases of the disorder are not diagnosed.[23]

The incidence of acute rheumatic fever in the United States has significantly declined since the beginning of the century. The morbidity and mortality caused by rheumatic carditis have decreased accordingly, except in some developing countries where rheumatic fever continues to be the leading cause of heart disease.[28] Recently there have been isolated reports of acute rheumatic fever outbreaks, suggesting a nationwide resurgence in the United States.[29]

The most widely accepted pathogenesis of acute rheumatic fever is that it is an auto-immune sequel to group A streptococcal upper respiratory infection. Occurring primarily in school-age children, acute rheumatic fever causes malaise, joint pain and swelling, and inflammatory changes in the three layers of the heart. The permanent heart damage of rheumatic fever results from valvular scarring and thickening as the endocardium heals. This scar tissue formation leads to valvular stenosis and regurgitation, primarily of the mitral and aortic valves.

Myocardial toxicity. Cardiotoxicity after exposure to the anthracycline antimetabolites doxorubicin (Adriamycin) and daunomycin has been reported in pediatric patients treated with these drugs. Anthracycline cardiotoxicity is usually dose dependent with an incidence of less than 1% in patients treated with cumulative doses of less than 500 mg/m^2. In patients receiving cumulative doses of 500 to 600 mg/m^2, the incidence of cardiomyopathy is 11%; if doses exceed 600 mg/m^2, the incidence of cardiomyopathy is 30%. Manifestations of anthracycline cardiotoxicity include early benign ECG changes with a progression to a frequently irreversible and sometimes fatal cardiomyopathy.[30]

Accidental poisoning, which affects 5 million children annually,[26] can cause heart failure if a cardiotoxic substance is ingested. Some of the cardiotoxic substances include the anticholinergics (antihistamines and tricyclic antidepressants)[26] and glycoside-containing plants (nerium oleander, thevetia peruviana, argemone mexicana, and digitalis purpurea).[22]

Ischemia. One of the most frequent causes of ischemic heart disease in infants and children is Kawasaki disease.[30] First described in 1967 as a benign mucocutaneous lymph-node syndrome prevalent in Japanese infants and young children, Kawasaki disease (KD) is a multisystem, febrile illness. The most salient feature of KD is a nonspecific, multiorgan panvasculitis. In the early, subclinical phase of the disease, endarteritis of the large vessels (especially the coronary arteries) leads to aneurysms, central obstruction, thrombosis, and embolization. Eventually, distal ischemia and infarction ensue with aneurysmal rupture and pancarditis that frequently involves the conduction system.

Kawasaki disease has been reported in adults, but it is predominantly a disease of young children, with 80% of its sufferers under 2 years of age. The heart is affected in approximately 40% of all KD cases. Of those children who die from KD, 1% to 2% of deaths result from primary cardiac involvement.[30,32]

Myocardial ischemia can develop in children with congenital heart disease and is most commonly seen in the defects subvalvular or valvular aortic stenosis, hypoplastic right or left ventricle, or anomalous coronary artery.[31] Myocardial injuries associated with pediatric chest trauma include myocardial contusions, concussions, and valvular and coronary artery damage. Ischemia resulting from these injuries can occur in the acute phase or in the long term from myocardial scarring, dysrhythmias, and ventricular aneurysms.[32] Bacterial endocarditis, which is more prevalent in infancy and childhood than in adults, can lead to myocardial ischemia and infarction from the migration of coronary emboli.[24] Myocardial infarction in infancy is an extremely rare finding. However, fatal myocardial infarction in a newborn with anatomically and histologically normal coronary arteries has been reported.[33] Causes of myocardial ischemia in the neonatal period include asphyxia neonatorum and conditions of increased myocardial oxygen demand (e.g., persistent fetal circulation, pulmonary hypertension due to respiratory distress syndrome, and meconium aspiration).[32]

Shock. Children suffering from any of the shock states may potentially experience myocardial dysfunction since cardiogenic shock or pump failure is the final "common pathway" of all types of shock.[31] However, direct myocardial depression has been described recently in patients with early septic shock. Myocardial depression occurring in sepsis is attributed to circulating myocardial depressant factor, which severely reduces the left ventricular ejection fraction and causes global depression of ventricular systolic function.[23,34]

Postoperative low cardiac output. Acute cardiac failure occurring in infants and young children after cardiac surgery has been termed postoperative low cardiac output syndrome (PLCO). Characterized by low cardiac index (2.0 to 2.5 L/min/m^2), poor organ perfusion, peripheral vasoconstriction, decreased urine output, extreme irritability or lethargy, and other signs of shock, PLCO is the most common cause of death after cardiac surgery in infants. Infants at the greatest risk for PLCO are those that are less than 4 to 6 kilograms or less than 3 months of age, those that have congestive heart failure before surgery, and those with complex cardiac defects.[35]

Postoperative low cardiac output may be caused by alterations in heart rate, preload, afterload, or contractility. Treatment of PLCO is aimed at correcting the underlying abnormality and providing supportive therapy (e.g., assisted ventilation, inotropic drugs). Unsuccessfully treated, PLCO can rapidly progress to postcardiotomy cardiogenic shock, a condition that has a high mortality rate.

Metabolic. Hypoglycemia, acidosis, and hypocalcemia can cause myocardial depression and dysrhythmias in the pediatric patient. Infants are especially at risk for developing hypoglycemia because they have high glucose needs due to a high metabolic rate but limited glycogen stores. The development of hypoglycemia is associated with cold stress, sepsis, and stress.

Acidosis develops more quickly in the child than in the adult and is less effectively compensated for because compensatory defense mechanisms are less well developed. Because the kidneys are immature, organic acids are not excreted as effectively and bicarbonate is absorbed and produced less efficiently than in adults.

Serum calcium values are the same from infancy to adulthood, but in infancy regulation of ionized calcium is less precise. Stress during infancy can cause hypocalcemia through the stimulation of the growth hormone secretion, which increases calcium deposition in bone. Infants and children who receive frequent blood transfusions are at risk for developing hypocalcemia from calcium binding to the citrate-phosphate-dextran anticoagulant used in bank blood.[23]

Systemic illnesses. Many of the pediatric systemic diseases that affect the heart have previously been discussed. In addition to those already addressed, cardiac failure can occur in the mucopolysaccharidosis of the Hunter's and Hurler's syndromes and in the neuromuscular disorders Duchenne's muscular dystrophy, myotonic dystrophy, and Friedreich's ataxia. In the Hunter's and Hurler's syndromes, heart failure is related to valvular involvement, although myocardial hypertrophy also occurs. In the neuromuscular disorders, a progressive degeneration of the cardiac muscle results in cardiomyopathy.

Pediatric dysrhythmias

Children typically experience a change in heart rate in response to hypoxia, fever, anxiety, and hypovolemia, but conduction defects in the pediatric patient are less common. Conduction defects in children are usually associated with an underlying cardiac defect, cardiac surgery, cardiomyopathy, electrolyte imbalances, or a critical illness that affects myocardial function.

Bradydysrhythmias. Bradydysrhythmias are the most common dysrhythmias of childhood. Although bradycardias are often well tolerated in the adult and older child, they can be particularly serious in the neonate, infant, and young child whose cardiac output is heart rate dependent. Because the neonate, infant, and young child have a very limited ability to increase stroke volume to compensate for bradycardia, cardiac output can fall precipitously from sinus bradycardia, sinus arrest, sick sinus syndrome, atrioventricular block, junctional rhythms, or AV dissociation.[23,35]

Tachydysrhythmias. Infants and young children increase their heart rate to compensate for a low cardiac output. Heart rate increases may also result from an increased sympathetic tone, conduction defects ("reentry phenomena"), or drugs. The most common pathologic tachydysrhythmia seen in pediatric patients is paroxysmal supraventricular tachycardia or paroxysmal atrial tachycardia. These tachydysrhythmias (with rates as great as 300 per minute in neonates and infants) may initially be well tolerated if episodes are short in duration. However, if episodes are frequent or prolonged, they may lead to heart and circulatory failure due to the decrease in diastolic filling time and subsequent low cardiac output.[23,31]

ADULT HEART FAILURE

The exact incidence of adult heart disease and failure is difficult to estimate because of inadequate reporting mechanisms for morbidity and mortality. Ischemic heart disease is most common in the industrialized nations of North America and Western Europe. In Africa, nutritional and infectious causes are more widespread. Hypertensive disease constitutes a major cause in Asia and the Pacific islands.[22,36] This section will discuss the most common causes of adult heart failure. The reader is referred to either Hurst or Braunwald for further information.[37,38]

Mechanical abnormalities

Heart failure may be caused by a number of mechanical or structural problems. These abnormalities can result in increased preload or afterload, decreased contractility, and/or impaired cardiac chamber filling. Injury to the heart from a traumatic event can also lead to dysfunction.

Congenital heart disease. The incidence of congenital heart disease is about 8 per 1000 live births. With improved techniques for diagnosing and treating life-threatening defects, as many as 60% of infants who would have otherwise died in the first year now survive. Bicuspid aortic valve is most likely the most common congenital defect seen in the adult population. The major defects have been previously discussed in this chapter.[22,39]

Valvular disease. Aortic stenosis, mitral stenosis, and tricuspid stenosis are commonly caused by rheumatic fever. Pulmonary stenosis is usually congenital in origin. Other, less common causes include atrial myxoma, thrombus, inflammatory lesions, and calcification. Aortic and pulmonary stenotic valves obstruct flow during systole, which increase left and/or right-sided afterload. The ventricle attempts to compensate for the increased pressure load by hypertrophing. In time, heart failure will develop secondary to this pressure overload. Mitral or tricuspid valve stenosis interferes with left or right ventricular diastolic flow. This obstruction increases left or right atrial pressure and volume, which may cause right ventricular hypertrophy (mitral stenosis), right atrial hypertrophy, pulmonary edema (mitral stenosis) and peripheral edema (tricuspid stenosis). Although tricuspid stenosis is not usually associated with heart failure by itself, it is mentioned because it very often accompanies mitral valve stenosis.[40-43]

Aortic, mitral, pulmonary, and tricuspid regurgitation can occur for many reasons. The incompetent valve allows backward flow either during systole (mitral and tricuspid) or diastole (aortic and pulmonary). A volume overload situation leading to eventual failure can develop. Some common causes include trauma, rheumatic fever, endocarditis, infarction, right or left ventricular dilatation (tricuspid and mitral) and tumor.[40-43]

The patient with a prosthetic heart valve (mechanical, porcine, pericardial, or human) can experience a number of problems that may lead to development of heart failure. Artificial valve dysfunction, thrombus formation, infection, fibrosis, calcification, and dehiscence of the base have been reported.[44]

Systemic arterial hypertension. Hypertensive cardiovascular disease is the most prevalent cause of heart failure worldwide. In the United States there is evidence that ischemic heart disease has become the leading cause.[4,22] Essential hypertension is the most common form. Other causes of hypertension include renovascular disease, renal parenchymal disease, primary aldosteronism, Cushing's syndrome, other types of mineralcorticoid hypertension, pheochromocytoma, and coarctation of the aorta. Chronic hypertension leads to a pressure overload (increased afterload). The result is hypertrophy of the ventricle, reduction of myocardial blood flow, reduction of available oxygen, and eventual heart failure if left untreated.[45,46]

Impairment of cardiac chamber filling. Constrictive pericarditis and cardiac tamponade are examples of a condition that may affect normal cardiac function. Diastolic function is affected when the ventricle is unable to fill to normal volume and pressure during diastole. This can be due to either increased pressure secondary to fluid buildup in the pericardium or noncompliant scar tissue. Ventricular diastolic pressure increases and cardiac output decreases because an adequate end-diastolic volume cannot be maintained. Trauma is the most common cause of acute tamponade. Other causes include viral pericarditis and neoplastic disease. Constrictive pericarditis has been associated as a posttrauma complication, postcardiac surgery complication, pericardial disease, tamponade, mediastinal radiation, and tuberculosis.[47]

Acute pulmonary embolism and neoplasms may also impair or obstruct flow and lead to failure.[48,49]

Traumatic injury. Trauma is one of the leading causes of death in the United States. A traumatic insult to the heart can be caused by either a penetrating wound or blunt trauma (nonpenetrating). Onset of heart failure may be sudden (e.g., from a projectile wound associated with major blood loss). Failure may develop later because of damage that is not immediately apparent, such as valve damage. Common injuries include damage to the percardium, myocardium, cardiac valves, and coronary arteries. In addition, conduction or rhythm disturbances secondary to the injury may develop and lead to failure.[50]

Myocardial abnormalities

Cardiomyopathies. Cardiomyopathy classification includes idiopathic or primary cardiomyopathy (unknown cause) and secondary cardiomyopathy (known cause). This is because there may be as few as 10% of the patients diagnosed who have an identifiable cause. The term "secondary cardiomyopathy" has been replaced lately by the use of "specific heart muscle disease."[51]

Dilated cardiomyopathy is the most common type of this group. It is characterized by poor myocardial systolic function. Ventricular contractility is decreased, which leads to a decrease in cardiac output and an increase in end-diastolic pressure and volume. Some identifiable diseases or risk factors associated with development of this cardiomyopathy include alcohol abuse, connective tissue disease, neuromuscular disorders, viral infection, parasitic infection, systemic arterial hypertension, cardiotoxic substances, infiltrative disease, pregnancy, progression of acute myocarditis to a chronic stage, and metabolic disorders. There may also be a genetic predisposition.[36,45,51-56]

Hypertrophic cardiomyopathy may account for 2% to 6% of all cardiomyopathy cases. It is characterized by poor left ventricular diastolic function due to reduced compliance. Left ventricular end-diastolic pressure is elevated and diastolic filling is impeded because of this poor compliance. Systolic dysfunction may also occur. The specific cause is unclear, and it is thought that an inherited abnormality may be responsible.[22,51]

Restrictive cardiomyopathy is the least common cardiomyopathy. It is characterized by varying degrees of systolic and diastolic dysfunction. Initially end-diastolic volume and ventricular stretch are affected. As the disease progresses, systolic function will decrease over time. It is more common in the tropics due to endomyocardial fibrosis (EMF). Suspected causes of EMF include malnutrition, serotonin, filariasis, lymphatic obstruction, and allergy. Restrictive cardiomyopathy may be idiopathic or associated with a disease process and includes amyloidosis, hemochromatosis, sarcoidosis, sclero-derma, neoplasm, and glycogen storage disease.[22,49,51,54-56]

Myocarditis. Myocarditis is an inflammatory process involving the myocardial wall. There are multiple causes (see the box on pp. 9-11) and they vary with age, geographic location, immunization, and sanitation. The majority of cases in the United States and Western Europe are of a viral etiology. In Central and South America a protozoal infec-tion causing Chaga's disease (*Trypanosoma cruzi*) is more prevalent. Cardiac dysfunc-tion is caused by either direct intrusion or toxicity on the cardiac cell structure. This leads to alteration of function and/or cell destruction. Ventricular involvement leads to end-diastolic pressure and volume overload. Dysrhythmias and conduction distur-bances that can adversely affect the heart's stroke volume can also occur. The more common causes of myocarditis include trypanosomiasis (protozoal), trichinosis (hel-minthic), echinococcosis (helminthic), Kawasaki disease, and acquired immune defi-ciency syndrome (AIDS).[22,52]

Metabolic deficiencies/disorders. Nutritional deficiencies (e.g., protein-calorie mal-nutrition), endocrine disease (e.g., diabetes mellitus, hyperthyroidism), and metabolic disorders (e.g., cardiac glycogenosis, hemochromatosis) can lead to the development of heart failure. There may be a primary or secondary cause depending on the problem. Protein-calorie malnutrition leads to pericardial fat depletion, cardiac muscle atrophy, and reduced cardiac output. The patient is at risk for sudden cardiac arrest. Diabetes mellitus is associated with an increased cardiac mortality due to an increased incidence of coronary atherosclerosis, development of cardiac autonomic defects, and a diabetic cardiomyopathy. Cardiac glycogenosis involves a carbohydrate mechanism disorder. Excessive quantities of glycogen accumulate in cardiac tissue and affect energy utili-zation. Increased myocardial glycogen has been seen in familial cardiomyopathy.[22,51,53]

Cardiotoxic/cardiac depressant effects. A number of agents including noncardiac drugs, animals, and plants can produce cardiotoxic or cardiac depressant effects when someone is exposed to them on either an acute or a chronic basis. Some of these agents include noncardiac drugs (e.g., tricyclic antidepressants), certain chemotherapeutic agents (e.g., Adriamycin), environmental accidents (electrical shock), poisonous plant ingestion (oleander), snake bite (rattlesnake), arthropod sting (bees), and environmental exposure (carbon monoxide). The exact mechanism for each type is different, but all can cause heart failure if not treated.[56]

Myocardial ischemia. Ischemic heart disease is the leading cause of mortality in the United States. It appears to be less prevalent in developing countries, which suggests that it is a disease of socioeconomic development.[2,22] The primary cause of myocardial ischemia is coronary atherosclerosis, which obstructs or narrows the vessel. Other causes include aortic valve disease, hypertrophic cardiomyopathy, coronary ostia stenosis, embolism, coronary inflammatory disease, coronary vessel spasm, or congenital defects. Major clinical presentations include angina, myocardial infarction, congestive heart failure, or sudden death. Ischemic events leading to dysfunction that does not result in necrosis may produce a "stunned" myocardium. Failure to wean from cardiopulmonary bypass or postcardiotomy low output syndrome are examples. Prolonged ischemia can lead to an infarction and/or development of a hypertrophied ventricle. Heart failure will ensue if the myocardial oxygen requirements are not able to be met.[57,58]

Other causes. Less frequent causes that may lead to heart failure are carcinoid heart disease, endocarditis, acute cardiac allograft rejection, Crohn's disease, chronic obstructive pulmonary disease, AIDS-related cardiomyopathy, cocaine induced heart disease, anaphylactic shock, and septic shock.[49,59,60,61]

Conduction system abnormalities

Dysrhythmias contribute to at least half of the mortality from coronary heart disease.[36] They may occur acutely as with an acute ischemic event (myocardial infarction) or from metabolic disturbance (acidosis). On a chronic basis they may be associated with cardiomyopathy, chronic ischemic heart disease, or conduction system disease (AV node disease).[62,63]

Bradydysrhythmias such as extreme sinus bradycardia and junctional rhythms, conduction disturbances such as high grade or complete heart block, and tachydysrhythmias such as ventricular tachycardia and atrial fibrillation can contribute to heart failure. A severe tachydysrhythmia can decrease diastolic filling time, which leads to inadequate coronary artery perfusion and further dysfunction. Sinus bradycardia may produce a state in which an inadequate stroke volume is produced. The atrium contributes up to 30% of total cardiac output (atrial kick). Atrial fibrillation can precipitate heart failure when there is no effective atrial contraction.

CONCLUSION

Cardiac failure is not a specific disease, but rather the potential outcome of a multitude of causes. All age-groups are affected, ranging from neonate to elderly. Some causes are restricted to certain parts of the world; others are seen universally. Although great strides have been made in medical therapies and cardiac mechanical assistance, these methods remain ineffective in successfully treating a large number of patients suffering from heart failure. Mechanical and biomechanical cardiac assist devices in use or in development will offer us additional temporary and permanent options in the battle against heart failure. Current approved and investigational uses of cardiac assist devices to treat severe heart failure are discussed in Part Two.

REFERENCES

1. Kahan BD: Preface: Pien Ch´iao, the legendary exchange of hearts, traditional Chinese medicine and the modern era of cyclosporine, *Transplant Proc* (suppl 2) 20(2):3, 1988.
2. Rutan PM: Mechanical support beyond the intraaortic balloon pump, *AACN Clinical Issues in Critical Care Nursing* 2(3):477, 1991.
3. Chiu CJ: *Biomechanical cardiac assist.* Mount Kisco, N.Y., 1986, Futura Publishing Company.
4. Teerlink JR, Goldhaber SZ, Pfeffer MA: An overview of contemporary etiologies of congestive heart failure. I, *Am Heart J* 121(6):1852, 1991.
5. Schlant RC, Sonnenblick EH: Pathophysiology of heart failure. In Hurst JW, ed: *The heart.* ed 7, New York, 1990, McGraw-Hill.
6. McElory PA, Shroff SG, Weber KT: Pathophysiology of heart failure, *Cardiol Clin* 7(1):25, 1989.
7. Weber KT, Janicki JS: Pathogenesis of heart failure, *Cardiol Clin* 7(1):11, 1989.
8. Parmley WW: Cardiac failure. In Rosen MR, Hoffman BF, eds: *Cardiac therapy.* The Hague, 1983, Martinus Nijhoff.
9. Rice V: Shock, a clinical syndrome: an update. I. An overview of shock, *Critical Care Nurse* 11(4):20, 1991.
10. Rice V: Shock, a clinical syndrome: an update. II. The stages of shock, *Critical Care Nurse* 11(5):74, 1991.
11. Shoemaker WC: Shock states: pathophysiology, monitoring, outcome prediction and therapy. In Shoemaker WC: *Textbook of critical care,* ed 2. Philadelphia, 1989, WB Saunders.
12. Ross J: Assessment of cardiac function and myocardial contractility. In Hurst JW, ed: *The heart,* ed 7, New York, 1990, McGraw-Hill.
13. Shub C: Heart failure and abnormal ventricular function: I. Pathophysiology and clinical correlation, *Chest* 96(3):636, 1989.
14. Shub C: Heart failure and abnormal ventricular function: II. Pathophysiology and clinical correlation, *Chest* 96(4):906, 1989.
15. Brozena S, Jessup M: Pathophysiologic strategies in the management of congestive heart failure, *Annu Rev Med* 41:65, 1990.
16. Grossman W: Diastolic dysfunction and congestive heart failure, *Circulation* (suppl 3) 81(2):1, 1990.
17. Leibovitch ER: Congestive heart failure: a current overview, *Geriatrics* 46(1):43, 1991.
18. Cosgrove JA: Atrial natriuretic peptide: a new cardiac hormone. *Heart Lung* 18(5):461, 1989.
19. LeJemtel TH, Sonnenblick EH: Nonglycosidic cardioactive agents. In Hurst JW, ed: *The heart,* ed 7. New York, 1990, McGraw-Hill.
20. Bristow MR, Hershberger RE, Port JD et al: Beta-adrenergic pathways in nonfailing and failing human ventricular myocardium, *Circulation* (suppl 1) 82(2):I12, 1990.
21. Morgan HE, Neely JR: Metabolic regulation and myocardial function. In Hurst JW, ed: *The heart,* ed 7. New York, 1990, McGraw-Hill.
22. Akinkugbe OO: Cardiovascular disease. In Strickland GT, ed: *Hunter's tropical medicine.* ed 7. Philadelphia, 1991, WB Saunders.
23. Hazinski MF: Cardiovascular disorders. In Hazinski MF, ed: *Nursing care of the critically ill child,* ed 2. St Louis, 1992, Mosby–Year Book.
24. Bruning MD, Schneiderman JU: Heart failure in infants and children. In Michaelson CR, ed: *Congestive heart failure,* St. Louis, 1984, CV Mosby.
25. Gerraughth AB: Caring for patients with lesions obstructing systemic blood flow, *Critical Care Nursing Clinics of North America* 1(2):231, 1989.
26. Thompson SW: *Emergency care of children.* Boston, 1990, Jones and Bartlett.
27. Cameron DE, Gardner TJ: Heart transplantation in children. In Baumgartner WA, Reitz BA, Achuff SC, eds: *Heart and heart-lung transplantation,* Philadelphia, 1990, WB Saunders.
28. Imamoglu A, Ozen S: Epidemiology of rheumatic heart disease. *Arch Dis Child* 63(12):1501, 1988.
29. Hosier DM, Craenen JM, Teske DW et al: Resurgence of acute rheumatic fever. *Am J Dis Child* 141:730, 1987.
30. Wetzel RL, Rogers MC: Unusual medical causes of pediatric heart failure. In Shoemaker WC: *Textbook of critical care.* ed 2. Philadelphia, 1989, WB Saunders.

31. Hazinski MF: Shock in the pediatric patient, *Critical Care Nursing Clinics of North America* 2(2):309, 1990.
32. Helfaer, MA: Myocardial ischemia and cyanosis. In Rogers MC, ed: *Handbook of pediatric intensive care,* Baltimore, 1989, Williams & Wilkins.
33. Iannone LA, Durtiz G, McCarty RJ: Myocardial infarction in the newborn: a case study complicated by cardiogenic shock and associated with normal coronary arteries, *Am Heart J* 89(2):232, 1975.
34. Jardin F, Brun-Ney D, Auvert B et al: Sepsis related cardiogenic shock. *Crit Care Med* 18(10):1055, 1990.
35. Johnson DL: Postoperative low cardiac output in infancy, *Heart Lung* 12(6):603, 1983.
36. Kannel WB, Thom TJ: Incidence, prevalence, and mortality of cardiovascular diseases. In Hurst JW, ed: *The heart,* ed 7. New York, 1990, McGraw-Hill.
37. Hurst JW, ed: *The heart.* ed 7. New York, 1990, McGraw-Hill.
38. Braunwald E, ed: *Heart disease: a textbook of cardiovascular medicine,* ed 3. Philadelphia, 1988, WB Saunders.
39. Nugent EW, Plauth WH, Edwards JE et al: The pathology, abnormal physiology, clinical recognition, and medical and surgical treatment of congenital heart disease. In Hurst JW, ed: *The heart,* ed 7. New York, 1990, McGraw-Hill.
40. Rackley CE, Edwards JE, Wallace RB et al: Aortic valve disease. In Hurst JW, ed: *The heart,* ed 7. New York, 1990, McGraw-Hill.
41. Rackley CE, Edwards JE, Karp RB: Mitral valve disease. In Hurst JW, ed: *The heart,* ed 7. New York, 1990, McGraw-Hill.
42. Rackley CE, Edwards JE, Wallace RB et al: Pulmonary valve disease. In Hurst JW, ed: *The heart,* ed 7. New York, 1990, McGraw-Hill.
43. Rackley CE, Edwards JE, Wallace RB et al: Tricuspid valve disease. In Hurst JW, ed: *The heart,* ed 7. New York, 1990, McGraw-Hill.
44. Rackley CE, Katz NM, Wallace RB: Artificial valve disease. In Hurst JW, ed: *The heart,* ed 7. New York, 1990, McGraw-Hill.
45. Dustan HP: Pathophysiology of systemic hypertension. In Hurst JW, ed: *The heart,* ed 7. New York, 1990, McGraw-Hill.
46. Hall WD, Wollman GL, Tuttle EP: Diagnostic evaluation of the patient with hypertension. In Hurst JW, ed: *The heart,* ed 7. New York, 1990, McGraw-Hill.
47. Shabetai R: Diseases of the pericardium. In Hurst JW, ed: *The heart,* ed 7. New York, 1990, McGraw-Hill.
48. Dalen JE, Alpert JS: Pulmonary embolism. In Hurst JW, ed: *The heart,* ed 7. New York, 1990, McGraw-Hill.
49. Hall RJ, Cooley DA, McAllister HA et al: Neoplastic heart disease. In Hurst JW, ed: *The heart,* ed 7. New York, 1990, McGraw-Hill.
50. Symbas PN, Arensberg D: Traumatic heart disease. In Hurst JW, ed: *The heart,* ed 7. New York, 1990, McGraw-Hill.
51. Wenger NK, Abelmann WH, Roberts WC: Cardiomyopathy and specific heart muscle disease. In Hurst JW, ed: *The heart,* ed 7. New York, 1990, McGraw-Hill.
52. Wenger NK, Abelmann WH, Roberts WC: Myocarditis. In Hurst JW, ed: *The heart,* ed 7. New York, 1990, McGraw-Hill.
53. Fleischer N, Fein FS, Sonnenblick EH: The heart and endocrine disease. In Hurst JW, ed: *The heart,* ed 7. New York, 1990, McGraw-Hill.
54. Healy BP: The heart and connective tissue disease. In Hurst JW, ed: *The heart,* ed 7. New York, 1990, McGraw-Hill.
55. Regan TJ: The heart, alcoholism and nutritional disease. In Hurst JW, ed: *The heart,* ed 7. New York, 1990, McGraw-Hill.
56. Crawley IS: Effect of noncardiac drugs, electricity and poisons on the heart. In Hurst JW, ed: *The heart,* ed 7. New York, 1990, McGraw-Hill.
57. Factor SM: Pathophysiology of myocardial ischemia. In Hurst JW, ed: *The heart,* ed 7. New York, 1990, McGraw-Hill.

58. Healy BP: Pathology of coronary atherosclerosis. In Hurst JW, ed: *The heart,* ed 7. New York, 1990, McGraw-Hill.
59. Rezkalla SH, Hale S, Kloner RA: Cocaine induced heart disease. I. *Am Heart J* 120(6):1403, 1990.
60. Durack DT: Infective and noninfective endocarditis. In Hurst JW, ed: *The heart,* ed 7. New York, 1990, McGraw-Hill.
61. Stewart JM, Kaul A, Gromisch DS et al: Symptomatic cardiac dysfunction in children with human immunodeficiency virus infection. *Am Heart J* 117(1):140, 1989.
62. Marriott HJL, Myerburg RJ: Recognition of cardiac arrhythmias and conduction disturbances. In Hurst JW, ed: *The heart,* ed 7. New York, 1990, McGraw-Hill.
63. Myerburg RJ, Kessler KM: Clinical assessment and management of arrhythmias and conduction disturbances. In Hurst JW, ed: *The heart,* ed 7. New York, 1990, McGraw-Hill.

CHAPTER 2

Overview of ventricular assist devices

Motomi Shiono, George P. Noon, Chris L. Coleman,
and **Yukihiko Nosé**

INTRODUCTION

Intraaortic balloon pumping (IABP) has been successfully used, and considerable experience has been obtained in patients with left ventricular power failure.[1] At the same time, however, limitations of this device in circulatory assistance have also been recognized.[2] Ventricular assist devices (VADs) and total artificial hearts (TAHs) have demonstrated clinical capabilities of far more profound circulatory support, with the potential of increasing use in recent years.[3] Mechanical circulatory assistance has also been employed to support a small number of hemodynamically deteriorating transplant candidates until a suitable donor heart has been obtained. These experiences have had a dramatic impact on specific patients who had dismal prognoses. As of December 1990 these devices have been used in more than 1400 patients with heart failure, according to the report in the International Registry supported by American Society of Artificial Internal Organs (ASAIO) and the International Society for Heart Transplantation (ISHT).[4] In this chapter we review and describe several devices that have been used clinically and discuss the results.

CLASSIFICATION OF MECHANICAL CIRCULATORY ASSISTANCE

All mechanical circulatory support systems have been used as an alternative when the patient becomes refractory to other conventional medical treatments. These supporting methods are classified into four main categories (see box on p. 26)[5]:

Series mechanical ventricular assistance
Parallel mechanical ventricular assistance
Mechanical replacement
Miscellaneous

_____ CURRENTLY AVAILABLE _____
MECHANICAL CIRCULATORY ASSISTANCE DEVICES

Series mechanical ventricular assistance

IABP
ECP; counterpulsation pants
Axial flow pump; hemopump (Nimbus), etc.

Parallel mechanical ventricular assistance

VADs; pulsatile pump, nonpulsatile pump, etc.

Mechanical replacement

TAHs; Jarvik-7 TAH (Symbion), etc.

Miscellaneous

Cardiomyoplasty, etc.

"Series" describes devices used in conjunction with the native heart and/or great arteries. Thus these devices use the entire left ventricular output that is ejected to the aorta and is used as a counterpulsation device. With its ease of use and effectiveness, IABP is the most common clinically applied device in this category. However, its effects are limited and it has been recognized that patients with profound heart failure could not be salvaged with IABP only. A salvage rate of 20% to 30% is expected.[6] External counterpulsator (ECP) is a noninvasive device that augments the diastolic blood pressure and is easy to apply.[7] However, the efficacy of this device is limited in profound heart failure. Hemopump (Johnson & Johnson) has a unique feature and is classified as an axial flow pump.[8] This intraaortic device can generate approximately 3 L/min of flow and decompress the failing left ventricle without applying counterpulsation. Pump flow rate is dependent on systemic circulation afterload. This type of axial flow pump is promising beyond IABP in more profound heart failure patients.

"Parallel" assistant devices include several systems that have recently been applied in many patients. They are grouped under the category of ventricular assist device (VAD).[9–13] A VAD is placed in parallel with the native ventricle and drains blood from the atrium or ventricle, which is returned to the great arteries. This device decompresses the failing ventricle and assists systemic or pulmonary circulation by generating 3 to 10 L/min of blood flow. VAD devices are divided into three categories according to their assisting method: (1) left ventricular assist devices (LVADs), (2) right ventricular assist devices (RVADs), and (3) combined biventricular assist devices (BVADs). Moreover, VADs are pulsatile and nonpulsatile, based on generated flow patterns. Currently available pusatile devices are pneumatic systems or electrical systems according to their driving source; they are classified as follows:

Pulsatile VADs

PNEUMATIC
Thoratec, Abiomed, TCI, Nippon Zeon,
Toyobo, Berlin, etc.
ELECTRICAL
Novacor

Nonpulsatile VADs

Roller pump, Centrifugal

Pulsatile VADs consist of a pump and cannulae (inflow draining cannula and outflow perfusion cannula). The draining cannula is inserted into the left atrium or left ventricle and the perfusion cannula into the aorta in a LVAD. Right atrium and pulmonary artery are used for inflow and outflow respectively in RVADs. Cannulation techniques are discussed in Part II.

Several devices of different sizes, shapes, and power sources have been developed to maintain both systemic and pulmonary circulation without native ventricles; this is called "mechanical replacement."[14] Various control modes have been developed to regulate pump output in response to changes in venous return, afterload, and left-right flow differences.[15] All total artificial hearts (TAHs) that have been used clinically are pneumatically-driven pulsatile systems; patients are tethered to the external driving console. The Jarvik-7 TAH (Symbion) has been the most frequently used and has contributed to a new field of clinical practice as a bridge-to-heart transplantation.[16]

APPLICATION AND ETIOLOGY

Clinical indications for mechanical circulatory assistance are as follows:

Postcardiotomy cardiogenic shock
Cardiogenic shock due to acute myocardial infarction
Endstage heart failure due to cardiomyopathy
Miscellaneous

The indications for circulatory support in the postcardiotomy setting have been divided into two categories: (1) unsuccessful weaning from cardiopulmonary bypass and (2) low output syndrome after cardiotomy. Postcardiotomy applications have been documented to be approximately 1% to 2% of all patients undergoing cardiac operations. Indications for circulatory support in conjunction with heart transplantation have been divided into three categories: (1) patients who have hemodynamic deterioration before orthotopic heart transplantation; (2) patients who have acute rejection after transplan-

Table 2-1. Selection of clinically applied VADs

VADs	Drive source	Name	Preferable assist period	Position
Pulsatile	Pneumatic	Thoratec, Abiomed	Short or intermediate term	Para-, extracorporeal
		Zeon, Toyobo, Berlin	Short or intermediate term	Para-, extracorporeal
		ThermoCardiosystems	Intermediate or long term	Intraabdominal cavity
	Electrical	Novacor	Intermediate or long term	Intraabdominal wall
Nonpulsatile	Roller pump		Short term	Extracorporeal
	Centrifugal	Biomedicus, Sarns	Short term	Extracorporeal

tation; (3) patients who have immediate donor organ failure after transplantation, considered not to be related to acute rejection.

Hemodynamic criteria

Hemodynamic criteria for application of the mechanical circulatory support have been proposed: (1) cardiac index of less than 1.8 L/min/m^2, (2) pulmonary capillary wedge pressure greater than 25 mm Hg, and (3) systolic arterial pressure less than 80 mm Hg despite maximal medical therapy including IABP.[17] The overall clinical impression is added to these parameters as an important criterion. Moreover, systemic vascular resistance of more than 2100 dynes/sec/cm^5 may be added in some institutions. Right ventricular assistance has been applied or added when a cardiac index of less than 2.0 L/min/m^2 and CVP more than 30 cmH$_2$O prevail after initiating left ventricular assistance. There have been many additional criteria and modifications in different clinical situations.

Device selection

The diagnosis of left, right, or biventricular failure is important in determining what type of device should be used (Table 2-1).[18] Etiology of the ventricular failure is also important in determining how long mechanical support should be continued. In most cases, left ventricular assist is initiated first and this may unmask right ventricular failure, necessitating right ventricular assistance. BVAD or a TAH is used to bridge a patient with biventricular failure to transplantation. If cardiac function is expected to be reversible, short-term (less than 1 week) or intermediate-term (1 week to 1 month) devices (i.e., centrifugal pump or pneumatic VADs), may be indicated. However, currently available mechanical devices are limited to use only in a few major institutions. To establish the management of profound ventricular failure, VAD usage must become much more widespread.

Table 2-2.   Clinical experience in The Methodist Hospital/Baylor College of Medicine

VAD/TAH	Cases	Weaned	Transplanted	Discharged
Centrifugal†				
LVAD	65	42	1	20 (31%)
RVAD	16	10	3°	3 (19%)°
BVAD	35	9	1	2 (6%)
Subtotal	116	61	5	25 (22%)
Novacor VAD	14	—	10 (71%)	9 (90%)
Symbion TAH	4	—	2 (50%)	0

° BioMedicus RVAD with Novacor LVAD.
†Data in centrifugal pumps include both postcardiotomy and bridge-to-transplant.

CLINICAL EXPERIENCE IN THE METHODIST HOSPITAL/BAYLOR COLLEGE OF MEDICINE

As of August 1991 VADs and TAHs have been applied in 134 patients for postcardiotomy ventricular support and bridge-to-transplantation (Table 2-2). Of the patients supported with the BioMedicus centrifugal device (including bridge-to-transplant) 53% have been successfully weaned. The mean survival rate is 22%. When BVADs are required for biventricular failure, survival rates reflect the severity of the ventricular failure and diminish compared with LVADs or RVADs setting (6%, 31% and 19% respectively). Novacor VAD (Baxter) and Jarvik-7 TAH (Symbion) have been used in 14 and 4 patients for bridge-to-transplantation, respectively. Of the patients who have been supported by a Novacor device, 71% have undergone successful transplants; the mean survival rate is 90%.

OVERALL RESULTS

Reasonable enthusiasm continues for the application of the devices, as evidenced by the International Registry data. In this report clinically applied devices are divided in two categories, postcardiotomy support and bridge-to-transplantation.[4]

Postcardiotomy support

Although VADs could salvage patients who would have died without such mechanical support, overall results in the postcardiotomy setting have been discouraging. As of December 1990, VADs have been used in 965 patients for postcardiotomy ventricular support. Device weaning rate is 45%, and the mean survival rate is 25% (discharged from hospital). Of all patients, 67% have been supported by centrifugal nonpulsatile devices; this is hypothesized to be due to limited availability of pulsatile devices. There are no statistical differences of survival rates between centrifugal and pneumatic

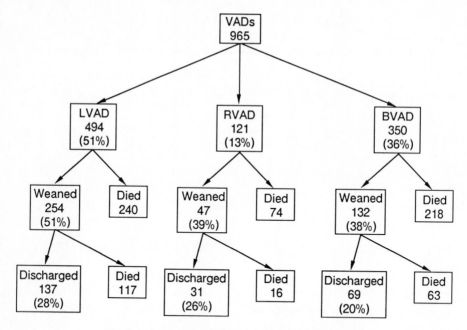

Fig. 2-1. VADs in postcardiotomy cardiogenic shock.

devices. Average supporting period is approximately 4 days in each LVAD, RVAD, and BVAD. When BVADs are required, survival rates reflect the severity of the ventricular failure and diminish compared with LVADs or RVADs setting (20%, 28%, and 26% respectively) (Fig. 2-1). A careful analysis of device selection and patient selection may significantly improve these results in the future.

Bridge-to-transplantation

Mechanical circulatory assistance has been employed to support deteriorating transplant candidates until a suitable donor heart has been obtained (i.e., bridge-to-transplantation or staged cardiac transplantation).[19,20] The most substantial development and establishment of treatment have been the application of mechanical circulatory support in this population. The early results are encouraging and have made a dramatic impact on this new clinical field. As of December 1990 VADs and TAHs have been used in 476 patients for bridge-to-transplantation. Of the patients who have been supported by mechanical circulatory assistance, 69% have been transplanted and the mean survival rate is 66%. Of 476 patients who received mechanical ventricular assistance, 26% received LVADs, 34% received BVADs, and 40% received TAHs. Univentricular RVADs are rarely indicated in this setting. The rates of subsequent transplantation are similar regardless of type of support used: 71% for LVADs, 65% for BVADs, and 71% for TAHs. The hospital discharge rate is significantly different among these groups:

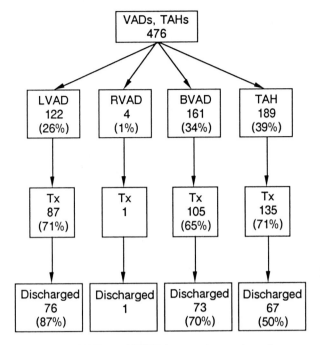

Fig. 2-2. VADs and TAHs in staged transplantation.

87% for LVADs, 70% for BVADs, and 50% for TAHs (Fig. 2-2). Patients receiving uni-ventricular LVADs approach the same actuarial survival rate as the standard heart transplant population. These results have been expected to be due to satisfactory results contributed by long-term (more than 1 month) devices and to complications. At present, availability of the devices is limited and only a few institutions have permission to implant a specific device. Thoratec pump (3M), Novacor, and TCI (Thermocardiac systems) devices have not been widely available. Average supporting period is approximately 31 days in LVADs, 20 days in RVADs, 15 days in BVADs, and 24 days in TAHs.

Complications

Complications are frequent in this critically ill group of patients.[21] Bleeding is the most common complication, occurring in 30% to 40% of all patients. Renal failure, infection, and poor cardiac output are also major complications encountered (Tables 2-3, 2-4).

DISCUSSION

In clinical applications of the devices, many problems have been encountered that should be solved (see the box on p. 32).

Table 2-3.   Major complications during postcardiotomy VADs

	Incidence	
Complication	Weaned cases (%)	Not weaned cases (%)
Bleeding/DIC	49	41
Renal failure	36	26
Biventricular failure	34	16
Cannula obstruction/low CO	21	9
Infection	7	19
Thromboembolism	9	12

Table 2-4.   Major complications associated with mechanical assistance in bridge use°

Complication	VAD (%) (N = 38)	BVAD (%) (N = 56)	TAH (%) (N = 54)
Bleeding	31	25	27
Biventricular failure	45	43	0
Renal failure	31	27	40
Respiratory failure	17	18	42
Infection	21	14	36
MOF†	0	11	29

° Precluding transplantation.
†Multiple organ failure.

PROBLEMS ASSOCIATED WITH MECHANICAL CIRCULATORY SUPPORTING DEVICES

Medical
    Patient selection
    Device selection and operative technique
    Management of patients in pre-, intra-, and postdevice situation
    Dependent patients, including multiple organ failure, etc.
Engineering
    Pump and connection parts: shape, size, position, fitting, antithrombogenicity, antihemolysis, durability, prevention of infection, etc.
    Driving mechanism: miniaturization, portability, ease in operation, automation, energy source, control algorithm, etc.
    Other parts: volume shifting device, energy transmission system, etc.
Socioeconomical

Patient selection and timing of the implantation are the most critical problems. In cases where mechanical assistance has been applied, poor preoperative cardiac function and latent organ failure have progressed to multiple organ failure by additional risks of surgical intervention and cardiopulmonary bypass. During mechanical assistance total cardiac index is maintained at 2.2 to 2.5 L/min/m^2 because a low output state already complicates the recovery from the latent injuries to the vital organs. An early application is essential to obtain a better result.

Selection of the appropriate device and implantation technique is important to consider. Centrifugal and external pulsatile devices can be used for left ventricular support with or without right ventricular support and can be used in either the atria or left ventricle. In postcardiotomy or postinfarction cardiogenic shock, left atrial cannulation is preferable because it avoids additional myocardial damage. In potential transplant candidates, left ventricular cannulation is preferred in order to obtain a sufficient pump flow. Positioning of both pump and cannulae should be considered carefully to obtain better hemodynamics and avoid complications (i.e., bleeding and infection). Results in the bridge-to-transplant population have been improved by clinical application of intermediate-term or long-term devices. As the number of heart transplants has increased, so has the longer waiting time for obtaining a suitable heart. Long-term devices, such as Novacor and TCI, have been applied for this specific population. Recent results of TCI implantation in 11 cases supported over a 30-day period as a bridge-to-transplant device have demonstrated a 100% survival rate after transplantation (Frazier OH and Noon GP, personal communication). However, clinical applications of these devices are restricted by the Food and Drug Administration as IDE (Investigational Device Exemption) in the United States. This leaves heart bypass systems or conventional ventricular assistance with short-term devices, such as Biomedicus or the Sarns centrifugal pump, as the only methods of support. Internationally there have been some commercially available devices, such as Nippon Zeon VAD system and Toyobo VAD system (Japan), and Berlin Assist Heart (Germany). The implantable LVADs have not been commercially available. Implantable devices have not been efficient in severe biventricular failure and a TAH would be necessary as a mechanical replacement device for intermediate-term or long-term assistance.

In the pre-, intra-, and postdevice patient care, special emphasis should be placed on maintaining other vital organ functions that impact the patients' prognosis. An anticoagulation regimen has been one of the essential treatments and almost all patients have received some type of anticoagulation during mechanical support. However, a uniform anticoagulation regimen has not been defined and established for any of these devices. At present, all devices require some degree of anticoagulant therapy to avoid thromboembolic complications. Bleeding is another major complication and is sometimes related to coagulopathy. Careful attention must therefore be given to implant procedures, anticoagulation therapy, and the monitoring of the coagulation system.

Infections are common during and after mechanical support. This complication is expected to be relevant to multiple organ failure in these critically ill patients. Device-centered infection is an important problem, especially in TAHs.[22] It is generally understood that the implantation of a device in the mediastinum (Jarvik-7) is not clinically feasible, whereas the devices implanted either inside the abdominal cavity or the abdominal wall are acceptable without causing infectious complications. It is, however, necessary to consider all the possible causes for the higher infection rate of Jarvik-7 TAH.[23] Prophylaxis is the only way to avoid this complication. Therefore arduous efforts must be undertaken to maintain the patient's general status quo condition.

At the present time, none of the devices mentioned here can be relied on to function without the possibility of thromboembolism. Many devices have been using polyurethanes as antithrombogenic material. It is also expected that biolization or endothelialization will be available as blood contacting surfaces in the future.[13,24] Engineering designs must consider antithrombogenicity and improvement of the pump, cannula, connection parts, prosthetic valve, and pump size and flow rate. Continuous development and modification are expected to be done on the existing parts of the devices.

It has been well documented that intensive care for patients requiring circulatory support is quite expensive, especially over long-term periods. How do we manage patients with multiple organ failure who cannot be weaned from assist devices? It has also been argued that mechanical assistance cannot increase the number of transplants in the limited situation of donor heart availability. Are more stable candidates excluded from transplant if supported patients with VADs have priority? Is the implantable long-term VAD really cost-effective? There are many arguments and problems that should be solved socially, economically, and ethically. They are presented in a subsequent chapter.

CONCLUSION

A number of patients requiring mechanical circulatory support have been identified in the last several years, and a new clinical field of bridge-to-transplantation has been introduced in the last decade. A variety of devices for circulatory support is under development. However, most of these devices are not clinically available. It is hoped that these devices will be simple to implant, cost-effective, and widely available in the future. After careful analysis of the results in the accumulated patient population, many problems encountered in the past might be resolved in the future. Continued efforts are required to further improve medical, engineering, and socioeconomical problems in accordance with the advances in ventricular assist devices.

REFERENCES

1. Sturm JT, McGee MG, Fuhrman TM et al: Treatment of postoperative low output syndrome with intraaortic balloon pumping: experience with 419 patients, *Am J Cardiol* 45:1033, 1980.
2. O'Connell JB, Renlund DG, Robinson JA et al: Effect of preoperative hemodynamic support on survival after cardiac transplantation, *Circulation* 78(suppl III):78, 1988.

3. Lefemine AA, Kosowsky B, Madoff I et al: Results and complications of intraaortic balloon pumping in surgical and medical patients, *Am J Cardiol* 40:415, 1977.
4. ASAIO-ISHT: American Society for Artificial Internal Organs-International Society for Heart Transplantation clinical registry of mechanical ventricular assist pumps and artificial hearts. Hershey, Pa, May 1991, Pennsylvania State University.
5. Ghosh PK: *3. Precedents and perspectives.* In Unger F, ed: *Assisted Circulation 3.* New York, 1989, Springer-Verlag.
6. Kantrowitz A, Wasfie T, Freed PS et al: Intraaortic balloon pumping 1967-1982: analysis of complications in 733 patients, *Am J Cardiol* 57:976, 1986.
7. Soroff HS, Cloutier CT, Giron F et al: Support of systemic circulation and left ventricular assist by synchronous pulsation of extramural pressure, *Surg Forum* 16:148, 1965.
8. Frazier OH, Macris MP, Wampler RK et al: Treatment of cardiac allograft failure by use of an intraaortic axial flow pump, *J Heart Transplant* 9:408, 1990.
9. Magovern GJ, Park SB, Maher TD: Use of a centrifugal pump without anticoagulants for postoperative left ventricular assist, *World J Surg* 9:25, 1985.
10. Pennington DG, Samuels LD, Williams G et al: Experience with the Pierce-Donachy ventricular assist device in postcardiotomy patients with cardiogenic shock, *World J Surg* 9:37, 1985.
11. Portner PM, Oyer PE, Pennington DG et al: Implantable electrical left ventricular assist system: bridge to transplantation and the future, *Ann Thorac Surg* 47:142, 1989.
12. Noon GP: Clinical complications with circulatory support. Presented at a US-USSR Joint Symposium on circulatory support and biomaterials, Houston, December 6-7, 1990.
13. Frazier OH: Clinical results with flocked surface. Presented at a US-USSR Joint Symposium on circulatory support and biomaterials, Houston, December 6-7, 1990.
14. Unger F, Semb BKH, Vasku J et al: *Part IV Total Artificial Heart.* In Unger F, ed: *Assisted Circulation 3.* New York, 1989, Springer-Verlag.
15. Snyder AJ, Rosenberg G, Landis DL et al: Introductory lecture on control. Presented at the second world symposium on the artificial heart, Berlin, July 3, 1984.
16. Joyce LD, Johnson KE, Pierce WS et al: Summary of the world experience with clinical use of total artificial heart as support devices, *J Heart Transplant* 5:229, 1986.
17. Pierce WS, Parr GVS, Myers JL et al: Ventricular assist pumping in patients with cardiogenic shock after cardiac operations, *N Engl J Med* 305:1606, 1981.
18. Pennington DG, Reedy JE, Swartz MC et al: Univentricular versus biventricular assist device support, *J Heart Transplant* 10:258, 1991.
19. Magovern JA, Pierce WS: *Mechanical circulatory assistance before heart transplantation.* In Baumgartner WA, ed: *Heart transplantation.* 1990, WB Saunders.
20. Pennington DG, Swartz MC: *Ventricular assistance as a bridge to cardiac transplantation.* In Hosenpud JF, ed: Cardiac transplantation: a manual for health care professionals. New York, 1990, Springer-Verlag.
21. Kriett JM, Kaye MP: The Registry of the International Society for Heart Transplantation: Seventh Official Report—1990, *J Heart Transplant* 9:323, 1990.
22. Gristina GG: Biomaterial-centered infection: microbial adhesion versus tissue integration. *Science* 237:1588, 1987.
23. Nosé Y: Intrathoracic cardiac prosthesis: is it really not clinically acceptable? *Artif Organs* 15:161, 1991.
24. Kambic H, Barenburg S, Nosé Y et al: Glutaraldehyde-protein complexes as blood-compatible coatings, *Trans Am Soc Intern Organs* 24:426, 1978.

CHAPTER 3

Total artificial hearts, ventricular assist devices, or nothing?

Willem J. Kolff

In 1957 Dr. Peter Salisbury, in his presidential address for the American Society for Artificial Internal Organs (ASAIO), described the possibility of a totally implantable artificial kidney and a totally implantable artificial heart. Encouraged by this speech, Dr. Tetsuzo Akutsu and I put an artificial heart in a dog in December 1957. It was the first such attempt in the Western world, although V. Demichov had done it in Russia in 1935. It was a good thing that we did not realize how long it would take before the artificial heart would finally come to clinical application.

The first electrohydraulic artificial heart was put into a dog in 1966. I showed a film at the annual meeting of the ASAIO, and it was fascinating to see how a bolus of contrast moved from the right ventricle to the lungs, from there into the left ventricle, into the aorta, and then to the greater circulation.

Dr. Domingo Liotta from Argentina, Dr. William Pierce now in Hershey, Pennsylvania, Dr. Frank Hastings, Dr. Bert Kusserow, Dr. Michael De Bakey, and Dr. C.W. Hall were among the early investigators of the artificial heart.

A special artificial heart device section was set up by the National Institutes of Health (NIH), and Dr. Frank Hastings became its first director. The Congress of the United States voted $12 million for the development of the artificial heart program, but the Director of the National Heart Institute of the National Institutes of Health took it upon himself to divert $5 million of that sum to the study of the natural history of heart disease. Although Dr. Hastings protested, he was powerless to do anything about it. This left him with only $7 million to set up a contract program to rapidly develop a totally implantable artificial heart. However, the fact that so much money was available for the contract program made it very difficult for other even well-established investigators to compete via the grant mechanism. With a wave of optimism, it was believed that within a 10-year period, an artificial heart could be on the market almost guaranteed to work for 10 years. This overoptimism led to a backlash from which we are still suffering.

Among physicians, and particularly among cardiologists, there is an inborn disbelief that the artificial heart will ever work. There is an unwillingness to accept the idea that the site of life, the symbol of love, and the habitat of the soul could be replaced by a simple pump. There certainly is a great unwillingness to part with the natural heart even if it does the owner "no good." This has led to a preference for a left ventricular assist device (LVAD) that leaves the natural heart in place.

There are certain advantages to the use of LVAD, although we already know that in 30% of the cases it has to be combined with a right ventricular assist device (RVAD). These advantages are most clearly demonstrated by an experience with the heterotopic heart transplantation or "piggyback" heart that was introduced by Dr. Christian Barnard in South Africa. A man living 3000 miles from Cape Town received a "piggyback" heart; he was suffering from a viral myocarditis from which he would probably have died. Whether or not he took any anti-rejection medicine, I do not know; but about a year later when he returned to Cape Town for a checkup, he had rejected his transplant (which was then removed). His own heart had recovered.

When an LVAD fails, as long as it is not a catastrophic failure, the natural heart can in many instances keep the recipient alive until something can be done about it. On the other hand, as long as the sick heart is left in place, the situation is never fully under control. An underlying heart disease is most likely progressive, and the existing heart can give rise to thromboses and emboli; it also takes up considerable space.

During the past few years the NIH has decided that preference should be given to assist devices rather than total artificial hearts. There is no scientific background for this assumption, particularly because the left ventricle is the difficult side. Since the right ventricle pumps only against low pressures, it is not as difficult to make.

The total artificial heart program was deferred, and most of the contract money, $5 million, was spent to develop totally implantable LVADs. Even now, large amounts of money are being spent to bring totally implantable LVADs to clinical application.

The advent of Cyclosporin A changed the entire situation. Suddenly the results of heart transplantation improved so that 95% of the patients survive 1 year, and a large number of those patients survive much longer. Thus the FDA changed the rules, and artificial hearts could now be applied only as a bridge-to-transplantation; whereas before, patients who were potential candidates for transplantation were specifically excluded.

In December 1982, such a patient, Dr. Barney Clark, received a total artificial heart implanted by Dr. William DeVries at the University of Utah. This artificial heart, called the JARVIK heart, was of the type developed at the University of Utah.

What did we learn from Dr. Barney Clark? We already knew that the circulation could be well sustained and that in animals all organs continued to function normally. What we learned was that the artificial heart inside the chest did not cause any pain or disagreeable feelings; that the noise of the driving system did not bother Dr. Clark; that he did not lose his desire to live or his considerable sense of humor; nor did he lose his love for his family or his desire to serve mankind. These observations have also been confirmed in many of the 160 people who have been recipients of the total artificial heart.

As I mentioned before, the FDA decreed that the artificial heart could henceforth be used only in patients as a bridge-toward-transplantation. However, when it was found that the average time patients were being sustained with the artificial heart was only 4 days, it undercut the justification for using either a total artificial heart or a totally implantable LVAD. Why spend $100,000 for equipment and $18,000 for the implantable pump if one could probably keep a patient alive for 4 days with any kind of blood pump used outside the body?

As of January 1991 the FDA has revoked the Investigational Device Exemption (IDE) of Symbion to provide additional artificial hearts. Dr. William Pierce in Hershey, Pennsylvania has an IDE to apply his devices only in his own hospital.

The NIH has given four contracts of about $5 million each to four centers to develop a totally implantable artificial heart. For others, it is very difficult to obtain financial support for artificial heart research and development through NIH grants. There are not enough peers interested in artificial heart research when a proposal comes up for a peer review; the money provided by the NIH is insufficient; only approximately 25% of all approved grants can be funded.

Our priorities are wrong. Research money is still being spent on Star Wars and on the continuation of nuclear explosions (financed via the Department of Energy) and in other ways relating to the waging of war.

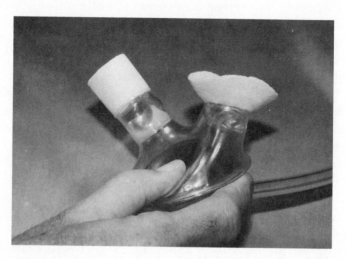

Fig. 3-1. Right ventricle and how it can be compressed. Tricusp semilunar valves and sinus valsalva can be clearly seen.

The FDA, forced by its mandate, requires assurances of the safety of artificial hearts, which small companies cannot afford. Venture capitalists and large corporations are not interested in providing funding for artificial heart research since the return on their investments would take more than 3 years. Large companies that were willing before to provide material to make artificial hearts are now refusing delivery for fear of liability and lawsuits.

What should an inventor of artificial hearts do in this country? In desperation, seek help from Japan or China? In the meantime, there are 33,000 people in the United States alone with irreparable heart diseases who die needlessly each year. A great number of them could be restored to a happy existence at least for some years, although no exact time can be guaranteed. The cost of an implantation with an inexpensive artificial heart would be less than the cost of dying slowly after repeated admissions to an intensive care unit. For that reason, I am concentrating on producing inexpensive artificial hearts of polyurethane by the technique of vacuum forming and radiofrequency welding (Fig. 3-1).

Whether a patient such as the one described above could be happy, we must remember Lief Stenberg who, 6 months after the implantation of his artificial heart, went to a restaurant outside Stockholm and served himself four times from a smorgasbord while carrying his Heimes' Drive System over his shoulder. No one in that restaurant realized that he had an artificial heart pumping inside his chest. Thereafter he sent a telegram to the United States stating "I am the happiest man in Europe."

PART TWO

CLINICAL APPLICATION OF PARTIAL AND TOTAL CARDIAC ASSIST DEVICES

CHAPTER 4

Roller pump ventricular assist device

Daniel M. Rose, Marguerite Corda, J.N. Cunningham Jr., and **F.C. Spencer**

INTRODUCTION

Although profound heart failure following cardiac surgical procedures requiring the utilization of ventricular assist devices is relatively infrequent, there have been a number of reports of increasing success with the use of these devices.[1-6] Furthermore, the role of ventricular assist devices has expanded with their utilization as a bridge-to-transplantation[7,9] and as a support device for patients with cardiogenic shock following myocardial infarction.[9] A variety of ventricular assistance devices have been utilized in these situations. We have used a roller pump-driven device since 1978, and this system is relatively effective, easy to use, and inexpensive. This chapter summarizes our experience with the use of a roller pump left heart assist device (LHAD) and right heart assist device (RHAD).

MATERIALS AND METHODS

From January 1978 to December 1990 at New York University Medical Center and from July 1982 to December 1990 at Maimonides Medical Center, Brooklyn, we have utilized a left heart assist device in 72 patients and a right heart assist device in 7 patients, following cardiac surgical procedures.

INDICATIONS
Left heart assist device

Indications for utilization of a left heart assist device were either an inability to discontinue cardiopulmonary bypass (57 patients), or cardiac arrest 1 to 12 hours postoperatively (15 patients). (See Table 4-1.) About one fourth of patients (15 of 57) who could not initially be weaned from cardiopulmonary bypass sustained a prebypass cardiac

43

Table 4-1.   Indications for insertion of ventricular assist device

Indications	LHAD° (open)		RHAD†
	Nonsurvivors	Survivors	Nonsurvivors
Inability to discontinue CPB‡	35	22	5
(Preop cardiac arrest)	(11)	(8)	(1)
Postop cardiac arrest	7	8	1
Cardiogenic shock following acute MI			1

°LHAD, left heart assist device.
†RHAD, right heart assist device.
‡CPB, Cardiopulmonary bypass.

arrest either during cardiac catheterization, attempted PTCA, or anesthetic induction. Standard techniques were employed in attempting to discontinue cardiopulmonary bypass in these patients. Techniques included volume loading, AV pacing, infusion of inotropic agents, and insertion of an intraaortic balloon. All patients demonstrated severe left heart failure with an elevated left atrial press (<25 mm Hg) and systemic hypotension (mean blood pressure < 50 mm Hg), and cardiopulmonary bypass could not be discontinued without the use of a left heart assist device.

Fifteen patients sustained a postoperative cardiac arrest either as a result of a graft spasm (six patients), refractory arrhythmias (six patients), or acute graft thrombosis (three patients). These patients required reinstitution of cardiopulmonary bypass to be resuscitated and insertion of a left heart assist device to be weaned from cardiopulmonary bypass.

Right heart assist device

In patients with isolated right heart failure (usually manifested by an elevated central venous pressure [> 20 mm Hg], a low left atrial pressure [< 6 to 8 mm Hg], systemic hypotension (systolic blood pressure [< 70 mm Hg], a low cardiac index [< 1.5 L/min/m²] and an elevated pulmonary vascular resistance), a trial of inotropic agents, pulmonary vasodilators, and systemic vasoconstrictors infused directly into the left atrium was usually attempted. In most patients an intraaortic balloon was also inserted. In five of the seven patients, cardiopulmonary bypass could not be discontinued without the use of right heart bypass (Table 4-1). In one other patient, acute right coronary graft thrombosis occurred 6 hours postoperatively; following graft revision, the patient had a right heart assist device inserted. Another patient with a large inferior wall myocardial infarction arrested during cardiac catheterization. This patient was placed on cardiopulmonary bypass, and a right heart assist device was inserted.

Preoperative clinical characteristics and operations performed

There were no major differences in the clinical characteristics of nonsurviving and surviving patients in whom a left heart assist device was inserted following cardiac sur-

Table 4-2.   Clinical characteristics of patients with ventricular assist devices

	Nonsurvivors	Survivors
LHAD		
Age	60.1 ± 2.0	59.8 ± 2.3
Preop CI (L/min/m^2)	2.17 ± 0.1	2.34 ± 0.10
EF (%)	40.7 ± 2.5	44.4 ± 2.6
Operation	31 CAB	24 CAB
	5AVR	3 AVR + CAB
	3 CAB + LV aneurysm + closure of VSD	2 CAB + LV aneurysm + closure of VSD
	3 MVR + CAB	1 MVR + CAB
AXC (min)	66.7 ± 8.1	73.6 ± 9.6
CPB (min)	236.1 ± 22.8	73.6 ± 28.1
VAD (hr)	36.4 ± 6.1	44.1 ± 4.6
RHAD		
Age	63.4 ± 3.1	
Preop CI (L/min/m^2)	2.2 ± 0.1	
EF (%)	38.5 ± 5.2	
Operation	3 CAB	
	2 CAB + closure VSD + LV aneurysm	
	1 MVR + CAB	
	1 acute RV infarction	
AXC (min)	52.3 ± 9.5	
CPB (min)	14.5 ± 30.6	
VAD (hr)	68.3 ± 10.1	

CI, cardiac index; *EF,* ejection fraction; *CPB,* cardiopulmonary bypass; *VAD,* ventricular assist device; *AXC,* aortic crossclamp time; CAB, coronary artery bypass; AVR, aortic valve replacement; VSD, ventricular septal defect; MVR, mitral valve replacement.

gery (see Table 4-2). The types of operations performed were also similar in both groups of patients as was the period of aortic occlusion.

Our impression in the last few years has been that more of the patients who require a ventricular assist device postoperatively have generally come to the operating room in profound cardiogenic shock (failed PTCA, left main coronary artery dissection, evolving myocardial infarction, ruptured ventricular septum, ruptured papillary muscle, etc.).

TECHNIQUE OF INSERTION
Left heart assist device

A 28-32 French venous cannula is inserted through a purse-string suture into the left atrium, either through the left atrial appendage or through the right superior pul-

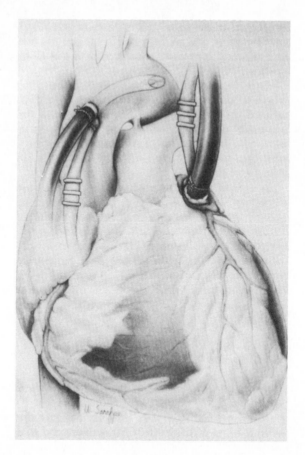

Fig. 4-1. Intracardiac location of aortic and left atrial cannulae.

monary vein. A 5 to 6 mm arterial cannula is inserted through a purse-string suture into the ascending aorta (Fig. 4-1). The tip is advanced beyond the left subclavian artery to decrease the potential for cerebral embolization. Cannulae exit through the sternotomy or through separate parasternal incisions (Fig. 4-2). The cannulae are connected to ⅜ × ¹⁄₁₆ silicone tubing (Dow Corning, Midland, Michigan) connected to a portable roller pump (Fig. 4-3).

With this device, maximal flow rates of 3.5 to 4.9 L/min can be attained. After insertion of the left heart assist device, flow rates of 2.0 to 4.0 L/min are provided to maintain adequate systemic perfusion and discontinue cardiopulmonary bypass. Left atrial pressure is maintained between 5 and 12 mm Hg, inotropic agents are used to augment right heart function, and an intraaortic balloon is used to provide counterpulsation.

When closing the chest, it is critically important to avoid cardiac compression and to open the pericardium widely. In some patients the sternum may not be closed with-

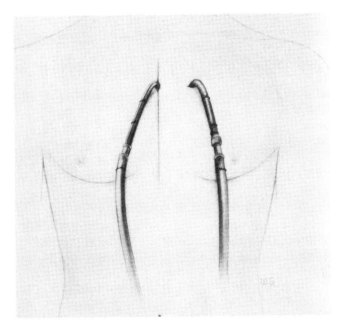

Fig. 4-2. Position of cannulae as they exit the sternum.

out compressing the heart; in these patients it is necessary to leave the sternum open and close only the skin. In some patients it may not be possible to close the skin; synthetic material may be used to cover the sternal defect.

Right heart assist device

The right heart assist device insertion technique is similar to that of the left heart assist device. A 28-32 French venous cannula is inserted into the right atrium through a purse-string suture. A small arterial cannula is inserted into the main pulmonary artery through a purse-string suture. Cannulae are connected to the silastic tubing, which is then connected to a portable roller pump.

Flow rates from 2.5 to 4.0 L/min are employed. Similar precautions concerning pericardial constriction and sternal compression are observed. Patients are generally placed on pulmonary artery vasodilators and inotropic agents to enhance myocardial function. Vasoconstrictors can be infused through a left atrial line. Patients are heparinized in a fashion similar to that used with the left heart assist device.

POSTOPERATIVE PATIENT CARE—NURSING MANAGEMENT
Early postoperative care

Patients with ventricular assist devices clearly require very intensive and thorough critical care nursing. The patient's heart rate, central venous pressure, pulmonary artery

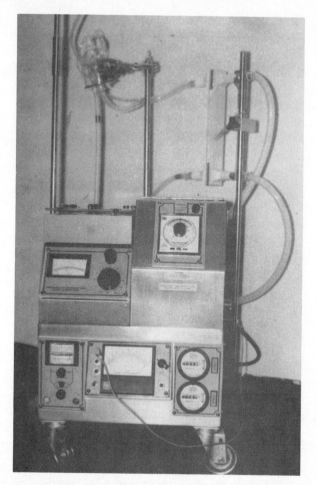

Fig. 4-3. Portable roller pump employed for ventricular assistance.

pressure, left atrial pressure, and systemic pressures are all continuously monitored. Cardiac output is determined with a balloon-tipped thermodilution pulmonary artery catheter. Left and right atrial pressures should be maintained in the range of 6 to 12 mm Hg to prevent air embolizaton.

If postoperative bleeding is not excessive (25 to 30 cc per hour), patients are given heparin (250 to 750 units per hour), 4 to 6 hours following surgery. The activated clotting time (ACT) is maintained between 150 and 250 seconds with this regimen. Aside from assessment of hemodynamics, it is also necessary to periodically evaluate pulmonary, renal, and neurologic function. Because there is a possibility of particulate or air embolization with these devices, other organ dysfunction may occur; and this may be due to embolization rather than primary organ dysfunction.

Hemodynamic deterioration in the early postoperative period (12 to 48 hours) in an otherwise relatively stable patient, may herald an occult cardiac tamponade rather than primary cardiac failure; this can only be adequately assessed by reexploration.

Patient family interaction

Ventricular assist devices are generally inserted during life-or-death situations, and often the family members may be overwhelmed by the severity of the patient's condition and the complexity of the information given. It is important for the nurse-clinician to provide reassurance and support to the patient and his or her family.

It is helpful for the nurse-clinician to reinforce the details presented by the physician. Diagrams are useful in enabling the family to "visualize" the interface of the assist device to the patient. The correct amount of information given to the family hinges on what they want to know or are ready to accept.

Once the patient is stabilized, the family can visit the patient for brief intervals. It is essential that the family receives adequate preparation regarding the patient's physical appearance and the myriad of machinery and personnel present at the bedside. Reassurance is provided to the waking patient that the operation is completed and that he or she is in the recovery area with nursing and medical personnel constantly in attendance to provide care. After a detailed neurologic assessment, sedation and pain medication may be administered as needed. Reiteration of relevant explanations before any intervention often allays many of the patient's anxieties.

Not to be lost in the mechanical complexity required to care for the patient with ventricular assist devices is the human component of touch. Holding the patient's hand and offering flavored mouth swabs are only a few of the nursing measures that enhance the patient's emotional well-being. The patient's sense of worth as a person and not just a receptacle for tubes and machinery must be stressed.

Weaning and removal of device

The ventricular assist device is usually run in collaboration with one of the cardiac perfusionists. Because of fatigue and wear to the tubing, it is necessary to rotate the tubing in the pump head every 4 to 6 hours depending on the flow rate. Failure to do this may lead to perforation of the tubing or excessive wear and particulate embolization. During rotation of the tubing, caution should be exercised not to reverse tubing direction, which would obviously have catastrophic results. Due to the length of the tubing exposed to ambient air temperature, there can be resultant heat loss to the patient. This can be minimized by wrapping the tubing in thermal insulation.

Periodic assessment of underlying hemodynamic function can be determined by lowering the flow rate on the assist device to 400 to 500 cc/min and then determining the patient's underlying cardiac output, systemic blood pressure, and left and right atrial pressures. It is usually apparent when the patient's own cardiac function begins to recover. At this time the flow rate on the assist device can be gradually decreased (200 to 400 cc/min) every 2 to 4 hours as the patient's cardiac function allows. Clearly, care should be taken not to wean the device prematurely.

Once the patient's cardiac output is satisfactory, flow rates can be maintained at 500 to 800 cc/min and the patient observed for a minimum of 12 hours. Maintaining a lower flow rate may result in tubing clot formation.

Once it has been determined that discontinuation of the assist device can be tolerated, the patient is returned to the operating room. Cannulae are removed and purse-string sutures snugly tied and oversewn. It has not been necessary, in our experience, to reinstitute cardiopulmonary bypass for cannulae removal; although if there are problems in repairing the atrial insertion sites, cardiopulmonary bypass can be reinstituted.

All foreign necrotic material should be removed, and the operative area should be generously irrigated before sternal reclosure. Soft drainage catheters are usually left in place for about 24 hours postoperatively, and patients are given prophylactic systemic antibiotics for 5 to 7 days thereafter.

RESULTS
Left heart assist device

Thirty patients (41.7%) were weaned from the left heart assist device 24 to 96 hours following insertion (Table 4-3). These patients had gradual recovery of their left heart function, allowing gradual discontinuation of the left heart bypass. Causes of death in the 42 nonsurviving patients included severe coagulopathy, refractory arrhythmias, biventricular failure, or massive neurologic injury. Often a combination of these factors was present, contributing to the patient's death.

Nine patients died 21 to 90 days postoperatively: seven as a result of sepsis and multisystem failure and two as a result of pulmonary embolism. Of the 21 long-term survivors, there were 2 late deaths, one 4 months and one 4 years postoperatively, both from cardiac causes. Of the 19 long-term survivors, 11 patients are New York Heart Association Class I, 7 patients are New York Heart Association Class II, and 2 patients are New York Heart Association Class III (Table 4-4). No preoperative or intraoperative patient factors appear to be predictive of patient survival.

Right heart assist device

Two patients were weaned from the right heart assist device 48 and 72 hours following insertion. One patient died 5 days postoperatively from multisystem failure and sepsis and one patient died 10 days postoperatively from pneumonia. Of the five patients who could not be weaned, three patients had profound coagulopathy, one patient had severe hypoxemia and "shock lung," and one patient had a massive neurologic injury and the right heart assist device was discontinued. Two of these nonsurviving patients had premature discontinuation of the right heart assist device; shortly following removal of the device, the patients had a rapid return of right heart failure and the

Table 4-3.   Clinical experience with roller pump ventricular assist devices

	Total patients	Early survivors	Late survivors
Left heart assist device (open)	72	30 (41.7%)	21(29.2%)
Right heart assist device (open)	7	2 (28.6%)	0

Table 4-4.   Status of patients weaned from LHAD

Results		Status	Patients
9	Early deaths:	Pulmonary emboli	2
	(21-90 days)	Sepsis (pulmonary, pancreatic, colon, renal)	7
2	Late deaths:	Sudden "cardiac" death	
	(4 mo-4 yr)		
19	Long-term survivors:	NYHA I	10
		NYHA II	7
		NYHA III	2

device had to be reinserted. Both of these patients developed profound coagulopathy and died postoperatively at 72 and 96 hours respectively.

DISCUSSION
Left heart assist device

Multiple factors can certainly produce profound postoperative cardiac failure. These include previous myocardial infarction with depressed ventricular dysfunction, active ongoing ischemia or infarction, inadequate myocardial protection, or incomplete myocardial revascularization.[10-12] In addition, coronary artery vasospasm in either the native coronary artery, vein graft, or internal mammary artery can produce significant myocardial failure and arrhythmias.[13,14]

It has been suggested that during the initial reperfusion period an oxygen supply and demand imbalance exists. Despite adequate reperfusion there may be cellular and metabolic abnormalities that could impair ventricular function,[15,16] causing the myocardium to act as if it has been "stunned," as has been suggested by Braunwald and Klouer.[17] As these investigators have shown, acute coronary artery occlusion for only 15 minutes can result in functional and metabolic abnormalities for as long as 7 days.[16] Thus despite adequate revascularization, some patients have persistent cardiac failure as a result of the myocardium being "stunned."

Previous experimental studies indicate that left ventricular bypass and left atrial bypass can effectively unload the left ventricle and arrest infarct expansion.[9,18,19] Thus marginally perfused ischemic tissue that could ultimately infarct may be salvaged with

LHAD Flow Rate

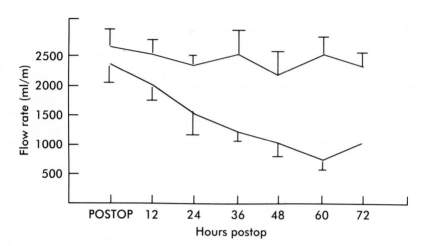

Fig. 4-4. Flow rates of nonsurviving and surviving patients. Note improvement of ventricular function in many patients as early as 12 hours postoperatively.

the utilization of left heart bypass. A critical determinant of ultimate survival is obviously the extent of irreversibly infarcted tissue compared with the amount of reversibly injured ischemic tissue; this ratio may be favorably affected with the use of the left heart bypass.

The optimal or necessary period of time left heart support should be provided is not clear. The device we have employed is not capable of providing flow rates as high as the device employed by Pierce and associates.[2] With the device we have utilized, surviving patients will demonstrate evidence of left ventricular recovery as early as 12 hours postoperatively, and most surviving patients will show improvement in left ventricular function within 48 hours postoperatively[1,9] (Fig. 4-4).

We have been reluctant to maintain flow rates in excess of 3000 ml/min for prolonged periods of time in our patients because we believed that this could produce significant hemolysis and destruction of blood elements. However, if larger arterial and venous cannulae were inserted, this most likely would not occur. The Hershey group[2] has supported patients with their left heart assist device for as long as 25 days (mean 6.8 days). Thus the optimal period of left heart support varies considerably with the type of assist device employed. The device that Pierce and co-workers have used is capable of providing flow rates of up to 6.5 L/min. Therefore it seems that with more complete left heart bypass, patients can be successfully supported for longer periods of time.

Right heart assist device

The cause of right heart failure can be similar to that of left heart failure (active ongoing ischemia or infarction, inadequate myocardial protection, incomplete revascularization, vasospasm, etc.).[20,21,22] In addition, right heart failure can be exacerbated or caused by increased pulmonary vascular resistance.[23] Often a combination of these factors (right heart ischemia and elevated pulmonary vascular resistance) will be present. Although we have not had any experience with pulmonary artery balloon counterpulsation, there have been some encouraging results with this modality.[24,25]

The effects of right heart bypass on pulmonary microcirculation and lung water formation have not been clearly elucidated experimentally. There is some recent experimental data suggesting that right heart bypass may have a deleterious effect on pulmonary function.[26] Thus this support device, in some instances, may create further pulmonary injury and elevate pulmonary vascular resistance, further impairing right heart function.

It is evident from experimental and clinical data that the right heart can often recover sufficiently to permit removal of the support device.[2,20,21] However, we have observed, quite dramatically, two patients in whom there was premature discontinuation of the right heart assist device, followed by the insidious return of profound right heart failure and cardiac arrest. The recurrence of right heart failure may be a result of an increase in the pulmonary vascular resistance that has gone undetected.

It is clear that in many patients there is evidence of biventricular failure[5]; however, there is often a preponderance of one chamber failure and thus either a right or a left heart assist device can be successfully employed. Our experience with biventricular assistance is minimal, although it seems from the experience of others that patients with severe biventricular failure will generally go on to cardiac transplantation if they are suitable candidates.[2,8]

CONCLUSION

As our data suggest, reasonably good results can be achieved with a roller pump type of ventricular assist device. Further experience obviously needs to be obtained in treating patients with acute evolving myocardial infarction. In the future, for roller pump ventricular assist devices to gain widespread use further refinement will be necessary to make them less complicated, more economical, and to contribute to enhanced patient survival.

REFERENCES

1. Rose DM, Laschinger J, Grossi E et al: Experimental and clinical results with a simplified left heart assist device for treatment of profound left ventricular dysfunction, *World J Surg* 9:11, 1985.
2. Pae WE, Pierce WS, Pennock JL et al: Long-term results of ventricular assist pumping in postcardiotomy cardiogenic shock, *J Thorac Cardiovasc Surg* 93:434, 1987.
3. Pennington DG, Bernhard WF, Golding LR et al: Long-term follow-up of postcardiotomy patients with profound cardiogenic shock treated with ventricular assist device, *Circulation* 72:206, 1985.
4. Park SB, Liebler GA, Burkholder JA et al: Mechanical support of the failing heart, *Ann Thorac Surg* 42:627, 1986.
5. Pennington DG, Merjavy JP, Swartz MT et al: The importance of biventricular failure in patients with postoperative cardiogenic shock, *Ann Thorac Surg* 38:16, 1985.

6. Zumbro GL, Kitchens WR, Shearer G et al: Mechanical assistance for cardiogenic shock following cardiac surgery, myocardial infarction, and cardiac transplantation, *Ann Thorac Surg* 44:11, 1987.
7. Hill JD, Farrar DJ, Hershon JJ et al: Use of a prosthetic ventricle as a bridge to cardiac transplantation for postinfarction cardiogenic shock, *N Engl J Med* 314:626, 1986.
8. Pennock JL, Pierce WS, Campbell DB et al: Mechanical support of the circulation followed by cardiac transplantation. *J Thorac Cardiovasc Surg* 92:994, 1986.
9. Rose DM, Grossi E, Laschinger J et al: Strategy for treatment of acute evolving myocardial infarction with pulsatile left heart assist device. Can this modality increase survival and enhance myocardial salvage? In Bregman D, ed: *Critical Care Clinics, New Techniques in Mechanical Support*. Philadelphia, 1986, WB Saunders.
10. Buda AJ, MacDonald IL, Anderson MJ et al: Long-term results following coronary bypass operation. Importance of preoperative factors and complete revascularization, *J Thorac Cardiovasc Surg* 82:383, 1981.
11. Hilton CJ, Beubl W, Acker M et al: Inadequate cardioplegic protection with obstructed coronary arteries, *Ann Thorac Surg* 28:323, 1979.
12. Kennedy JW, Kaiser GL, Fisher LD et al: Clinical and angiographic predictors of operative mortality from the collaborative study in coronary artery surgery (CASS), *Circulation* 63:793, 1981.
13. Buxton AE, Goldberg S, Harken A et al: Coronary artery spasm immediately after myocardial revascularization. Recognition and management, *N Engl J Med* 304:1249, 1981.
14. Lockerman ZS, Rose DM, Cunningham JN Jr et al: Reperfusion ventricular fibrillation during coronary artery bypass surgery and its association with postoperative enzyme release, *J Thorac Cardiovasc Surg* 93:247, 1987.
15. Klouer RA, Ellis ST, Lange R et al: Studies of experimental coronary artery reperfusion: effects on infarct size, myocardial function, biochemistry, ultrastructure and microvasculature damage, *Circulation* 68 (suppl I):1, 1983.
16. Ellis SB, Henschke CI, Sandor T et al: Time course of functional and biochemical recovery of myocardium salvaged by reperfusion, *J Am Coll Cardiol* 11:1047, 1983.
17. Braunwald E, Klouer RA: The stunned myocardium—prolonged, postischemic ventricular dysfunction, *Circulation* 66:1146, 1982 (editorial).
18. Pennock JL, Pae WE, Pierce WS et al: Reduction of myocardial infarct size. Comparison between left atrial and left ventricular bypass, *Circulation* 59:275, 1979.
19. Grossi EA, Laschinger JC, Cunningham JN Jr et al: Time course in myocardial salvage with left heart assist in evolving myocardial infarction, *Surg Forum* 35:322, 1984.
20. Dembitsky WP, Daily PO, Raney AA et al: Temporary extracorporeal support of the right ventricle, *J Thorac Cardiovasc Surg* 91:518, 1986.
21. O'Neill MJ, Pierce WS, Wisman CB et al: Successful management of right ventricular failure with the ventricular assist pump following aortic valve replacement and coronary bypass grafting, *J Thorac Cardiovasc Surg* 87:106, 1984.
22. Cohn JN: Right ventricular infarction revisited, *Am J Cardiol* 43:666, 1979.
23. Vlahades GJ, Turley K, Hoffman JIE: The pathophysiology of failure in acute right ventricular hypertension. Hemodynamic and biochemical correlations, *Circulation* 63:87, 1981.
24. Spence PA, Weisel RD, Easdown J et al: The hemodynamic effects and mechanism of action of pulmonary artery balloon counterpulsation in the treatment of right ventricular failure during left heart bypass, *Ann Thorac Surg* 39:329, 1985.
25. Symbas PN, McKeown PP, Santora AH et al: Pulmonary artery balloon counterpulsation for treatment of intraoperative right ventricular failure, *Ann Thorac Surg* 39:437, 1985.

CHAPTER 5

Centrifugal ventricular assist devices

Lyle D. Joyce, Carol Toninato, and **Jane B. Hansen**

INTRODUCTION

It is well documented that pulsatile flow is not the only acceptable way to support the circulation. Barcroft used a centrifugal pump in 1933 during the early development stages of a pump for cardiopulmonary bypass.[1] De Bakey and others perfected this and the nonpulsatile roller pump eventually became the pump of choice for cardiopulmonary bypass. Early attempts at supporting left ventricular function in the postcardiotomy period utilized the roller pump.[2] Although there was some limited success with this approach, development of centrifugal pumps markedly improved results of postcardiotomy support. Centrifugal pumps were considered for circulatory assist and replacement devices as early as the 1950s.[3,4] Some of the advantages were described by Sexton in 1960.[7]

Three types of centrifugal pumps are commercially manufactured (Fig. 5-1): Biomedicus, Sarns, and St. Jude Medical. Although approved by the FDA for use during cardiopulmonary bypass only, the clinical success from use of these devices for temporary postcardiotomy ventricular support appears to have secured them a definite position in the list of mechanical devices presently available for short- to long-term mechanical circulatory support.

PATIENT SELECTION

The most frequent use of centrifugal pumps for ventricular support is in that group of patients who are unweanable from cardiopulmonary bypass. However, these devices have been utilized multiple times for bridging to cardiac transplantation and in attempts to quickly resuscitate patients in acute cardiogenic shock who have potentially salvageable myocardium.

The hemodynamic criteria for use of ventricular assist devices (VAD) after cardiopulmonary bypass or during cardiogenic shock have been well documented by other authors.[5] Patients generally have a cardiac index of less than 2 L/min/m^2 with a mean arterial pressure of 60 mm Hg despite inotropic support and use of the intraaortic bal-

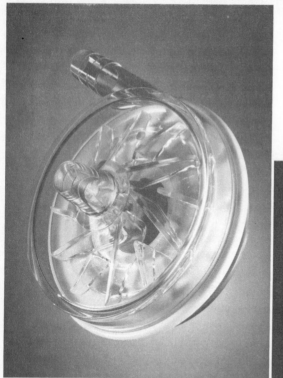

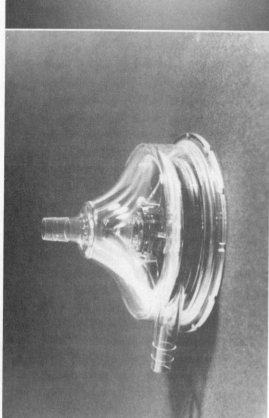

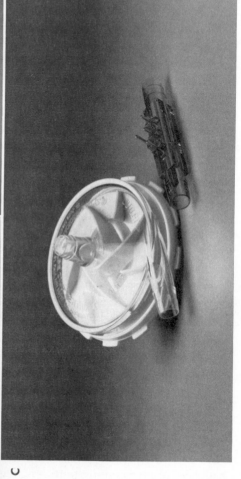

Fig. 5-1. A, Medtronic Biomedicus centrifugal pump head; **B,** Sarns 3M centrifugal pump head;

loon pump, with volume loading to a pulmonary artery wedge pressure of greater than 25 mm Hg.

In the case of inability to wean successfully from the cardiopulmonary bypass machine, patients are generally given at least an additional hour of "resting" on the cardiopulmonary bypass machine with repeated attempts to wean, before proceeding with insertion of a ventricular assist device.

Use of univentricular or biventricular devices is based on the observed hemodynamics for each ventricle. If it appears that there is single ventricular failure, this device is inserted initially and the second ventricle then evaluated carefully. However, if there are beginning signs of biventricular failure with filling pressures on the nonsupported side greater than 25 mm Hg or evidence of hypoxia and/or acidosis, biventricular support is indicated.

There are no absolute contraindications to the use of a device, other than advanced age (greater than 75 years), evidence of major neurologic injury, uncontrollable disseminated intravascular coagulation, or complete loss of vascular tone during cardiopulmonary bypass despite the use of various alpha agents.

INSERTION TECHNIQUES

Various cannulation techniques for biventricular support have been reported.[6] All patients received right atrial to pulmonary artery bypassing during right ventricular support. Some surgeons prefer direct right ventricular cannulation via the apex of the right ventricle. For left ventricular support, inflow cannulae were inserted into the left atrium through the left atrial appendage, left atrium dome, or (most frequently) the right superior pulmonary vein. Others have used left ventricular apical insertion for direct ventricular cannulation. The left ventricular assist device outflow cannula was inserted into the ascending aorta in all instances.

The greatest limiting factors in surgically implanting one of the centrifugal ventricular assist devices have been (1) inadequate cannulae for convenient and secure cannulation of the heart, and (2) the lack of a means of maintaining complete hemostasis at the cannulation sites. Multiple manufacturers have now developed cannulae that have made positioning of the inflow and outflow ports much easier to carry out, thus allowing less impedance when attempting to maintain higher flows.

Each of the cannulae is initially secured into the heart's various chambers and great vessels through the use of two concentric purse-string sutures; teflon pledgets are used to buttress tissue against the cannula wall.

Initial experience included transition of the cannulae through the sternum or anterior chest wall. With the cannulae now available, each of the four cannulae can be transferred retrosternally to the subxyphoid area and brought out through separate stab-wound incisions in this area. This allows much better device security and perhaps would even allow patient ambulation. Fibrin sealant is frequently used to assist in maintaining even greater hemostasis at the cannulation sites.

Date	Nurse ✓	

Minneapolis Heart Institute
Postop right and/or left ventricular assist device orders

Primary physician _____

Height: _____ Weight: _____

Allergies: _____

A. Hemodynamic management
   1. Brand of assist device _____

      Placement of: inflow cannulae LVAD _____
                      inflow cannulae RVAD _____
                      outflow cannulae LVAD _____
                      outflow cannulae RVAD _____

   2. Call surgeon if the following parameters are not maintained by protocols listed below:
      a. Pulse maintained from _____ to _____
      b. Blood pressure maintained from _____ to _____
      c. PAD/LA maintained from _____ to _____
      d. RA/CVP maintained from _____ to _____

   3. Autotransfuse chest tube losses
      _____ Yes _____ No

   4. If BP is low and filling pressures are low, give:
      a. _____ FFP, _____ 5% Albumin, _____ Hespan   If Hgb greater than 10.0
      b. If Hgb less than 10.0, give RBCs
      * If giving Hespan, call if greater than 1500 cc replacement is needed.

   5. If any of the following IV medications are infusing, keep within the dosages listed. Do not start any of the following medications without first contacting the physician.
      Dopamine _____ mcg/kg/min
      Dobutamine _____ mcg/kg/min
      Epinephrine _____ mcg/min
      Inocar _____ mcg/kg/min
      Nitroglycerin _____ mcg/min
      Nitroprusside _____ mcg/kg/min

   6. Maintenance IV of D5 electrolyte #2 @ _____ cc/hr.
      Total all IVs

   7. Infuse all IV chronotropic, inotropic, and vasoactive drips via an infusion pump. Run all pressors via a central line.

   8. VAD flow rates and RPMs to be adjusted by the surgeon or perfusionist.

(Continued)

Fig. 5-2. Postoperative right and/or left ventricular assist device orders. Courtesy Minneapolis Heart Institute.

Date	Nurse
	✔

9. Heparin to be started by R.N. when blood loss is less than _____ .
    Heparin dose determined and ACTs managed by surgeon or perfusionist.
    * If flow rate greater than 2 L/min, maintain ACT at 180-200 sec.
    * If flow rate 1-2 L/min, maintain ACT at 350 sec.
    * If flow rate less than 1 L/min, maintain ACT at 480 sec.

10. IABP _____ 1:1 _____ 1:2 _____ 1:3
    _____ % augmentation

11. If pacemaker present, set _____ on _____ off
    _____ demand _____ fixed

    Atrial MA _____
    Ventricular MA _____
    Ventricular rate _____
    Ventricular sensitivity _____
    AV interval _____

12. Defibrillate according to VAD defibrillation protocol.

13. Add patient to Dr. Love's census.

B. General nursing care
    1. Admit to station 10 from OR.
        Protective isolation _____ Yes _____ No

    2. VS, cardiac and hemodynamic monitoring per ICU routine q 15 minutes HR
        and BP while on any titrated inotropic, chronotropic, or vasoactive infusion.

    3. Bedrest. May elevate head of bed 15 degrees. Flat for pressure readings. May
        tilt slightly from side to side.

    4. Range of motion to hands and feet only.

    5. Kinair bed with scale.

    6. Daily weight (bed weight only). Do not use sling.

    7. NG to continuous suction, if placed. May irrigate with 30 cc NS prn. May D/C
        after extubation.

    8. Dietician to consult regarding nutrition on 1st postop day.
        _____ Yes _____ No

    9. NPO while intubated. Sips of water 2h after extubation.

    10. Advance diet as tolerated to:
        _____ 2 gm Sodium   _____ ADA
        _____ Calorie restriction _____ Low cholesterol
        _____ NAS   _____ Regular
        Check for BS, abdominal distention, nausea, etc.

    11. I&O. Discontinue when off IV x 24 hours.

(Continued)

Date	Nurse ✔	
		12. Chest tubes to suction @ 20 cm/H_2O negative pressure. Strip prn. Record output.

12. Chest tubes to suction @ 20 cm/H_2O negative pressure. Strip prn. Record output.

13. Foley catheter. Measure output every 1 hour.

14. No TED stockings until VAD removal.

15. Change chest dressings per VAD procedure, only after consulting with surgeon.

16. Soft restraints if not receiving paralytic agents.

C. Respiratory care

1. Oximeter to keep SaO_2 greater than _____

2. Oxygen per face mask after extubation.

3. IS 10-15 times, q1-2h while awake x 24h, then q 2-4h. Progress volume.

D. Medications

1. Protamine sulfate _____ mg IV upon arrival to ICU.

2. Vancomycin 12 mg/kg IV loading dose in OR.
Begin Vancomycin in ICU per pharmacy protocol.
Notify Dr. Love of patient's arrival in ICU.

3. Sedation and control of paralytic agents by MDA/surgeon.

4. Acetaminophen (Tylenol) 650 mg po/R q 3h prn if temp greater than 38.4 C, or for mild discomfort.

5. Furosemide (Lasix) _____ mg IV prn for urine output less than
_____ ml/h x 2h, if filling pressures are adequate. May increase to
Furosemide (Lasix) _____ mg IV if response is less than _____ ml in 1st hour after dose.

6. KCl (Potassium chloride) 10 mEq IV x 3h for K^+ less than 4.0. Repeat K^+ after KCl infused. If less than 4.0, repeat protocol. If greater than 5.2 and urine output greater than 20 cc/h, recheck K^+ in 1h. If still greater than 5.2, change IV to D51/3NS. Give half dose of KCl if patient is less than 40 kg.

7. Lidocaine 1 mg/kg IVP prn for greater than 8 PVCs/min, couplets, multifocal or V-Tach. If arrhythmia recurs, rebolus and begin IV drip @ 2 mg/min. Check K^+ if indicated.

8. For pain:
MS04 1 - 2 mg IV q 1h prn while intubated.
MS04 4 - 10 mg IM q 3-4h prn after extubation.
Tylenol #3 or #4, 1 tab q 3-4h prn x 48h when tolerating po.

9. Halcion (Triazolam) 0.125 mg po hs prn when tol po fluids. May repeat x 1 if age less than 65 years. Do not give if systolic BP is less than 100.

(Continued)

Date	Nurse ✔	

10. Early am 1st postop day:
    If LAP greater than _____, weight greater than _____ kg from preop, and BP greater than _____
    a. give salt poor albumin 12.5 g
    b. give Lasix 20 mg IV

11. _____ Yes _____ No Heparin _____ 2500 U _____ 5000 U SQ q 12h x 3 days, or until ambulatory. Start after chest tubes removed. Do not give for redos.

12. Lasix _____ mg in _____ 250 cc _____ 500 cc 20% mannitol.
    Infuse @ _____ cc/h.

13. Zantac _____ mg IV q _____ h.

14. Maalox _____ cc NG q _____ h.

E. Laboratory

1. Immediately postop and daily until assist device is removed:
   Hgb (L9450), plasma free Hgb (L9131), ABG (L9196), SMA 7.

2. DIC screen II (L9494) upon arrival to ICU and before removal of VAD.

3. Calcium (L9056) & Magnesium (L9175) upon arrival to ICU.

4. ABGs q 6h x 24h and during weaning of VAD.

5. CXR _____ Yes _____ No
   Obtain permission from surgeon before obtaining CXRs.

6. Daily T & S while assist device is in. Keep 4 u of RBCs on hand.

7. First postop day SGOT, CPAN, & EKG.

8. Second postop day SGOT & CPAN.

9. Fourth postop day Hgb.

10. Fifth postop day EKG, CXR _____ Yes _____ No

11. PCXR 1h after removal of pleural chest tube.

12. PT daily on valves.

13. K^+ prn for increased ventricular ectopy or induced diuresis greater than 200 cc/hr x 1.

14. ABGs prn for evidence of hypoxia or respiratory alkalosis/acidosis.

15. Notify surgeon if Hgb less than 10.0.

16. Notify MDA regarding respiratory status, vent settings, and related treatments. Check for pulmonary consult if still intubated on third postop day.

17. Notify cardiologist regarding cardiac status, glucose greater than 250, oral anticoagulation orders, and protimes.

_____ M.D.

PATIENT TRANSPORT

Management of the transport of patients with ventricular assist devices has been simplified primarily by the evolution of the devices themselves. All ventricular assist devices are currently equipped with batteries to drive the system for a minimum of 2 hours. This allows flexibility in the transporting of patients from the operating room to the intensive care unit or to radiology. The patients are kept sedated and paralyzed from the time of insertion until the period of weaning from the device, with the exception of periodic emergence for neurological evaluation. Cannulation of the great vessels predisposes the patient to hemorrhage if the cannulae should inadvertently be displaced. Therefore great care must be exercised in transport. Disconnection of the tubing from the device can occur, requiring that clamps be available to occlude the inflow and outflow cannulae in a position most proximal to the patient. Transport is accomplished with the assistance of nurses, perfusionist, and other ancillary personnel.

POSTOPERATIVE MANAGEMENT

Management of ventricular assist device patients requires the coordinated efforts of physician, ICU nurse, and perfusionist. The Minneapolis Heart Institute has standard orders for this group of patients (Fig. 5-2). Ventricular assist device flows are maintained at 2 to 2.5 L/min/m². Attempts are made to discontinue intravenous inotropes, with the exception of those needed to maintain systemic vascular resistances within normal limits. Filling pressures are maintained at 10 mm Hg.

Patients are periodically allowed to awaken to evaluate their neurological status, with subsequent activity dependent on the degree of stability that the physician believes he or she has maintained through VAD cannula placement.

NURSING CARE

A nursing care plan for the centrifugal VAD patient is presented in Table 5-1.

ANTICOAGULATION

Varying protocols for anticoagulation have been used; however, there is no real need for heparinization until flows drop below 1.5 to 2.0 L/min. If there is no evidence of significant bleeding, prophylactic heparinization is begun even at greater flows.

POTENTIAL COMPLICATIONS

Because of the critical illness of these patients at the time of device implant, complications during circulatory support are frequent and multiple. The International Registry analysis[7] indicated that bleeding, disseminated intravascular coagulation, renal failure, biventricular failure, cyanosis secondary to a patent foramen ovale, inadequate

Table 5-1.   Nursing care plan for the centrifugal VAD patient

Nursing diagnosis	Expected outcome	Interventions
Decreased cardiac output related to myocardial dysfunction, requiring centrifugal VAD support	Cardiac output is adequately maintained as evidenced by: (1) adequate VAD flow, (2) vital signs normal, (3) adequate urine output, (4) skin warm, pink, and dry, (5) no dysrhythmias, and (6) normal cerebral function	Monitor BP, RAP, P/A, PAWP hourly Monitor indicators of perfusion: (1) urine output, (2) skin color and temperature, (3) rhythm, and (4) sensorsium Monitor VAD flow (1/minute) and communicate with VAD team regarding any S/S of VAD dysfunction Compute TDCO for LVAD patient and FICK CO for RVAD patient every 4 hours Observe for volume depletion and replace as ordered with blood, fluid, and colloids Observe VAD atrial line for "chatter" suggesting that flow needs to be decreased Observe for S/S of cardiac tamponade Assess patient's intrinsic VAD function daily with VAD team Monitor indicators of perfusion as needed when VAD flow is decreased Observe arterial pressure waveform for documentation of dicrotic notch for LVAD patient and P/A dicrotic notch for RVAD patient
Impaired gas exchange related to atelectasis, V/Q mismatch, immobility, and sedation	Satisfactory oxygenation and respiratory status maintained	With patient intubated and mechanically ventilated, follow unit procedure for vent checks, arterial blood gases, and mixed venous O_2 measurements Verify endotracheal tube placement by chest x-ray Instill saline and suction every 2 hours, and as needed Auscultate breath sounds every 2 hours
Bleeding related to blood component traumatization from VAD and cardiopulmonary bypass	Hemostasis with normalization of blood-clotting factors	Observe for bleeding from any source (chest tubes, urine, stool, GI tract) Observe dressing sites for bleeding Complete daily hemotologic profile: CBC, prothrombin time, partial thromboplastin time, activated clotting time, reticulocyte count, fibrinogen, and fibrin split products Keep extra set of VAD tubing and clamps at bedside

Continued

Table 5-1. Nursing care plan for the centrifugal VAD patient—cont'd

Nursing diagnosis	Expected outcome	Interventions
High risk for injury and thrombi related to VAD use	No evidence of thrombi formation	Be aware that patient is susceptible to thrombi formation if VAD flows are decreased. Check with physician regarding anticoagulation before decreasing flows Observe pumphead every hour for evidence of thrombi formation Administer anticoagulation protocol as ordered
High risk for infection related to multiple invasive lines	Absence of infection as evidenced by: no sign of redness or drainage from VAD cannulae and invasive lines and normal temperature and leukocyte count	Assess for S/S of infection (increased leukocyte count, fever, redness, swelling, and/or drainage from VAD cannulae and invasive lines) Aseptic technique when changing VAD lines, pumphead, and dressings Place patient in reverse isolation

Modified from Quaal SJ: Centrifugal VAD. *AACN's clinical issues in critical care nursing,* 2:515, 1991.

cardiac output, and inlet cannula obstruction were statistically associated with inability to wean a patient from circulatory support regardless of the type of support (right, left, or biventricular). When these variables were analyzed according to type of device used in relationship to ability to wean, only bleeding became a significant factor. This complication was most frequently associated with the centrifugal pump group.

Infection rates in patients receiving ventricular assist devices listed by the International Registry ranged from 15% to 30%. In our group of patients 18% developed infections; however, this had little effect on the overall survival rate (60% in patients with infections).

A major concern that continues with the use of VADs is the potential for cerebral vascular accidents (CVA). As many as 20% have been reported in some series; however, we had no documented CVAs secondary to the use of the Sarns VAD.

With the present centrifugal ventricular assist devices, a persistent buildup of an amorphous material occurs at the shaft/seal interface, which can cause the impellers to freeze from time to time, necessitating a quick pump change. Thus it is important to check the seals at least every 8 hours; pump heads should be changed when seepage begins.

WEANING FROM THE DEVICE

Once VAD insertion is completed, the patient is given maximum cardiac support for a minimum of 24 hours before any efforts are made to determine the native myocardium's status. At that point, flows are temporarily turned down over 30 to 60 minutes to determine if there is any evidence of myocardial function with and without intraaortic balloon pump assistance. If there is no evidence of returnable myocardial function, the flows are immediately returned to maximum levels and the patient receives additional support for another 24-hour period. This reassessment is carried out on a daily basis until the patient is deemed either unsalvageable or weanable. If believed to be weanable, a formal weaning process is then carried out over a 12-hour period, during which time flows are reduced approximately 500 ml/min every 2 to 4 hours until decreased to 1 to 1.5 L/min. At this point the patient is fully heparinized and the pumps are turned off for a minimum of 30 minutes before returning to the operating room. If the patient continues to maintain good cardiac support, with only moderate pressor agents and intraaortic balloon pump support, the patient is then taken back to the operating room and the devices are removed.

CLINICAL SUCCESS

Drs. Walter Paye and Bill Pierce periodically report on the International Registry of Clinical Use of Ventricular Assist Devices.[7,8] This is a voluntary registry and is therefore certainly somewhat incomplete.

The registry now includes the use of various types of ventricular assist devices for postcardiotomy cardiogenic shock in 965 patients. Approximately 45% of the patients were weaned from temporary circulatory assistance, and 25% were discharged. Results were equal whether nonpulsatile centrifugal or pulsatile pneumatic devices were utilized for support.

As of January 1990 the registry contained 544 patients who had been supported with ventricular assist devices or total artificial hearts in conjunction with heart transplantation.[11] Three categories of patients were included in this registry: (1) patients deteriorating before transplantation (436), (2) patients with acute rejection following cardiac transplantation (40), (3) patients with immediate donor organ failure after heart transplantation considered not to be related to acute rejection (68).

Results for the immediate donor organ failure group of patients were very similar to those for postcardiotomy and cardiogenic shock following other cardiac procedures. Of the 68 patients, 29% were weaned from circulatory support and 19% were discharged from the hospital.

For patients requiring left ventricular support, the rates of transplantation and hospital discharge were similar with electric, pneumatic, or centrifugal devices. There was a trend in patients supported with centrifugal devices to fare less well overall. However, with only 26 patients in this group, the numbers were too small to be of any statistical significance.

Although many patients have had biventricular support using hybrid-type systems, where the left side was supported pneumatically and the right side was supported with centrifugal pumps, the results of these hybrid systems were inferior to those in patients who received either two concomitant pneumatic or centrifugal devices.

We have previously reported our experience with use of the Sarns VAD for post-cardiogenic shock.[6] The overall weanability was 71% with a 50% discharge rate.

Of the 12 patients that the Minneapolis Heart Institute has bridged to cardiac transplantation,[9] 5 had centrifugal pumps used for circulatory assistance; however, 2 patients were converted to a total artificial heart because of the suspected long-term wait for a donor heart.

MORBIDITY AND MORTALITY

Cause of death is most frequently persistent cardiac failure of one type or another. More sophisticated techniques for determining myocardial viability in the intraoperative period are needed to identify the subgroup of patients who would not benefit from use of a VAD. A more aggressive approach to device insertion may lead to fewer deaths secondary to multiple organ failure. Renal failure requiring dialysis could also be avoided in most patients by earlier VAD insertion.

CONCLUSION

The success with the use of the centrifugal pumps and any other ventricular assist device depends largely on good patient selection, early recognition of the need for a device, efficient and accurate insertion techniques, maximum cardiac support while on the device, appropriate use of anticoagulation and antibiotics, and appropriate timing of weaning and removal.

REFERENCES

1. Barcroft H: Observations on the pumping action of the heart, *J Physiol* 78:186, 1933.
2. De Bakey ME: Left ventricular bypass for cardiac assistance: clinical experience, *Am J Cardiol* 27:3, 1971.
3. Wesolowski SW, Welch CS: Experimental maintenance of the circulation by mechanical pumps, *Surgery* 31:769, 1952.
4. Wesolowski SA, Fisher JH, Welch CS: Perfusion of pulmonary circulation by non-pulsatile flow, *Surgery* 33:370, 1953.
5. Norman JC, Cooley DA, Igo SR et al: Prognostic indices for survival during post cardiotomy intra-aortic balloon pumping, *J Thorac Cardiovasc Surg* 74:709, 1977.
6. Joyce LD, Kiser JC, Eales F et al: Experience with the Sarns centrifugal pump as a ventricular assist device, *ASAIO Trans* 36(3):M619, April 1990.
7. Pae WE, Miller CA, Pierce WS: Ventricular assist devices for post cardiotomy cardiogenic shock: a combined registry experience, *J Thorac Cardiovasc Surg,* accepted for publication, 1992.
8. Oaks TE, Pae WE, Miller CA et al: Combined registry for the clinical use of mechanical ventricular assist pumps and the total artificial heart in conjunction with heart transplantation: fifth official report, *J Heart Lung Transplant,* 10(5):621, 1991.
9. Joyce LD, Emery RW, Eales F et al: Mechanical circulatory support as a bridge to transplantation. C. Walton Lillehei Surgical Symposium, October 1988.

CHAPTER 6

Thoratec ventricular assist device

S. Jill Ley and **J. Donald Hill**

INTRODUCTION

Mechanical cardiac assistance with pneumatic or air-driven ventricular assist devices (VADs) began in the 1960s, when De Bakey and associates first used a sac-type blood pumping system to support the failing circulation.[1] The Thoratec VAD (Berkeley, California) was first used successfully in 1982 at St. Louis University for a patient suffering from cardiogenic shock. San Francisco's Pacific Presbyterian Medical Center followed with the first bridge-to-transplant procedure in 1984.[2] Since those initial operations, over 100 patients have been long-term survivors following Thoratec VAD support.

THEORY OF OPERATION

Thoratec pneumatic VADs use pulses of air to alternately compress and empty a blood pumping sac, thus delivering pulsatile blood flow. Paracorporeal prosthetic ventricles are utilized, consisting of seamless polyurethane blood sacs enclosed within rigid casings and tilting disk inlet and outlet valves for unidirectional blood flow (Fig. 6-1). A thin hose carries compressed air from the driver to the pump's air chamber, with adjustments in pressure and vacuum made via console controls (Fig. 6-2). Blood is diverted from a failing ventricle to inflow cannulae that provide pump filling with return aortic or pulmonary artery perfusion via outflow cannulae, thus ensuring systemic or pulmonary perfusion despite severe ventricular dysfunction.

Ventricular support can be provided in any of three different modes of operation: volume (full-to-empty), R-wave synchronous, or asynchronous. The **volume** mode is preferred in most clinical situations because VAD rate and output will automatically adjust to venous return. In this mode, activation of a Hall effect switch occurs when the blood sac is full, thus triggering ejection of a complete 65 cc stroke volume. This mode offers optimal ventricular support and completely washes the blood sac, thereby decreasing thrombus formation. The **R-wave synchronous** mode allows counterpulsation or timing of VAD systole during natural heart diastole. Weaning can be accom-

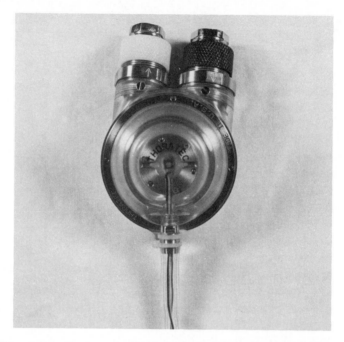

Fig. 6-1. Thoratec prosthetic ventricle. (Courtesy Thoratec Laboratories, Berkeley, Calif.)

plished in this mode, similar to an IABP by decreasing VAD emptying from every R-wave (1:1) to every second or third R-wave (1:2 or 1:3). The **asynchronous** mode allows VAD emptying at any programmed rate and is asynchronous with intrinsic heart rates. This mode is also used for VAD weaning, but allows more gradual decreases in VAD support than the R-wave method.[3]

The Thoratec VAD is capable of delivering flow rates of 6.5 L/min, although flows of 4 to 5 L/min are usually adequate to maintain organ perfusion.[4] Appropriate prosthetic ventricle filling and emptying requires a drive line pressure of 200 mm Hg or 75 mm Hg above the patient's systolic blood pressure (SBP), and an adequate systolic ejection time (usually >300 msec). The perfusionist sets these parameters, which then require minimal adjustment during volume mode support. VAD console displays include peak ejection pressure (mm Hg), percent ejection (%), VAD rate (bpm), output (L/min), and vacuum pressure (−mm Hg). Continual flashing of the green "FILL" light and AC power light indicate appropriate VAD pumping status.

PATIENT SELECTION

Three groups of patients have been identified as potential VAD candidates: (1) patients who cannot be weaned from cardiopulmonary bypass after a cardiac surgical

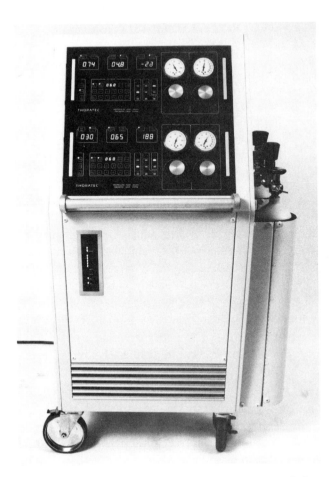

Fig. 6-2. Dual drive console for the Thoratec VAD. (Courtesy Thoratec Laboratories, Berkeley, Calif.)

procedure, (2) patients who have had an acute myocardial infarction (MI) resulting in cardiogenic shock, and (3) patients with end-stage cardiomyopathy who need VAD support as a bridge-to-transplant until a suitable donor heart can be found. The box on p. 70 lists the hemodynamic criteria for initiation of VAD support. Although intraaortic balloon pumping is usually initiated before insertion of a VAD, this step may be eliminated if it is obvious that more aggressive support is needed for patients who are decompensating rapidly.

Exclusion criteria for VAD support remain controversial and vary with different patient categories. There is general agreement that VADs should not be used for patients with active malignancy, recent cerebrovascular event, sepsis, hepatic or multiorgan failure, or massive hemorrhage.[5-7] Additional inclusion criteria for postcardi-

---

HEMODYNAMIC CRITERIA FOR INITIATION OF VAD SUPPORT

Cardiac index < 2 L/min/m^2
Mean arterial pressure < 60 mm Hg
Systolic blood pressure < 90 mm Hg
Atrial pressure > 20 mm Hg
Systemic vascular resistance > 2100 dynes/sec/cm^5
Urine output < 20 cc/hr
Presence of above despite:
Optimum preload
Maximal pharmacological therapy

---

otomy patients include a technically correct surgical repair. Patients in this group, as well as the MI group, should also be given a reasonable chance of ventricular recovery before VAD insertion. Irreversible myocardial damage ($>40\%$) generally precludes VAD weaning.[8] Debate continues regarding VAD use for patients with renal failure, advanced age, or active infection. Bridge-to-transplant patients must also meet institutional criteria for heart transplantation (see the box on p. 71). High levels of preformed cytotoxic antibodies are an additional consideration in these patients, because this limits the number of suitable donors and can dramatically prolong VAD support before transplantation.

In isolated right ventricular failure (central venous pressure [CVP] > 20 mm Hg with left atrial pressure [LAP] ≤ 10 mm Hg), univentricular right-sided support is indicated. In left ventricular failure, however, criteria for the use of univentricular left vs. biventricular support remain controversial. Although signs of left heart failure may dominate the clinical picture, addition of a right-sided VAD (RVAD) must be considered intraoperatively, because severe right ventricular (RV) failure occurs eventually in up to 36% of patients receiving only left-sided support.[3,9] However, several authors have demonstrated that even profound RV dysfunction may be reversible once univentricular LVAD assistance is initiated.[10,11] Biventricular support should be considered if signs of acute RV failure develop intraoperatively following LVAD insertion or when the likelihood of lethal dysrhythmias is high. Farrar et al.[12] showed that hemodynamic compromise was avoided in patients experiencing prolonged asystole or ventricular fibrillation when they were supported with biventricular assist devices. Fig. 6-3 demonstrates this phenomenon in a patient who was in ventricular fibrillation for several weeks before undergoing successful cardiac transplantation.

INSERTION TECHNIQUES

Univentricular or biventricular heterotopic prosthetic pumps are always implanted using general anesthesia through a median sternotomy incision. Although it is theo-

---

**ADDITIONAL EXCLUSION CRITERIA FOR VAD SUPPORT IN
THE BRIDGE-TO-TRANSPLANT GROUP**

Active infection
Recent pulmonary embolism
Recent gastrointestinal hemorrhage
Significant peripheral vascular disease
Pulmonary hypertension (PVR $\geq$ 480-640 dynes/sec/cm^5)
Inadequate psychosocial support

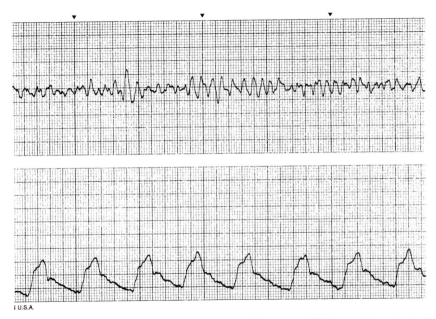

Fig. 6-3. ECG and arterial pressure tracings from BVAD patient. VADs provide pulsatile flow, and MAP = 66 mm Hg despite ventricular fibrillation.

retically possible to put a univentricular pump on the left side through a lateral thoracotomy incision, this approach would limit right ventricular access should it fail during surgery. The devices can be implanted without going on extracorporeal circulation. This depends on patient morbidity and site of left inflow cannulation.

Return flow from the left prosthetic pump is always directed to the ascending aorta via a 12 mm preclotted woven Dacron graft. This anastamosis requires a continuous running suture of 4-0 prolene. There are three choices for removing blood from the left heart using a 16-18 mm cannula: left atrial appendage, *reflected interatrial groove* adjacent to the right superior pulmonary vein, or left ventricular apex (Fig. 6-4). When

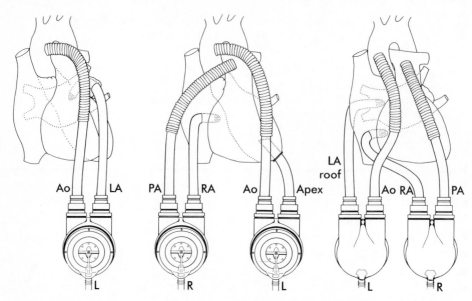

Fig. 6-4. Cannulation approaches for univentricular (**A**) or biventricular (**B** and **C**) support. In flow cannulation from the left heart is via the left atrial appendage (**A**), left ventricular apex (**B**), or LA roof via the interatrial groove (**C**), with return blood flow to the aorta. Right heart cannulation is from the right atrium to the pulmonary artery (**B** and **C**). (From Farrar DJ, Hill JD, Gray LA Jr et al: *N Engl J Med* 318:333, 1988.)

a right interatrial groove site is used, it is possible to implant the pump without extracorporeal circulation. This site is attractive when there are preexisting left-sided vein grafts that might be compressed by a cannula in the left atrial appendage. The LV apex provides the largest and most complete pump filling. This site is commonly used when it is certain that a transplant will be required and sacrificing a portion of the ventricular apex will not be a concern. The right-sided outflow conduit is anastamosed to the pulmonary artery in the same fashion as the aorta. The right pump inflow is via a large bore (16-18 mm) cannula into the right atrium.

The cannulae are brought out percutaneously, inferior to the wound, and attached to the prosthetic ventricle(s). The pumps are deaired before weaning from cardiopulmonary bypass onto prosthetic ventricle support. When only a univentricular left-sided pump is used, one must watch carefully for RV dysfunction because left-sided function is then totally dependent on right-sided performance. Protamine is given for complete reversal of heparin; platelets and fresh frozen plasma can be given as required. The sternal wound is always completely closed after placement of 2 to 3 chest tubes in the mediastinum and/or left pleural space.

POTENTIAL COMPLICATIONS

Bleeding, infection, and end-organ failure are the most frequent complications of VAD assistance.[4,6,13] Ongoing assessment for these potential complications is critical to patient survival.

Bleeding

Bleeding is the most prevalent and devastating early complication of mechanical circulatory support, warranting reoperation in 22% to 73% of reported cases.[4,13] Factors that contribute to postoperative coagulation abnormalities include: (1) preoperative hepatic congestion, (2) prolonged cardiopulmonary bypass (CPB) times, (3) multiple cannulation sites, and (4) platelet interaction with biomaterial surfaces. Interaction between blood and the pump oxygenator results in a decrease in platelet number and effectiveness, with normalization of platelet function within 30 minutes after bypass is discontinued.[14] Hemodilution of coagulation factors also contributes to hemostatic abnormalities. Bypass times, and therefore bleeding tendency, are greatest in postcardiotomy patients who have undergone multiple attempts at CPB weaning before VAD insertion. At our center we have not experienced severe problems with bleeding, probably because of a responsive blood bank and a policy of keeping patients in the operating room until bleeding is well controlled.

Assessment for bleeding complications includes strict monitoring of chest tube (CT) output, hematocrit (HCT), and coagulation tests, as well as noting signs of excessive bleeding from line sites and incisions. Packed red cells and fresh frozen plasma (FFP) are administered to maintain a desired HCT, prothrombin time (PT) and partial thromboplastin time (PTT) respectively. If bleeding is excessive, platelets may be administered despite a relatively normal laboratory count to counteract platelet dysfunction. Cryoprecipitate and vitamin K are generally avoided because of potential thrombus formation after device insertion.[15] Desmopressin (DDAVP) has been shown to decrease bleeding effectively, but its short duration of action (30 to 60 minutes) requires careful timing to achieve maximum effectiveness.[14] Reexploration should be considered if CT output exceeds 200 cc/hr for 2 consecutive hours after clotting factors have been restored. Autotransfusion of CT drainage either immediately after collection or after additional washing procedures is carried out according to institutional policy.[7]

Infection

Infectious complications in VAD patients have been reported as high as 61%, most commonly caused by pneumonia in this early report.[16] However, the total series of Thoratec VAD patients has not implicated any specific site or organism as contributing to this complication. Predisposing factors to infection include invasive monitoring lines and catheters, sternotomy wounds, and ventilatory support. A decrease in circulating T-cell levels has been noted following CPB, leaving VAD patients with impaired host defense mechanisms during the immediate postoperative period.[16,17] Avoidance of infection is a primary goal for all patients but achieves special significance in transplant candidates. Even a minor infection could warrant removal from the transplant waiting list, thus delaying or even precluding organ transplantation.

Measures to decrease infection include frequent handwashing, strict aseptic technique during contact with invasive lines, prompt removal of lines and catheters, and use of sterile technique during VAD dressing changes. Prevost et al. found no correlation between the number of infection control measures utilized and 1 year survival rates in cardiac transplant recipients when they surveyed transplant centers around the country.[18] Although protective isolation is advocated by some centers, its use for VAD patients warrants additional study. Early extubation and mobilization of VAD patients and aggressive pulmonary hygiene measures are instituted to prevent pneumonia. Routine antibiotic prophylaxis is discontinued after 3 days, with resumption of organism-specific antibiotics as needed based on positive culture results. Surveillance for infection includes daily leukocyte counts and temperature assessment every 4 to 8 hours.

End-organ failure

Multiorgan failure occurs in as much as 42% of VAD patients and is the most frequent cause of death in patients who could not be transplanted.[4,9] Profound shock before VAD pumping often leads to this fatal complication, although many patients experience a reversal of organ failure once tissue perfusion is restored following VAD insertion. Renal failure requiring dialysis occurred in 12% of patients in one series, with 56% of these patients undergoing successful transplantation and restoration of renal function.[4] Treatment of coagulopathies with massive transfusion may result in "shock lung," pulmonary hypertension, and irreversible respiratory failure.[9] Neurologic events related to embolism have occurred in 7% to 8% of VAD patients, with half of these patients being discharged alive.[4,13] In patients with sepsis, the risk of stroke increases and survival rates are poor. Efforts to avoid end-organ failure should focus on prompt control of coagulopathies, avoidance of sepsis, and earlier identification of candidates with initiation of VAD support before irreversible organ dysfunction develops.

ANTICOAGULATION

Anticoagulation is initiated once initial bleeding has been controlled, in order to avoid thrombus formation on biomaterial surfaces. Protocols using either heparin or low molecular weight dextran have been effective in limiting embolic complications to 7% to 8% of reported cases.[4,13] Heparin is administered as a continuous infusion to maintain activated clotting times (ACTs) between 140 to 160 seconds. The ACT is monitored every 4 to 6 hours until values remain stable, then once daily. An alternative regimen includes dextran at 25 cc/hr for 24 to 36 hours, followed by heparin infusion or dipyridamole 100 mg tid, plus warfarin to maintain the PT at 1.5 times control.[15] Daily coagulation studies serve as a basis for adjustments in anticoagulation. Although Thoratec

VADs have not resulted in significant hemolysis, plasma free hemoglobin levels are monitored routinely. An elevation $>$ 40 mg/dl (normal 2 to 7 mg/dl) indicates the presence of red cell lysis.[15]

MORBIDITY AND MORTALITY

As of April 1992 Thoratec VADs have been placed in 95 postcardiotomy patients with 37% of these patients being weaned from the devices, and with a 57% survival after VAD removal.[2] Pennington et al. reported biventricular failure as their most frequent complication, occurring in 80% of postcardiotomy patients (21/30 patients had received univentricular support).[19] Severe RV failure occurring during univentricular LVAD support is treated initially with isoproterenol and volume resuscitation.[4,9] However, reoperation for RVAD placement should be considered if the cardiac index (CI) remains $<$ 2 L/min/m^2 with a CVP $>$ 17 to 20 mm Hg despite these nonmechanical therapies.[9,20] Factors known to adversely affect survival in postcardiotomy patients include perioperative MI and renal failure, which have been reported to have a 75% and 90% mortality respectively.[19]

The largest group of patients to receive Thoratec VAD support is the bridge-to-transplant group, with 172 patients supported as of April 1992. Of these, 66% ultimately received a transplant (8 are still waiting on the devices as of this writing); 82% of these recipients were discharged home.[2] One year actuarial survival posttransplant is 81%, identical to conventional cardiac transplantation without the use of assist devices.[4] Multiorgan failure and sepsis were the complications that most frequently precluded transplantation in this group.[4,13] Results following pneumatic VAD support are continuing to improve, primarily as a result of improved patient selection and earlier use of mechanical assistance.

PATIENT TRANSPORT

Transport of patients with pneumatic VAD systems is safe and simple, facilitating patient ambulation during support. Thoratec's dual drive console contains internal air compressors and automatic battery activation on disconnection from an external power source, providing up to 40 minutes of VAD driver support. Prosthetic ventricles should be secured with telemetry pouches or Montgomery straps before physical activity, with care taken to avoid compression of pneumatic lines during ambulation. Some centers have transferred these patients from an intensive care environment and encourage nurse-supervised ambulation outside the hospital.[15]

WEANING FROM PNEUMATIC VADS

Weaning from assist devices is initiated after patient stability is maintained for at least 24 hours, with minimal requirements for inotropic therapy. Native heart recovery

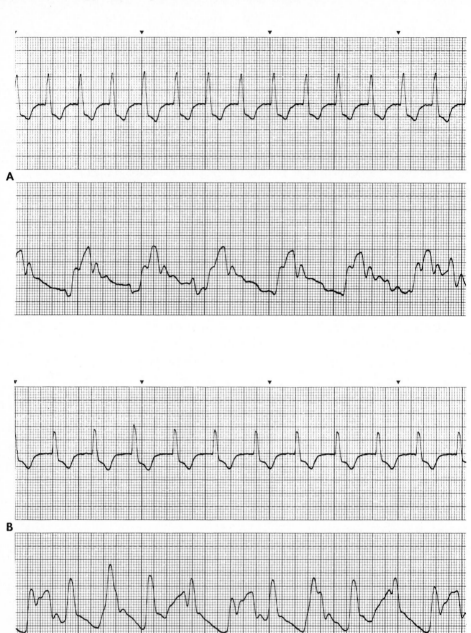

MADE IN U.S.A.

Fig. 6-5. A, ECG and arterial pressure tracings immediately after LVAD placed, showing small, intermittent pulsations from native LV (asynchronous mode, rate 55). **B,** Improved LV function noted 4 days later by return of native pulsations on arterial tracing (asynchronous mode, rate 55).

_____ **PROTOCOL FOR LVAD WEANING** _____

Operate in asynchronous mode
Decrease LVAD rate by 5 beats/min q 6-8 hr
Discontinue weaning and return to 55 beats/min for the following:
  MAP < 70 mm Hg
  LAP > 20 mm Hg
  CI < 2 L/min/m^2
  Svo$_2$ < 50%
  Ventricular ectopy

is demonstrated by improved hemodynamics and perfusion, as well as increased arterial waveform pulsations during natural heart systole. Fig. 6-5 shows arterial pressure tracings on the day of LVAD placement in a postcardiotomy patient and again 4 days later, with return of native pulsations signalling ventricular recovery. Weaning may be accomplished in either R-wave synchronous or asynchronous modes, as described earlier in this chapter. The box above lists one protocol that can be used to gradually wean VAD support. Weaning in the R-wave synchronous mode is accomplished by decreasing VAD ejection to 1:2, then 1:3 if diminished mechanical support is tolerated.

During weaning, attention to anticoagulation is paramount to avoid thrombus formation during periods of decreased flow through the device. Additional heparin is given to maintain an ACT of 160 to 170 seconds. Hemodynamic data obtained during a brief pump-off period allows assessment of native heart function without VAD support. Pennington warns against clamping of VAD cannulae during these trials to avoid thrombus formation.[13] A return to surgery is necessary for VAD removal once the hemodynamic picture on minimal support is satisfactory, usually 16 to 24 hours after weaning began.

NURSING MANAGEMENT

Nursing care of VAD patients requires an understanding of the unique circulatory pathway and its impact on hemodynamic monitoring parameters. Nurses are responsible for assessing the adequacy of pumping and noting potential complications, as well as remaining prepared for emergency troubleshooting procedures. Several alarm conditions require nursing troubleshooting maneuvers. An alarm sounds on interruption of AC power and the VAD automatically switches to an internal battery (battery console light illuminates). Console illumination of "low battery" means that power will remain for less than 30 minutes. If complete loss of power occurs, the drive line should immediately be disconnected from the console and connected to a bulb syringe for hand pumping at a rate of 60 bpm until power can be restored.

Table 6-1.   Hemodynamic assessment during VAD support

	CVP (mm Hg)	LAP (mm Hg)	MAP (mm Hg)	CI (L/min/m²)
Adequate pumping	10-15	10-15	>60	>2
Hypovolemia	<10	<10	<60	<2
Check LVAD pump	10-15	>20	<60	<2
Check RVAD pump or RV failure (LVAD patient)	>20	<10	<60	<2
Check both pumps or cardiac tamponade	>20	>20	<60	<2

Inadequate VAD filling during volume mode support causes another alarm condition and the appearance of an -E- display for VAD output. If the fill signal from the Hall switch remains lost, an automatic change to asynchronous mode occurs (an alarm sounds and the red "sync" light illuminates), delivering a variable stroke volume at a preset backup rate. Signs of an impaired cardiac output (CO) can develop quickly if this output differs significantly from previous settings. Poor VAD filling is commonly due to inadequate preload or kinking of VAD cannulae (either externally or internally) with position changes. Less common causes include thrombus or cardiac tamponade. Hemodynamic monitoring offers additional cues for diagnosing potential problems during VAD support.

Initially after VAD placement, both right and left-sided filling pressures and mixed venous oxygen saturation (Svo$_2$) are continuously monitored. A unilateral problem such as failure of an unsupported ventricle or a kinked cannula is indicated by decreased output and Svo$_2$, elevated pressures on the side of the problem and decreased contra-lateral pressures. Hypovolemia is a common problem that is evidenced by decreased right *and* left-sided filling pressures and is associated with low CO and Svo$_2$. Left-sided filling pressures should be maintained at 10 to 15 mm Hg to optimize VAD filling and organ perfusion.[4,6,21] Cardiac tamponade is uncommon but potentially life-threatening, resulting in impaired filling of the heart and both assist devices. Hemodynamic parameters for these potential complications are listed in Table 6-1.

Thermodilution cardiac outputs are complicated by placement of an RVAD because an alternate pathway for thermodilution injectate exists, making this method invalid.[6,8] The Fick formula must be used for CO estimates in RVAD patients. However, thermodilution CO is accurate for LVAD patients, allowing for assessment of VAD vs. native LV flow rates. By subtracting VAD flow from a thermodilution or "total" CO, the patient's contribution to perfusion can be estimated. In many cases complete systemic output is provided by the LVAD, and console flows are therefore an accurate estimate of total body perfusion.

Invasive monitoring lines are discontinued as soon as hemodynamic stability and extubation are achieved, usually within 48 to 72 hours after VAD placement. Physical

Table 6-2.   California Pacific Medical Center division of nursing standard of care

Care of patient receiving ventricular assist device (VAD) support	
Standard of care	**Standard of practice**
The patient's hemodynamic status will be optimized through the use of a ventricular assist device.	The nurse will: 1. Assess the following every 15 minutes × 4 → q 30 min × 2 → and then q 1 hr until stable: VS, Svo₂, CVP, PA pressures, SVR, and PVR (note: both CVP and PA waveforms will be continuously displayed). Assess thermodilution CO q 1 to 2 hr only if patient does *not* have an RVAD (CO inaccurate with right assist, use LVAD CO to calculate PVR/SVR). 2. Titrate inotropes, vasodilators and/or vasopressors to maintain pressures within ordered parameters. 3. Assess tissue perfusion, skin color, temperature, capillary refill, and peripheral pulses every 1 hr initially, then q 2 to 4 hr and PRN.
The patient's fluid balance will be optimized.	The nurse will: 1. Measure and record I&Os q 1 hr. 2. Obtain daily weight. 3. Administer albumin to maintain desired filling pressures (LAP/PCWP ≥15 mm Hg initially) PRN per volume replacement protocol. 4. Administer diuretics as ordered.

Complications of inadequate ventricular assistance will be minimized.	The nurse will:
	1. Assess hemodynamic status for S&Ss of potential problems.
	2. Observe for S&Ss of vital organ dysfunction (i.e., change on LOC, ↓ peripheral perfusion, decrease in UO, rise in LFTs).
	3. Assess for proper VAD function:
	  a. Monitor right and left VAD flow (CO), vacuum (−20), and ejection pressure (110 to 180 mm Hg) on VAD console q 1 hr and record on nursing flowsheet.
	  b. Assess console for continuous flashing of fill light and absence of battery light and document q 1 hr on nursing flowsheet.
	  c. Notify perfusionist and MD of abnormal findings.
	  d. Emergency procedure in event of VAD failure: disconnect L, then R drive lines from back of console and connect to bulb syringes. (Drive lines should be labeled R and L at all times). Squeeze bulbs manually at rate of 60/min. Then call a perfusionist and MD STAT.

Continued.

Table 6-2.   California Pacific Medical Center division of nursing standard of care—cont'd

| Care of patient receiving ventricular assist device (VAD) support | |
Standard of care	Standard of practice
The patient's oxygenation will be optimized.	The nurse will: 1. Verify ETT placement on chest x-ray and reposition per protocol; note abnormal x-ray findings. 2. Maintain ventilator settings as ordered—wean and extubate per protocol. 3. Assess breath sounds q 1-2 hr. 4. Suction prn and document type of secretions; observe for changes in VS with suctioning. 5. Provide adequate oxygen per ventilator, mask, or NP to maintain $Sao_2 \geq 92\%$ or as ordered. 6. Observe for changes indicative of hypoxia; assess nail beds and mucous membranes for cyanosis. 7. Turn, and encourage cough and deep breathing q 1-2 hr and prn using pillow to support chest; incentive spirometer q 1-2 hr.
The patient's high risk for injury from bleeding problems related to CPB, VAD, and/or IABP will be minimized.	The nurse will: 1. Monitor VS, hemodynamics, I&O q 1 hr for signs of hypovolemia. 2. Check coag panel and administer blood products as indicated. (Note: only CMV neg blood administered to transplant candidates.) 3. Measure chest tube drainage q 1 hr—notify MD of >150 cc/hr × 2 hr. 4. Assess for abnormal bleeding tendency: ecchymosis, petechiae, oozing at line sites or oral cavity, heme positive stools, endotracheal secretions, nasogastric bleeding, or hematuria. 5. Notify MD of ↑ plasma-free Hgb—*may* order ↓ pressure/vacuum. 6. Assess lab values as ordered, including daily: plasma Hgb, antithrombin III, fibrinopeptide A, coag panel, H/H, platelets, and FSP. 7. Ensure that clamps remain at bedside at all times; use in event of cannulae disconnection *only!*
The patient's high risk for mural or VAD thrombus formation will be minimized.	The nurse will: 1. Check coagulation studies and administer anticoagulation therapy as indicated. 2. Administer *only* beef lung heparin per MD order after initial bleeding controlled. (Obtain from pharmacy.) Adjust to maintain desired ACT: 140 to 150 sec for Thoratec VAD. 3. Inspect pump and tubing with flashlight q 4 hr and PRN; notify MD of fibrin, air, or clot formation. If present, do *not* clamp tubings.

Table 6-2.   California Pacific Medical Center division of nursing standard of care—cont'd

| Care of patient receiving ventricular assist device (VAD) support | |
Standard of care	Standard of practice
The patient's risk of infection is minimized.	The nurse will: 1. Record rectal/core temperature q 1 hr. Decrease temp with antipyretics and/or cooling blanket PRN. 2. Obtain B, U, S cultures PRN temp spike or suspicious clinical findings. 3. Draw daily CBC and note ↑ WBC. 4. Encourage good handwashing by all personnel and family. 5. Maintain aseptic technique with all dressings, line insertions, and site procedures. 6. Perform sterile dressing change to VAD sites q 12 to 24 hr per protocol with hibiclens. 7. Change all IV and transducer tubings q 48 hr. 8. Permit no visitors with potential infection. 9. Allow no flowers/plants in room. 10. Perform pulmonary hygiene measures as appropriate for patient. 11. Assess for early signs of sepsis: ↑ HR, ↑T, ↓BP, hot dry skin, bounding pulses, ↑CO, ↓SVR, ↑Svo$_2$.
The patient's nutritional status will be optimized.	The nurse will: 1. Follow intake and output closely—obtain dietary consult PRN ↓ intake. 2. Administer tube feedings or parenteral nutrition as ordered if po intake is inadequate. 3. Supplement po intake with Ensure as tolerated. 4. Follow weight qd and calorie count PRN. 5. Check electrolyte and protein levels as ordered. 6. Encourage regular diet and food from home as tolerated.
The patient's risk of skin breakdown will be reduced.	The nurse will: 1. Advance activity as tolerated per MD orders: turn q 2 hr, passive-active ROM, dangle on side of bed, physical therapy (exercycle). 2. Support VAD and tubing with telemetry pouch/ montgomery straps to avoid kinking or dislodgement during activity. 3. Use Kin-air bed, heel, and elbow protectors as needed. 4. Maintain proper body alignment. 5. Apply foot board to bed PRN footdrop.
The patient will receive optimal pain relief.	The nurse will: 1. Assess type, degree, location, and duration of discomfort. 2. Provide back care and reposition as needed. 3. Provide reassurance and explain all events to patient. 4. Medicate with analgesics as needed, then evaluate and document effect. 5. Observe for symptoms of pain, such as increased anxiety, restlessness, and facial gestures.

Continued.

Table 6-2.   California Pacific Medical Center division of nursing standard of care—cont'd

Care of patient receiving ventricular assist device (VAD) support	
Standard of care	**Standard of practice**
Patient and family coping mechanisms will be optimized.	The nurse will: 1. Maintain open communication with patient and family. 2. Answer all questions honestly at the appropriate level of patient understanding. 3. Provide explanations and information in clear, simple terms. 4. Prepare patient and family for procedures by explaining purpose and procedure before their occurrence. 5. Give appropriate reassurance. 6. Allow and encourage family visits. 7. Provide nursing care conferences as appropriate per individual patient. 8. Involve social worker early to arrange visits from other VAD patients and work with patient and family. 9. Encourage family participation in patient care as appropriate.

VS, vital signs; *Svo$_2$,* mixed venous oxygen saturation; *CVP,* central venous pressure; *PA,* pulmonary artery; *SVR,* systemic vascular resistance; *PVR,* pulmonary vascular resistance; *CO,* cardiac output; *RVAD,* right ventricular assist device; *LVAD,* left ventricular assist device; *I&O,* intake and output; *LAP,* left atrial pressure; *PCWP,* pulmonary capillary wedge pressure; *S&S,* signs and symptoms; *LOC,* level of consciousness; *UO,* urine output; *LFT,* liver function tests; *ETT,* endotracheal tube; *CXR,* chest x-ray; *Sao$_2$* arterial oxygen saturation; *CPB,* cardiopulmonary bypass; *IABP,* intraaortic balloon pump; *CMV,* cytomegalovirus; *Hgb,* hemoglobin; *H/H,* hemoglobin/hematocrit; *FSP,* fibrin split products; *ACT,* activated clotting time; *BUS,* blood, urine, sputum; *CBC,* complete blood count; *WBC,* white blood cell count; *IV,* intravenous; *HR,* heart rate; *T,* temperature; *BP,* blood pressure; *ROM,* range of motion.

assessment findings are validated with hemodynamic data before line withdrawal. Signs of adequate end-organ perfusion include appropriate mentation and neurologic status, urine output > 20 cc/hr, palpable peripheral pulses, warm and dry skin, clear breath sounds, and laboratory values within established parameters. A nursing diagnosis framework is useful in assessing for potential complications and developing an appropriate plan of care for VAD patients. The Standard of Care for VAD patients from California Pacific Medical Center is included in Table 6-2.

Nursing Diagnosis #1: Decreased cardiac output related to decreased preload, inappropriate afterload, or device malfunction

An impaired CO in VAD patients is usually due to factors other than impaired contractility because the device assumes responsibility for the heart's pumping function. Physiologic principles apply, however, in that VADs cannot deliver an adequate stroke volume when underfilled or when ejecting against increased resistance. After ensuring proper device function and adequacy of filling pressures, ventricular afterload should be assessed as a cause of low CO. An increased LV afterload related to vasoconstriction is noted by an elevated systemic vascular resistance (SVR), decreased pulses, cool and clammy skin, cyanotic nailbeds, and hypertension (although hypotension occurs if pump ejection is severely impaired). Right ventricular afterload is assessed by calculation of pulmonary vascular resistance (PVR), which should be <240 dynes/sec/cm.[5] Vasodilators such as nitroglycerin, nitroprusside, or angiotensin converting enzyme inhibitors are indicated for excessively high afterload. A severely low afterload is rarely seen during VAD support, but massive vasodilation may accompany sepsis. Vasoconstrictive agents such as neosynephrine or levophed are used in this situation to restore vascular tone and increase mean arterial pressure (MAP).

Nursing Diagnosis #2: Impaired gas exchange related to atelectasis, sedation, immobility, or intracardiac shunt

The paracorporeal nature of this device allows complete sternal closure, avoiding prolonged intubation due to chest wall instability. Extubation is accomplished when hemodynamics stabilize and anesthesia effects subside, usually within 48 hours after insertion. Hypoxemia in the initial postoperative period may be caused by pulmonary edema or by the adult respiratory distress syndrome, following aggressive intraoperative fluid resuscitation or hypotensive episodes. Severe hypoxemia associated with an elevated CVP and a normal chest x-ray may be indicative of a patent foramen ovale with right to left shunting.[5] After identifying the cause of respiratory compromise, appropriate interventions are initiated to maintain a $Po_2 > 75$ mm Hg, $Pco_2 < 45$ mm Hg, and $Sao_2 > 95\%$.[21]

Nursing Diagnosis #3: Inadequate nutritional intake related to decreased caloric intake with increased metabolic demands

Nutritional support is initiated within 48 hours of VAD insertion to facilitate wound healing, decrease risk of infection, and promote physical recovery. Tube feedings offer less risk of infection than parenteral methods, but may be poorly absorbed in the immediate postoperative period.[7] Nutritional support with either method requires assessment of patient tolerance to an increased volume load and may require diuretics to achieve a desired intake of 3000 calories per day. Following extubation, patients are progressed rapidly to a regular diet with nutritional supplements, and favorite foods from home are encouraged.

Nursing Diagnosis #4: Alteration in mobility related to preoperative disability, surgical trauma, and VAD instrumentation

Sternal closure enables aggressive mobilization for most patients, beginning with frequent turning and range-of-motion (ROM) exercises shortly after surgery. Transplant patients may sit up within 24 hours after extubation and progressive ambulation is encouraged, as tolerated.[15] A stationary bike or light exercise weights are additional

	(23)	00	01	02	03	04	05	06
LVAD CO	5.9	6.1	5.8	6.0	6.3	6.1	5.9	6.0
EJECT/VACUUM	180/-21	182/-20	180/-22	183/-20	179/-21	182/-20	183/-21	179/-20
FILL+/BATT-	+/-	+/-	+/-	+/-	+/-	+/-	+/-	+/-
RVAD CO	4.8	4.9	5.1	4.7	4.9	5.2	4.8	5.1
EJECT/VACUUM	126/-22	128/-20	127/-21	125/-22	128/-20	126/-21	125/-20	128/-22
FILL+/BATT-	+/-	+/-	+/-	+/-	+/-	+/-	+/-	+/-
P.A. Syst/Diast		32/13		34/14		30/12		33/13
P.A. MEAN		21		22		20		22
(PA)/LAP WEDGE		14		13		13		14
CVP		8		8		7		8
C.O./C.I. NA								
SVO2		68		69		70		69
PVR/SVR		1.6/1032		1.4/992		1.5/1012		1.6/989

Fig. 6-6. Nursing documentation during biventricular support with Thoratec VAD.

adjuncts for physical conditioning, but routine sternal precautions must be maintained. Increased physical activity offers potential benefits of reversing cardiac disability, preventing complications from immobility, and improving physical status before undergoing cardiac transplantation. Pennington cites the benefits of increased mobility as "one of the most important lessons we have learned."[13] A less aggressive approach is warranted for short-term support in a recovery patient; ROM exercises and frequent repositioning are initiated when hemodynamic stability is achieved. Reconditioning efforts following VAD removal include participation in the inpatient cardiac rehabilitation program offered to all patients recovering from cardiac surgery or myocardial infarction, with modifications as needed based on existing physical limitations.

DOCUMENTATION DURING VAD SUPPORT

In addition to vital signs and hemodynamic parameters, data pertinent to proper VAD function are documented hourly on nursing flowsheets. Right and left VAD parameters and indicator lights for filling and battery use are noted from the VAD console. Fig. 6-6 is an example of nursing documentation during VAD support shortly after implant. The LVAD flow rate is used to calculate pulmonary and systemic resistance when a right-sided device is in place. Additional documentation including relevant clinical information and laboratory values are collected by a clinical investigator for completion of Thoratec data requirements.

PSYCHOSOCIAL ISSUES

The acute nature of cardiogenic shock limits advance preparation of patients and their families to very basic information regarding mechanical VAD assistance. Support and information are provided at a level appropriate to their knowledge and emotional state. Anxiety related to dependence on life-support is decreased when nurses appear confident with the equipment and can explain its function and backup safety measures. The uncertain nature of waiting for a donor heart is an additional stress that can be overwhelming for patients and families. Visits from clergy, social workers, or patients who were previously bridged to transplant are arranged as needed. Nurses promote adequate coping by encouraging ventilation of feelings and allowing patients as much control over their environment as possible. A daily schedule keeps patients active during daylight hours, with adjustments as needed based on patient input. Sleep is promoted by providing a dark and quiet environment, uninterrupted rest periods, and the timely administration of sleeping medications. Promoting an atmosphere of patient control and preserving out-of-hospital routines can make a tremendous difference in the patient's outlook during an extended wait for a donor heart.

Family members often fear that death of their loved one is imminent and are fearful to leave the bedside. An open visitation scheduled is instituted, but families are reminded to attend to their own needs and take periodic breaks away from the intensive care environment. Establishing a trusting relationship with the nursing staff can enable families to leave their loved one without undue anxiety.

Ruzevich and co-workers evaluated psychological effects of mechanical circulatory support in 12 VAD patients.[22] Seventy-five percent stated they had a brighter outlook on life since their illness, 66% returned to a normal lifestyle, and the same number said they would consent to have another device, if needed. Although 80% of the spouses surveyed believed that appropriate people were available to answer their questions, only 40% believed they were prepared for what to expect. Physicians and nurses caring for VAD patients must make every effort to answer questions and provide feedback regarding patient progress during mechanical circulatory support.

CONCLUSION

Clinical applications of circulatory support technology have made a dramatic impact on outcomes for critically ill cardiovascular patients. Survival rates for postcardiotomy VAD patients have risen from 15% during early trials to approximately 40% in 1990.[2] Bridge-to-transplant patients continue to experience survival rates identical to patients transplanted without mechanical circulatory assistance.[4] Considering the dismal prognosis for these patients without VAD support, this represents a significant breakthrough in the management of profound cardiac failure. As selection criteria are refined and the number of centers using Thoratec VADs increases, it is hoped that the 1990s will see even greater numbers of patients given this final chance to survive "end-stage" heart disease.

REFERENCES

1. De Bakey ME: Left ventricular bypass pump for cardiac assistance, *Am J Cardiol* 27:3, 1971.
2. Farrar DJ, Litwak P, eds:100 VAD survivors, *Thoratec's Heartbeat* 5(2):1, 1991.
3. Farrar DJ, Compton PG, Lawson JH et al: Control modes of a clinical ventricular assist device, *IEEE Engr Med Biol* 5:19, 1986.
4. Farrar DJ, Lawson JH, Litwak P et al: Thoratec VAD system as a bridge to heart transplantation, *J Heart Transplant* 9:415, 1990.
5. Pennington DG, Joyce LD, Pae WE et al: Panel 1: patient selection, Circulatory Support Symposium: Society of Thoracic Surgeons, *Ann Thorac Surg* 47:77, 1989.
6. Barden C, Lee R: Update on ventricular assist devices, *AACN Clin Issues Crit Care Nurs* 1:13, 1990.
7. Ruzevich SA, Swartz MT, Pennington DG: Nursing care of the patient with a pneumatic ventricular assist device, *Heart Lung* 17:399, 1988.
8. Mulford E: Nursing perspectives for the patient receiving postoperative ventricular assistance in the critical care unit, *Heart Lung* 16:246, 1987.
9. Pierce WS, Gray LA, McBride LR et al: Panel 4: Other postoperative complications, Circulatory Support Symposium: Society of Thoracic Surgeons, *Ann Thorac Surg* 47:96, 1989.
10. Kormos RL, Borovetz HS, Gasior T et al: Experience with univentricular support in mortally ill cardiac transplant candidates, *Ann Thorac Surg* 49:261, 1990.
11. Pennington DG, Reedy JE, Swartz MT et al: Univentricular versus biventricular assist device support, *J Heart Lung Transplant* 10:258, 1991.
12. Farrar DJ, Hill JD, Gray LA et al: Successful biventricular circulatory support as a bridge to cardiac transplantation during prolonged ventricular fibrillation and asystole, Circulation 80(suppl III):147, 1989.
13. Pennington DG, Kanter KR, McBride LR et al: Seven years' experience with the Pierce-Donachy ventricular assist device, *J Thorac Cardiovasc Surg* 96:901, 1988.
14. Copeland JG, Harker LA, Joist JH et al: Panel 3: Bleeding and anticoagulation, Circulatory Support Symposium: Society of Thoracic Surgeons, *Ann Thorac Surg* 47:88, 1989.
15. Reedy JE, Ruzevich SA, Noedel NR et al: Nursing care of the ambulatory patient with a mechanical assist device, *J Heart Transplant* 9:97, 1990.
16. McBride LR, Ruzevich SA, Pennington DG et al: Infectious complications associated with ventricular assist device support, *Trans Am Soc Artif Intern Organs* 33:201, 1987.
17. Reedy JE, Swartz MT, Raithel SC et al: Mechanical cardiopulmonary support for refractory cardiogenic shock, *Heart Lung* 19:514, 1990.
18. Prevost S, Lange SS, Lewis P et al: Infection control in cardiac transplant patients, NTI Poster Presentation, 1990.
19. Pennington DG, McBride LR, Swartz MT et al: Use of the Pierce-Donachy ventricular assist device in patients with cardiogenic shock after cardiac operations, *Ann Thorac Surg* 47:130, 1989.
20. Starnes VA, Oyer PE, Portner PM et al: Isolated left ventricular assist as bridge to cardiac transplantation, *J Thorac Cardiovasc Surg* 96:62, 1988.
21. Teplitz L: Patients with ventricular assist devices: nursing diagnoses, *DCCN* 9:82, 1990.
22. Ruzevich SA, Swartz MT, Reedy JE et al: Retrospective analysis of the psychologic effects of mechanical circulatory support, *J Heart Transplant* 9:209, 1990.

CHAPTER 7

Johnson & Johnson HEMOPUMP
Temporary Cardiac Assist System

W. Donald Rountree, Ronald N. Barbie, Jeffery N. Neichin, and **Maura L. Neichin**

INTRODUCTION

Clinical investigation of the HEMOPUMP Temporary Cardiac Assist System, manufactured by Johnson & Johnson Interventional Systems, began in April 1988. Several centers in the United States and abroad continue to participate in trials with this unique device, designed to provide left ventricular assistance for a failing heart. This system has demonstrated its role as a life-saving device and as a myocardial-saving device. As clinical trials continue, the goal is to prove that a significant number of lives can be saved if a HEMOPUMP is inserted into the circulatory system faster and that HEMOPUMP complications are fewer than with traditional ventricular assist devices.

THEORY OF OPERATION

The HEMOPUMP system (Fig. 7-1) consists of an inner cannula that contains a pump assembly, purge fluid system, and control console. When properly placed in the left ventricle (Fig. 7-2) the device's axial flow concept is designed to provide up to 3.5 L/min of continual, nonpulsatile flow.

The pump assembly (Fig. 7-3) consists of a curved inflow cannula, pump housing, flexible drive sheath, and motor magnet housing. The inflow cannula is 25 cm in length and 7 mm (21 French) in diameter with a flexible beveled tip of silicone rubber. It is reinforced with a coil spring to maintain flexibility and prevent kinking. This cannula is fixed to the pump, forming an integral pump/cannula assembly.[1]

The pump is contained within a cylindrical housing. Pump axial flow configuration is achieved by rotating blades and stationary blades with a seal dividing the two (Fig. 7-4). A rotating speed of almost 25,000 RPM draws blood from the left ventricle and pumps it into the systemic circulation. Nonrotating or stationary blades provide a unidirectional flow of blood.

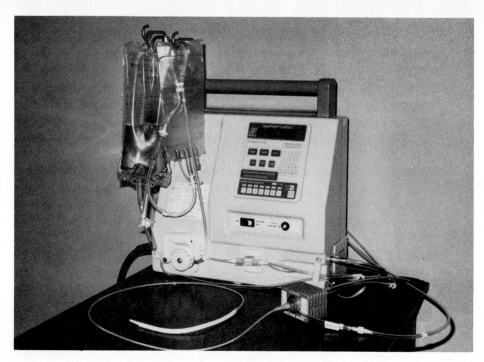

Fig. 7-1. The HEMOPUMP system.

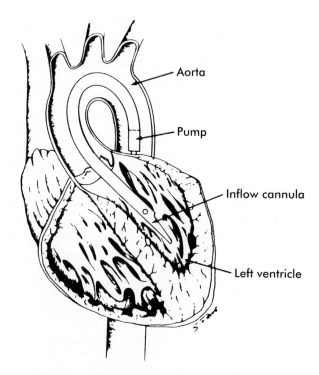

Aorta

Pump

Inflow cannula

Left ventricle

Fig. 7-2. HEMOPUMP positioned in left ventricle.

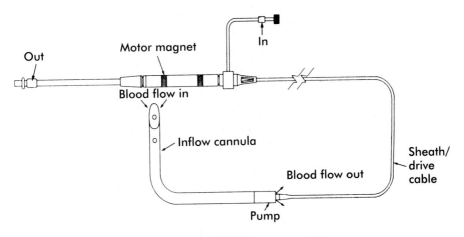

Fig. 7-3. HEMOPUMP pump assembly.

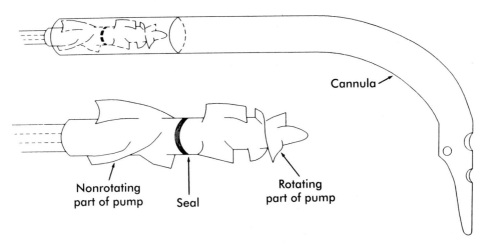

Fig. 7-4. HEMOPUMP cannula/pump assembly.

A flexible drive shaft housed in the inner lumen of a catheter-like sheath drives the pump. This drive shaft is connected to the pump at one end and the motor magnet housing at the other. Magnet housing, which is seated in the motor's bore, turns the drive shaft, which then turns the pump blades. Outer sheath lumens carry the 40% dextrose lubricating fluid to and from the pump seal.[1]

Pump motor magnet housing is inserted in a small motor that is externally applied to the patient. When placed through the motor bore, console power causes the motor to generate an alternating magnetic field that turns the magnet. A flexible drive shaft

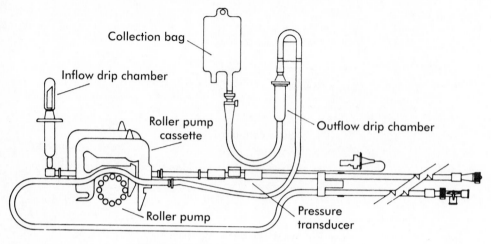

Fig. 7-5. HEMOPUMP purge set assembly.

connects the magnet to the pump. Magnet rotation is imparted to the drive shaft, turning the pump blades.

The purge set assembly (Fig. 7-5) is divided into delivery and collection sides. The delivery side carries $D_{40}W$ to the pump for seal lubrication. Some of this fluid is released into the patient's circulation; the remaining fluid is returned to a collection bag on the control console. Purge fluid is propelled through the system by roller pumps that are connected to the control console. Roller pump speeds are controlled to deliver a specific amount of fluid per hour. A pressure transducer monitors the amount of pressure required to deliver lubricating fluid throughout the system.[1]

The console is a lightweight (approximately 25 pounds) electronic controller that incorporates all of the power, control, and diagnostic alarm systems required to operate the pump. Motor power required to rotate the pump is obtained from this control console. The console also includes the roller pump that controls purge fluid delivery and collection. Backup power is provided by two rechargeable batteries.[1]

The physiologic effects of HEMOPUMP support do not differ greatly from any ventricular assist device. Basic concepts are a reduction in preload, afterload, and ventricular wall stress, all of which lead to decreasing myocardial oxygen consumption (MVO_2). Coronary and systemic perfusion is maintained while allowing the ventricle time to rest and recover from insult or injury. The imbalance between myocardial oxygen supply and demand is at least partially corrected by device support.[2,3]

PATIENT SELECTION

For the first 3 years of clinical investigation, patient selection was based on three categories: (1) cardiogenic shock as a result of an acute myocardial infarction; (2) failure to successfully wean from cardiopulmonary bypass following cardiac surgery or developed low cardiac output syndrome in the immediate postoperative period; and (3) patients who met hemodynamic criteria but did not fall into the first two diagnostic groups. These patients were typically diagnosed with cardiomyopathy, myocarditis, or acute rejection of cardiac allografts. Certain hemodynamic criteria also had to be met. These included (1) systolic blood pressure of less than 90 mm Hg; (2) pulmonary capillary wedge pressure greater than 18 mm Hg; (3) cardiac index less than 2.0 L/min/m^2; and (4) patient refractory to drug and volume therapy.

Phase I of clinical investigations occurred during the first 3 years. Phase II protocol has been developed and submitted to the FDA for approval. It includes limiting device use to postcardiotomy patients who fail to wean from cardiopulmonary bypass. It is hoped that the more restricted patient population will enable investigators to fully evaluate device effectiveness. A comparative trial with other circulatory assist devices will possibly demonstrate the safety and advantages of the HEMOPUMP over other modes of treatment. In addition, recent pump design changes have been made and the Phase II transthoracic pump will have a 5.0 L/min flow capability.

The HEMOPUMP experience abroad was different from that in the United States. Because there were no federal regulations in effect, patient selection was more liberal. Device placement was not limited to emergent conditions, but also included nonemergent situations. Four primary indications were cardiogenic shock, failure to wean from bypass, high risk PTCA, and as a bridge-to-cardiac transplant. The HEMOPUMP cannot be used in the United States as a bridge-to-transplant. A total of 30 centers in Germany, France, Belgium, Holland, and England were involved with use of the HEMOPUMP. Other exclusion criteria for use of the HEMOPUMP are listed in the box below.[4]

INSERTION TECHNIQUES

Lengthy implantation procedures for conventional ventricular support systems may produce a high risk of postoperative complications in patients whose hemodynamic sta-

---

EXCLUSION CRITERIA FOR USE OF THE HEMOPUMP[8]

Significant blood dyscrasias
Awaiting cardiac transplantation
Recipient of a prosthetic aortic valve
Participating in another cardiovascular clinical trial (drug or device)
Known aortic wall disease
Known or suspected thoracic or abdominal aneurysm or dissection
Severe aortic valve stenosis and/or insufficiency
End-stage terminal illness
Severe aortoiliac disease (relative contraindication)

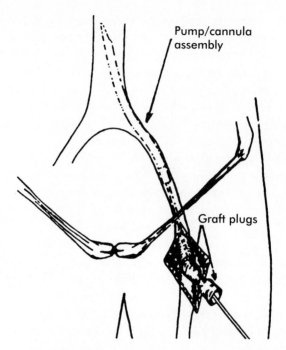

Fig. 7-6. HEMOPUMP placed in Dacron graft.

tus is already compromised. The HEMOPUMP is designed to permit rapid device placement with minimal surgical intervention. In Phase I of the clinical trials the most frequently used technique is a retrograde approach through the femoral artery, with placement guided by fluoroscopy. The arteriotomy site is prepared by suturing a length of 12 mm woven Dacron tubular graft to the incisional orifice through which the entire pump and cannula assembly is introduced and contained (Fig. 7-6). Threaded through a silicone plug, the device cable anchors the distal end of the graft and seals the unit to prevent bleeding. The pump's 7 mm diameter sheath allows insertion in all but the most marginally sized arteries.[5]

In patients with severe femoral/iliac and abdominal aorta atherosclerotic disease, or for those who cannot be weaned from cardiopulmonary bypass, a thoracic approach has been used. A 10 cm short cannula that can be inserted through a longitudinal ascending aorta arteriotomy into the left ventricle, although not presently utilized, is under further laboratory trials. This is the proposed approach for Phase II of the clinical trials. The tubular Dacron graft is anastomosed to the aorta at a 60 degree angle to receive the HEMOPUMP assembly as it is advanced substernally from a supraclavicular incision. Fluoroscopy is used to ensure accurate positioning at the base of the left ventricle. If a radiographic examination is not possible, the pump position may be verified by palpation.[6]

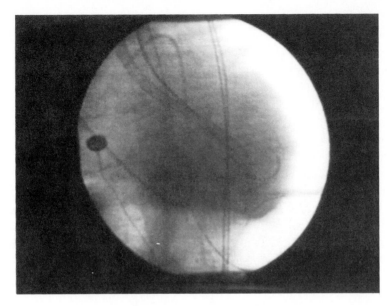

Fig. 7-7. X-ray film of the HEMOPUMP in position.

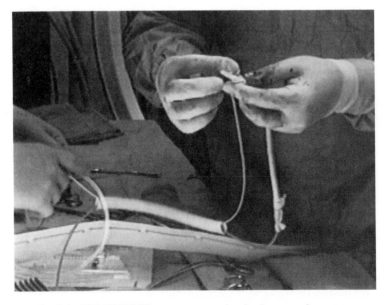

Fig. 7-8. HEMOPUMP pump preparation in the operating room.

HEMOPUMP insertion through the distal abdominal aorta or common iliac artery may be necessary in patients with small femoral arteries. A flank incision permits retroperitoneal access to the aorta, which is heparinized before being clamped, while a longitudinal aortotomy is made. Tubular Dacron graft anastamosis is similar to the femoral artery approach. Cannula and drive cable are sealed within. The drive cable is maintained through its closed incision extension.

Problems encountered during insertion may include inability to transverse the aortic arch or valve. Therefore it is sometimes necessary to pass the HEMOPUMP cannula over a pig-tailed cardiac catheter for position in the left ventricle apex (Fig. 7-7). This has been necessary in several HEMOPUMP insertions.

To accomplish this, the artery must be large enough to introduce a 7 mm HEMOPUMP plus a 2 mm catheter (Fig. 7-8). If the arterial diameter will not accommodate these dimensions, the catheter must be cannulated after the pump is introduced into the descending thoracic aorta. The guidewire, pigtail, and HEMOPUMP are then carefully advanced up the descending thoracic aorta, over the arch, and into the left ventricle, where proper position is identified under fluoroscopy (Fig. 7-7).

POTENTIAL COMPLICATIONS

HEMOPUMP complications are similar to those of other circulatory assist devices. These include vascular injury, valvular injury, thrombus formation, ventricular arrhythmias, bleeding, infection, myocardial and endocardial injury, pump dependence, and death.[8]

ANTICOAGULATION

Because of the risk of thrombus formation, all patients must be anticoagulated. Before pump insertion, patients are given a 10,000 unit bolus of heparin. The patient then receives a continual heparin infusion beginning at 1000 units per hour with a follow-up Partial Thromboplastin Time (PTT). The desired PTT level is 1.5 to 2 times control. Below this range the patient is at risk for thrombus formation, especially at HEMOPUMP flows less than 1.5 L/min. A rebolus of heparin may be required to increase the PTT.

MORBIDITY AND MORTALITY

The box on p. 95 lists some statistical data from the first 3 years of clinical investigation.[3] Since the number of study patients is limited (129), further data is needed to support the position that the HEMOPUMP is a safe and effective circulatory assist device.

Successful insertions numbered slightly more than 78%. Most failed insertions were

_____ **CLINICAL TRIAL RESULTS** _____

Number of patients included in the study: 129
Successful insertions: 78.3%
   Myocardial infarction: 30.7%
   Failure to wean from bypass: 31.7%
   Low cardiac output syndrome: 15.8%
   Other: 21.8%
Patients weaned from HEMOPUMP support: 40.2%
30-day survivors: 25.3%

due to severe aortoiliac disease in which the cannula could not be inserted beyond the iliac artery. Patients in which the device could not be implanted were all nonsurvivors, despite maximum pharmacological support and/or another circulatory assist device such as the IABP.

More than 40% of the patients were successfully weaned from the device with an average implant time of more than 50 hours. Of the patients who were HEMOPUMP-supported, 30-day survival rate was slightly more than 25%. Although this rate does not seem extremely high, one must examine the patient's physiological state when the device was inserted, as well as the overall cardiogenic shock mortality rate, which is nearly 90%.

Causes of death for nonsurviving patients generally fall into three categories: (1) irreversible left ventricular failure, (2) multisystem organ failure, and (3) biventricular failure.[9] If aggressive interventions are to be employed for patients with cardiogenic shock/low cardiac output syndrome, these measures must be entertained earlier in the patient's management.

PATIENT TRANSPORT

Patient transport from the operating room or the cardiac catheterization laboratory to a critical care unit is usually accomplished without difficulty. As previously mentioned, the HEMOPUMP console is lightweight. It can be mounted either on a stand that rolls easily or it can be mounted to the foot portion of most hospital beds.

Two batteries supply power to the console for approximately 30 minutes each. When the unit is plugged into an AC outlet, the batteries are continuously charged.

WEANING FROM THE DEVICE

In an attempt to determine the patient's readiness to wean, several factors must be considered and evaluated. Patient hemodynamic stability must be the first consideration. Cardiac output, pulmonary capillary wedge pressure, arterial blood pressure, amount of vasoactive support required to maintain adequate tissue perfusion, and return of arterial pulsatility, indicating the amount of left ventricular ejection must be assessed. Echocardiography is extremely useful to determine ejection fraction and overall left ventricular function. These evaluations could be considered as early as 24 hours postinsertion. Other factors to evaluate include pulmonary status, renal function, neurological state, and hematological status of the patient.

A speed reduction or on-off trial may be conducted at 24 or 48 hours to determine the patient's readiness to wean. Complete hemodynamic and echocardiography studies can be obtained with the device at very low flows (0.5 L) or turned off for a short period of time. This requires careful coordination by the entire staff.

Once the decision to begin weaning has been made, the entire process takes approximately 24 hours. The amount of support is reduced by 0.5 L/min every 4 hours. This slow weaning allows the ventricle time to become adjusted to its now increased work load. During the weaning process, careful attention must be paid to invasive and noninvasive tissue perfusion measurements. Overall patient clinical status is carefully evaluated with each speed reduction and then reevaluated to determine intervention tolerance. When weaning is completed, the patient is taken to the operating room for device removal. This can be accomplished under local anesthesia.

DATA COLLECTION/DOCUMENTATION

Additional documentation over and above routine for any critically ill patient is not excessive. Three important HEMOPUMP parameters must be monitored closely and documented. These include motor current, purge pressure, and seal flow.

Motor current is a measure of electrical energy required to make the pump spin and move blood. Purge pressure is a measurement of pressure built up in the system. Normal purge pressures are required to ensure proper seal flushing. Seal flow is the amount of 40% dextrose that crosses the seal and flows into the patient's vascular system. Seal flow is controlled by the roller pump located on the control console.[2]

Special laboratory studies may be required to evaluate the degree of hemolysis. Plasma free hemoglobin, serum haptoglobin, and fibrin split products are collected at regular intervals. Routine vital signs and hemodynamics are also collected and documented on a special form. Nurse investigators or study coordinators usually collect any additional data so nursing time is not taken away from patient care.

NURSING MANAGEMENT

Nursing management of the HEMOPUMP patient does not differ significantly from any critically ill patient. A nursing plan of care should be developed based on the identified nursing diagnoses outlined in the box on p. 97.[3]

NURSING DIAGNOSES

Alteration in cardiac output: decreased
Alteration in tissue perfusion
Impaired gas exchange
Alteration in comfort
Potential for injury
Potential for infection
Anxiety/fear
Altered nutrition: less than body requirements
Sleep pattern disturbance
Powerlessness

Important concepts include oxygenation and ventilation, hemodynamic stability, tissue perfusion, and renal function. Neurological and gastrointestinal systems must also be carefully evaluated and appropriate nursing interventions selected.

Laboratory values must be closely monitored and potential complications related to the device must be prevented. Other nursing interventions include prevention of infection, prevention of skin breakdown, and an adequate nutritional status.

The psychosocial issues that stem from being placed on a ventricular assist device must also be addressed. Often we place our emphasis on the physiological status and put emotional needs of the patient and family at a lower priority. Anxiety, fear, and knowledge deficits should be identified and interventions selected. An important and often forgotten nursing diagnosis in these patients is powerlessness. The dependence upon a mechanical device to sustain life must be an overwhelming thought process to overcome. It is the critical care nurse who can diagnose and treat all of these patient and family needs.

Although there are many similarities among patients, there are also some unique and specific variations in this patient population. The device's nonpulsatile flow may eliminate systolic and diastolic components of the arterial waveform. For that reason, mean arterial pressure should be used for monitoring and titration of pharmacological agents.[3] Pulmonary artery pressures and waveforms should not be affected because the HEMOPUMP is a left-assist device; however, critical care nurses must also closely monitor for impending right ventricular failure.

Monitoring of mixed venous oxygen saturation (Svo_2 monitoring) can be extremely useful to assess tissue perfusion. Other noninvasive measurements of tissue perfusion are just as important. Color, temperature, motion, sensitivity, and capillary refill of extremities should be used. Sao_2 monitoring and peripheral pulse checks may be difficult, secondary to the nonpulsatile flow. Ausculation of heart sounds is affected and sometimes difficult because of HEMOPUMP noise and because the cannula crosses the aortic valve. As the ventricle recovers, there should be a changing intensity of heart sounds and an increasing pulse pressure with return to a more normal arterial waveform.[2]

Prevention of device-related complications can be minimized or avoided by careful attention to the system parameters of motor current, purge pressure, and seal flow, as previously described. Because the femoral artery is cannulated, keeping the leg straight and immobilized, as well as not elevating the head more than 30 degrees, are important nursing functions.

CONCLUSION

Early trial results on the use of the HEMOPUMP cardiac assist system are encouraging. Certainly a larger patient population is needed to further prove its effectiveness and its safety and efficacy. The advantages of HEMOPUMP support over traditional and more invasive assist devices bring forth a new potential in providing ventricular assistance to patients in cardiogenic shock from diverse causes.

REFERENCES

1. HEMOPUMP Temporary Cardiac Assist System: directions for use, Rancho Cordova, Calif., 1988, Nimbus Medical, Inc.
2. Rountree WD: The HEMOPUMP Temporary Cardiac Assist System, *AACN Clin Issues Crit Care Nurs* 2:3, 1991.
3. Rountree WD, Rutan RM, McClure AL: The HEMOPUMP Cardiac Assist System: nursing care of the patient, *Crit Care Nurs* 11:4, 1991.
4. Rutan PM, Rountree WD, Myers KK et al: Initial experience with the HEMOPUMP, *Crit Car Nurs Clin N Am* 1:3, 1989.
5. Fraizer OH, Wampler RK, Duncan JM et al: First human use of the Hemopump, a catheter-mounted ventricular assist device, *Ann Thorac Surg* 49:299, 1990.
6. Duncan JM, Frazier OH, Radovancevic B et al: Implantation techniques for the Hemopump, *Ann Thorac Surg* 48:733, 1989.
7. Duncan JM, Burnett CM, Vega JD et al: Rapid placement of the Hemopump and hemofiltration cannula, *Ann Thorac Surg* 50:667, 1990.
8. Rutan PM, Riehle RA, Julian TE: HEMOPUMP training course: management of the patient with the Nimbus Hemopump, Rancho Cordova, Calif., 1989, Nimbus Medical, Inc.
9. Butler KC, Moise JC, Wampler RK: The Hemopump—a new cardiac prosthesis device, *IEEE Transactions on Biomedical Engineering* 37:2, February 1990.

CHAPTER 8

Novacor ventricular assist system

Julie A. Shinn and **Philip E. Oyer**

INTRODUCTION

In the past decade notable progress has been made in the development and clinical application of implantable circulatory support devices that are capable of long-term support. Clinical investigation of the Novacor, an electrically powered, left ventricular assist system (LVAS), has been underway since 1984. Trials are being conducted in over 12 major centers in the United States and in several European centers. Major successes have been achieved using this device for support of patients whose condition has deteriorated while waiting for heart transplantation. Bridging-to-heart transplant is the primary indication for use of the Novacor LVAS. It has, however, been used for postcardiotomy support on a limited basis. An eventual goal of this system is to provide long-term support for selected patients with end-stage heart failure who do not have transplantation as an option. Data from current clinical trials are establishing the efficacy of long-term support.

As of May 1992, 116 patients have been supported with the Novacor LVAS while waiting for heart transplant.[1] Of those patients, 3 continued to wait on support and 67 (59%) were successfully bridged-to-transplant. Of those, 62 (93%) were alive 2 days to 92 months following transplant.[1] This chapter will review the operation of the Novacor LVAS, patient selection, insertion techniques, patient care issues, and device management issues. Future long-term support goals will also be outlined.

OPERATION OF THE DEVICE

The Novacor LVAS is an electrically driven, totally implantable pump with an externally located console. The pump consists of dual pusher plates that are bonded to a cylindrical, seamless, polyurethane pump sac. When energized, the pusher plates compress the pump sac, providing symmetrical deformation. This configuration results in optimal flow characteristics that provide good washing with no areas of blood stasis.[2] The pusher plates are powered by a solenoid that converts electrical energy received from the control console to the mechanical energy required to compress the plates and

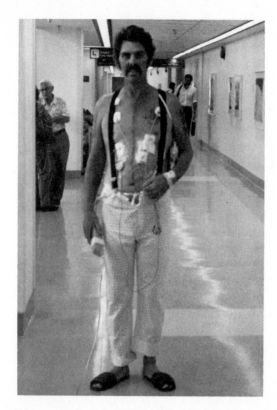

Fig. 8-1. A patient walking approximately 18 feet behind the Novacor console. (From Shinn JA: *AACN Clinical Issues* 2(3):575, 1991.)

propel blood from the pump. Unidirectional flow is maintained with inflow and outflow bioprosthetic valves. A percutaneous vent tube provides electrical energy to the pump and returns control signals from displacement transducers located at the pusher plates and solenoid. Transducer signals provide information about filling volumes, pump output volume, pump rate, and energy usage. Both the power lead and the cable carrying pump transducer signals are attached to a 20-foot extension cable that is secured to the external console. The extension cable provides patients with considerable mobility away from the console. Fig. 8-1 shows a patient standing approximately 18 feet away from the console.

Support of circulation is achieved by placing the pump in series with the patient's circulation. It is positioned in a pocket in the left upper abdominal quadrant just anterior to the posterior rectus abdominis sheath. Woven Dacron conduits direct blood to and from the pump. A semirigid plastic cannula is placed in the left ventricular apex and is connected to the inflow conduit, which traverses the diaphragm before connecting to the implanted pump. Blood is returned to circulation via the outflow conduit, which

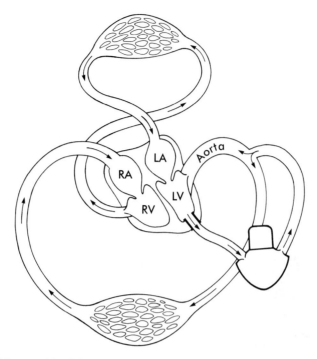

Fig. 8-2. The Novacor LVAS is positioned in series with the patient's heart. The left ventricle fills the LVAS, and systemic pressures are generated by the LVAS. *RA,* right atrium; *RV,* right ventricle; *LA,* left atrium; *LV,* left ventricle. (From Shinn JA: *AACN Clinical Issues* 2(3):575, 1991.)

traverses the diaphragm and is anastomosed to the ascending aorta. Fig. 8-2 illustrates the pump position in series with the native heart. When properly timed, the ventricle is decompressed and serves as a low-pressure filling chamber for the implanted systemic pump, much like the atria function for normal ventricles. All blood flows from the left ventricle to the pump at less than systemic pressure, so the aortic valve remains closed.

The external console houses two separate pump controllers and standby batteries. The second controller is immediately available if problems should develop with the controller in use. A monitor that displays signals from the pump's volume transducers is located in the console. In addition, the patient's electrocardiogram signal and arterial and left ventricular pressures are displayed. Pump timing controls are located on the face of the console, allowing clinicians to make adjustments to maintain synchrony between the native heart systole, pump filling, and ejection.

Consistent synchrony between the pump and left ventricle decreases left ventricular wall tension and myocardial oxygen consumption. Synchrony also ensures that total left ventricular volume is diverted to the pump and that the aortic valve remains closed.

The primary principle governing pump timing is that the pump is ready to fill at the beginning of left ventricular systole. As the ventricle contracts, blood flow follows the path of least resistance toward the implanted pump, which fills with a minimum pressure gradient of 10 mm Hg. Pump ejection subsequently occurs during left ventricular diastole. Aortic pressure reaches its peak during pump ejection, which corresponds to the diastolic period of the normal cardiac cycle. At completion of pump ejection, the LVAS is ready to receive blood from the next left ventricular contraction.

Timing of pump ejection is achieved by one of three methods: (1) triggering from an electrocardiogram signal, (2) triggering from changes in rate of pump filling, or (3) by using a fixed rate setting. Use of the QRS complex from the electrocardiogram signal as a trigger can effectively maintain synchrony. A timing delay following the QRS must be set so that the pump ejection does not occur until the corresponding native left ventricular ejection has filled the pump. This ejection delay, determined by the heart rate, can be set by the clinician. This trigger mode is not ideal when frequent, large changes in heart rate occur and it is dependent on maintenance of a good electrocardiogram signal. It also becomes less practical to use as patients begin to ambulate.

Under most circumstances the change in rate of LVAS filling during native left ventricular systole is preferred as the trigger for pump ejection. The initial rapid rate of pump filling decreases toward the end of left ventricular contraction. Clinicians determine the percentage decrease in the rate of filling that corresponds most closely to the end of the left ventricular contraction. When the LVAS fill rate falls below the selected threshold, pump ejection occurs. A delay can be introduced following this threshold, if necessary, to maintain optimum synchrony. This maneuver may be necessary with large stroke volumes. Using this trigger mode, synchrony can be maintained over a wide range of heart rates. The pump responds appropriately to physiologic changes in heart rate during rest or exercise.

A third choice of trigger, fixed rate, will allow the pump to operate asynchronously, independent of native heart action. Therefore it is rarely used clinically. It may have some usefulness during ventricular fibrillation to maintain pump output and systemic blood pressure, but use of the fill-rate trigger can usually provide the same function.

Table 8-1. Patient age, body surface area, cardiac index preimplant, and during support and duration of support in 90 bridged-to-transplant

	Age (yr)	BSA m^2	CI preimplant L/min/m^2	CI on LVAS L/min/m^2	Duration[°] (days)
Mean	45	1.94	1.91	2.99	46
Maximum	67	2.70	2.87	4.56	370
Minimum	15	1.54	0.68	1.12	1
Median	47	1.90	1.90	3.06	30

[°]Nine operative deaths are excluded; all were supported less than 12 hours. *BSA,* body surface area; *CI,* cardiac index. Data from Novacor Division, Baxter Healthcare Corporation, Oakland, Calif.

Current pumps in clinical use hold a maximum volume of 70 ml. After ejection, the pump is never completely empty. Residual volumes normally range from 2 to 6 ml, providing stroke volumes of 64 to 68 ml per beat. Total pump output will be determined by the patient's heart rate and volume status. As patient requirements for output increase such as with exercise, the LVAS can respond to subsequent increased frequency of left ventricular contractions and stroke volume to increase pump output as required.

Long-term support capabilities of the Novacor LVAS have been well documented. Range of support has been 1 day to 370 days.[1] Table 8-1 outlines capabilities of long-term support and the range of cardiac indices achieved with the Novacor LVAS.

Any LVAS used for long-term support should be capable of doing so with minimal blood trauma and minimal requirements for anticoagulation. Serious hemolysis or thrombocytopenia have not been major problems associated with the Novacor LVAS. Anticoagulation is maintained with heparin early postoperatively, with eventual conversion to warfarin. The box below outlines a sample anticoagulation protocol. Some centers utilize dextran therapy for the first postoperative week before commencing with warfarin.[3] In this sort of protocol, patients may be started on coumadin directly without using intravenous heparin. Antiplatelet agents may be used in conjunction with warfarin.

PATIENT SELECTION

All patients selected for Novacor LVAS insertion for bridge-to-transplantation must meet the criteria for heart transplantation at the time of LVAS insertion. These criteria include (1) age less than 65 years, (2) absence of infection, (3) no fixed pulmonary hypertension, (4) no recent pulmonary infarction, (5) no renal or hepatic dysfunction that can not be reversed with adequate cardiac output, and (6) no other chronic systemic illness. The National Institutes of Health Study Group has determined other exclusion criteria to be utilized when making patient selection.[4] These criteria are outlined in the box on p. 104. Chronic conditions of this nature would not be reversed by LVAS support and would jeopardize successful transplantation. If right ventricular failure is present, it

---

SAMPLE ANTICOAGULATION PROTOCOL USED FOR LONG-TERM SUPPORT

1. Dextran at 25 ml/hr when chest tube drainage <100 cc/hr for 3 to 4 consecutive hours°
2. Continuous heparin infusion within 6 to 24 hours of implant, titrated to maintain a partial thromboplastin time 1.5 times the preoperative value or activated clotting times between 150 to 200 seconds
3. Switch to oral warfarin therapy when the patient is eating, at a dose that maintains a prothrombin time of 20% to 30% of the preoperative value

---

°Dextran may not be used in all centers. Duration of dextran infusion varies.

```
_____ EXCLUSION CRITERIA FOR LVAS INSERTION _____
DEVELOPED BY THE NATIONAL INSTITUTES OF HEALTH STUDY GROUP[4]

Blood dyscrasia
Cancer with metastasis
Chronic renal failure
Diffuse, severe peripheral vascular disease
Severe hepatic disease
Severe pulmonary disease associated with pulmonary arterial hypertension
Severe bacterial infection not responsive to antibiotic therapy
```

must be carefully evaluated. Following LVAS insertion the right ventricle must be able to maintain left heart preload. If this function is impaired, LVAS pump filling and subsequent pump output will not be optimum. Right ventricular function improves with restored left-sided output in most patients. Patients may often require inotropic support of the right ventricle and pulmonary vasodilatation for afterload reduction for several days following insertion. However, these medications are usually unnecessary after the first week. Temporary right ventricular circulatory assistance has been used when right ventricular failure is severe. However, the need for right ventricular support has been associated with less satisfactory outcomes.[5]

Hemodynamic criteria for the use of the Novacor LVAS is uniform regardless of the cause of end-stage heart failure. Before considering insertion, attempts should be made to correct hypovolemia, acidosis, and any blood gas abnormalities. Patients being considered for LVAS support generally must be in cardiogenic shock that has proven unresponsive to conventional therapy, including maximal pharmacological support and intraaortic balloon pump (IABP) therapy. A trial of IABP support may be bypassed if it appears that the patient will not derive significant benefit from it. Specific hemodynamic criteria for considering LVAS insertion include (1) mean arterial blood pressure less than 60 mm Hg, (2) left atrial or pulmonary capillary wedge pressure greater than 20 mm Hg, (3) urine output less than 20 ml/hr, and (4) a cardiac index of less than 2.0 L/min/m^2 despite the therapeutic measures just described.[3,4] Systemic vascular resistance of 2100 dynes/sec/cm^{-5} is also used as a criteria by some centers.[3]

Patient size must be considered when an LVAS system is implanted vs. using an extracorporeal system. There must be adequate room in the left upper abdominal quadrant to house the pump. The smallest patient supported by the Novacor LVAS had a body surface area of 1.54 m^2.[1] Table 8-1 outlines the ranges of body surface areas of patients who have been supported by the Novacor LVAS. Patients with body surface areas of less than 1.5 m^2 are excluded as candidates for LVAS insertion. Even patients who meet this criteria but are small and short-waisted may be excluded because of lack of adequate space in the left upper abdominal quadrant.

PUMP INSERTION

A median sternotomy incision is used to retract the sternum and expose the heart. This incision is extended down the abdomen to the umbilicus. An abdominal pocket is created to house the pump in the previously described area. The patient is then placed on cardiopulmonary bypass. The woven Dacron pump outflow conduit is preclotted and anastomosed to the ascending aorta, following which the pump is placed in its pocket. The pump inflow graft is placed through the left diaphragm into the pericardium. Priming of the pump is achieved with normal saline. The inflow conduit is then anastomosed to the ventricular apex, and all air is evacuated from the system. LVAS support is then initiated, and cardiopulmonary bypass is discontinued. Heparin anticoagulation is reversed with protamine. Before closing the chest, a Millar pressure transducer may be placed in the left ventricle for monitoring purposes. Chest tubes and temporary epicardial pacemaker wires are also secured before closing the chest. Jackson-Pratt drains are placed in the abdominal pocket before closing the incision.

POTENTIAL COMPLICATIONS
Bleeding

Bleeding is a common complication following LVAS insertion.[3,5] Extensive surgical dissection, multiple cannulation sites, anticoagulation, and cardiopulmonary bypass all contribute to the potential for bleeding.[3,6,7] Close monitoring of the patient's hematologic status is essential. When the patient is admitted to the intensive care unit, it is important to obtain a complete hematologic profile that includes a complete blood count, partial thromboplastin time (PTT), prothrombin time (PT), thrombin time, platelet count, and fibrinogen and possibly fibrin split products. Results will guide decisions about fresh frozen plasma, blood, and platelet administration. Use of human lymphocyte antigen type-specific platelets and type-specific blood products will minimize the possibility of antibody formation that could make matching a donor heart more difficult later.[6]

Cardiac tamponade, abdominal bleeding, or continued excessive blood loss may all be indications for reexploration of the chest or abdomen. Monitoring for cardiac tamponade requires close monitoring of central venous pressures, pulmonary artery pressures, and pump output. Restriction to filling of the right side of the heart will be evidenced by elevation of right heart pressures. Pump output will fall as pump filling from the right heart is impaired. It will be important to distinguish cardiac tamponade from signs and symptoms of right ventricular failure. Tamponade should always be considered in a bleeding patient. Excessive blood loss that persists after coagulation status is under control may indicate bleeding from a cannulation site or large vessel that will require reexploration for control.

Abdominal bleeding is not as frequently seen, nor has it been life threatening. Generally a reexploration of the abdominal wound is undertaken when the patient is hemodynamically stable; usually 24 to 48 hours after implant. The procedure is undertaken to remove accumulated clot and locate any vessels that continue to ooze.

Alteration in cardiac output

Before implanting the Novacor LVAS, all patients are in severe heart failure or cardiogenic shock. In addition, they are dependent on pharmacological support of cardiac function. Surgical placement of the pump and coring of the left ventricular apex will likely result in a transient increase in impairment of myocardial function. Even though the LVAS will take over left ventricular performance, the pump is still dependent on right ventricular function to sustain optimal output. Impaired LVAS filling postoperatively can be the result of inadequate circulating volume or persistent right ventricular failure.

Any condition that impairs venous return to the right ventricle can result in inadequate preload for the pump, causing output to decrease. Optimal filling pressure will vary with individual patients, but generally central venous pressure is maintained at 8 to 15 mm Hg and pulmonary capillary wedge pressure is maintained at 10 to 15 mm Hg. Concomitant decreases of both right and left-sided filling pressures associated with a fall in pump output usually indicates a need for volume therapy. Vasodilatation with rewarming, diuresis, or blood loss may all result in hypovolemia and subsequent decreased pump output.

Elevation of central venous pressure associated with decreased left-sided pressures and pump output requires investigation of potential deterioration of right ventricular function. Right heart failure results in decreased forward flow to the left heart and thus the LVAS. Serious, but usually transient, right ventricular failure has been reported to develop in as many as 20% to 30% of patients requiring a left ventricular assist device following surgery.[8] In the first 70 patients supported with the Novacor LVAS, 16 patients required right ventricular support with an assist device for a period of half an hour to 16 days.[1] Since right ventricular dysfunction is almost always caused by profound left ventricular dysfunction, right heart performance can be expected to improve over time with the restoration of normal left-sided output via the pump. Inotropic drug support will likely be used for several postoperative days to augment right ventricular function. Prostaglandin E_1 is frequently used to dilate the pulmonary vascular bed and provide right ventricular afterload reduction. Once the patient is hemodynamically stable, drug support is gradually weaned. Pressure lines are removed when the patient's weight and fluid balance are stable.

Infection

Potential development of infection is a great concern for any patient being bridged-to-transplantation because infection could preclude transplantation. These patients are at increased risk for infection because of their preoperative debilitated state, the surgical intervention, and multiple invasive lines.

Nutritional status is usually impaired before implant because of profound heart failure. Inadequate absorption, hypoperfusion of the gastrointestinal tract, and anorexia are factors that contribute to poor nutrition in heart failure patients. Parenteral nutrition, if not already started, is begun within 24 to 48 hours of implant. Nutritional recovery is important to minimize risk of infection and to promote wound healing. Parenteral nutrition is discontinued once oral intake provides adequate caloric intake. Some of these patients have required smaller meals and more frequent snacks because of an inability to eat large amounts at any one sitting.

Routine prophylactic antibiotic coverage with cephalosporin is used for 3 to 4 days postoperatively. Antibiotics are not used again unless specific organisms are cultured. Some centers routinely house these patients in protective isolation.[3,7] Our practice has been to place patients in semiprivate rooms with other clean surgical patients. We depend on good hand washing and strict aseptic technique for all dressing changes. Invasive lines, chest tubes and Jackson-Pratt drains are removed as soon as possible to eliminate as many portals of entry as possible. Nurses also need to be vigilant about monitoring wounds, line insertion sites, and the percutaneous vent tube exit site for any signs of infection.

Potential device-related complications

Important mechanical malfunction of the Novacor LVAS has not been reported. All nursing personnel caring for these patients are trained in emergency procedures should problems arise with the controller. The LVAS console contains two controllers so that one is always immediately available as a backup. A third separate controller is always kept in the patient's room. Problems with the extension cable that delivers power to the pump and returns transducer signals to the console have occurred in patients supported for prolonged periods (greater than 1 to 2 months). A spare extension cable is kept with the patient in the event problems occur. Nurses need to know how to switch to backup controllers and change the extension cable in an expedient manner. In the event of power failure, there are 40 minutes of battery time in a fully charged controller. The system switches to battery operation immediately upon disruption of power. Patients must be well grounded during walks with the console. There have been incidents where patients have built up enough static electrical charge to cause pump interference. Proper grounding prevents the problem in most cases.

NURSING MANAGEMENT

All patients are admitted to the intensive care unit directly from surgery. Patients are monitored similarly to any other cardiac surgery patient with a radial arterial pressure line and a pulmonary artery pressure line. The side port of the pulmonary artery catheter and a peripheral intravenous line are used for volume replacement. A second central venous line is utilized for drug administration. It is our practice to use a left

Table 8-2. Nursing care plan

Nursing diagnosis	Expected outcomes	Interventions
1. High risk for injury: bleeding related to cardiopulmonary bypass and extensive surgical dissection.	1. Prevention of bleeding demonstrated by control of postoperative bleeding, normal coagulation studies, and no cardiac tamponade.	1. Monitor coagulation studies daily Monitor for signs of excessive wound and chest tube drainage Notify MD of sudden changes in chest tube drainage or coagulation status Monitor for signs of cardiac tamponade Administer blood component therapy guided by coagulation studies and hematocrit Observe for guiac positive NG drainage and stool Monitor for signs of petecchi and extensive bruising.
2. High risk for injury: thromboembolism related to the LVAS	2. Patient will have adequate tissue perfusion demonstrated by warm extremities, normal peripheral pulses, normal level of consciousness with normal motor and sensory function.	2. Maintain ACT greater than 150 seconds Administer antiplatelet drugs as ordered Assess neurological system at least every 4 hours Assess peripheral perfusion (pulses, skin temperature, color, and capillary refill) every 4 hours.
3. Alteration in cardiac output: decreased related to right ventricular failure or inadequate preload.	3. Maintenance of cardiac (pump) output between 4-8 L/min with normal hemodynamic pressures, improved urine output, and adequate peripheral perfusion.	3. Record pump output hourly and with any change in therapy Compare right ventricular cardiac output measured with pulmonary artery catheter and LVAS output Administer inotropic drugs, volume therapy, and afterload reduction to achieve optimal right ventricular performance Monitor renal function via BUN and serum creatinine daily Monitor peripheral perfusion at least every 4 hours.
4. Alteration in cardiac output: decreased related to LVAS malfunction.	4. Prevention of any malfunction or prompt correction with no negative patient sequelae.	4. Maintain backup extension cable and console in patient room Monitor nursing staff for retention of skills for emergency procedures Monitor cable connections for wear and loose connections Properly ground the patient before ambulation with the LVAS.

Table 8-2.   Nursing care plan—cont'd

Nursing diagnosis	Expected outcomes	Interventions
5. High risk for infection related to debilitated state and multiple invasive lines.	5. Patient will remain a febrile with WBC within normal limits. Wound healing will be normal and free of purulent drainage or erythema.	5. Maintain aseptic technique for all dressing changes and insertion site care Monitor temperature and WBC for elevation Administer prophylactic antibiotics as ordered Remove all invasive lines as soon as possible Initiate restoration of nutrition as soon as possible Assess skin at percutaneous vent site, LVAS pocket, and sternal incision for signs of drainage, swelling, or erythema every 8 hours.
6. Activity intolerance related to debilitated state and surgical procedure.	6. Increases strength as demonstrated by increased mobility, activity tolerance, and frequency of exercise.	6. Maintain adequate analgesia for activity Initiate assisted exercise as soon as possible Initiate physical therapy as soon as possible Encourage frequent activity Allow for periods of rest Secure extension cable to prevent undue discomfort or stress to surrounding tissue Develop an exercise plan to include time of day, activity, and activity duration.
7. High risk for sensory alteration related to noise and vibration from the LVAS.	7. Patient demonstrates normal uninterrupted sleep and verbalizes acceptance of LVAS.	7. Monitor patient's sleep patterns and provide uninterrupted sleep during night Encourage patient and family to verbalize feelings and perceptions about the LVAS Provide accurate information about the LVAS Encourage socialization and normal activities Provide diversional activities Provide for privacy for patient.

Modified from Shinn JA: Novacor left ventricular assist system, *AACN Clinical Issues* 2(3):580, 1991.

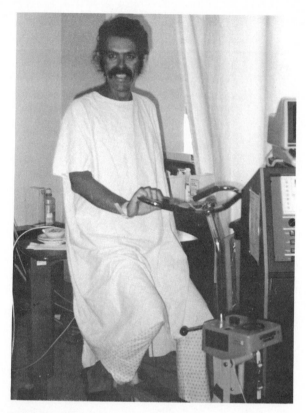

Fig. 8-3. This patient is exercising on a stationary bicycle on the tenth postoperative day. (From Shinn JA: *AACN Clinical Issues* 2(3):575, 1991.)

ventricular pressure transducer to monitor left ventricular function directly.

Routine inotropic support consists of dopamine hydrochloride (3 to 8 μg/kg/min) and low dose epinephrine (less than 100 ng/kg/min). The patient's right ventricular function will determine the degree of inotropic support required. Afterload reduction and blood pressure control are achieved with sodium nitroprusside. Elevated pulmonary vascular resistance that compromises right ventricular function is treated with prostaglandin E_1. These drugs will be gradually weaned during the first week, depending on patient condition.

In addition to monitoring for the potential complications described, nursing management also focuses on activity progression and the psychosocial needs of the patient. Table 8-2 outlines a standard plan of care that incorporates all of these issues.

Activity progression is an immediate priority following extubation. Most patients are able to be extubated by 48 hours after surgery. Patients who are more debilitated or who have persistent right ventricular dysfunction may require longer periods of intubation. Activity begins within 24 hours of extubation with sitting on the side of the bed. As soon as this is tolerated, patients are encouraged to sit in a bedside chair as often as three times a day. Physical therapy is instituted at this point. Initially, patients receive passive exercise that is gradually progressed to resistance exercise. When walking about the bedside in the room is well tolerated, patients begin walking in the hallways. Usually, by 2 weeks, patients begin stationary bicycle riding under the supervision of the physical therapist. Fig. 8-3 shows a patient on an exercise bicycle on the tenth postoperative day. Cycling to resistance is gradually increased and patients are encouraged to bicycle ride twice a day in addition to hallway walks. This aggressive approach to activity is also advocated by other centers.[3] Care must be taken during exercise to secure and support the device extension cable so that the weight of the cable does not cause tension or traumatize tissue surrounding the percutaneous vent tube exit site.

Initially, some patients will be disturbed by the noise or vibration of the pump. As a result these patients may have problems related to sensory overload and sleep disruption. Gradually, patients adapt to these sensations. Some have stated the noise provides comfort and reassurance that they are alright. Nurses caring for these patients need to recognize the significance of the cable and console to the patient. In particular, patients may come to view the cable as an extension of themselves or as a sort of "umbilical cord." The cable needs to be treated as respectfully as the patient's body is treated. Many patients will have very specific ideas as to how it should be handled and secured.

Some patients will have difficulty dealing with their dependency on the pump. Expression of this conflict may take the form of depression or need for control. It is important to find opportunities for patients to have control of their situation, such as letting them plan mealtimes, exercise activities, and private time with family members. Providing them with such opportunities will minimize the risk that they will attempt to control their situation by being noncompliant with important issues such as taking medications.

Long periods of waiting for a donor heart, their uncertain future, and lack of privacy are all potential sources of discouragement. Patients may require assistance to maintain their spirits. Diversional activities can be planned with the assistance of occupational therapists and family members. Teaching about posttransplant life-style and medications may also provide a more hopeful outlook. Patients can be taken out of the unit for meals in the cafeteria with family or to garden benches outside the hospital. See Fig. 8-4. The nurse can stay near the console while the patient can have privacy with family members up to 20 feet away. These activities help to provide a break in normal routines and to maintain patient spirits.

PATIENT OUTCOMES

As of May 1992, 59% of patients were successfully transplanted following support with the Novacor LVAS. Of the 46 patients not transplanted, 26% died within 12 hours

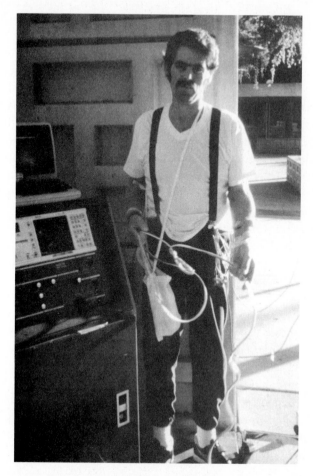

Fig. 8-4. Patient during an excursion outside the hospital. An outdoor power outlet was used while the patient enjoyed a visit with his family and some sunshine.

of implant and were considered operative deaths. In the remaining patients, mortality was primarily attributed to infection, multisystem organ failure, or severe right heart failure. In the patients who survived to transplant, 93% were alive at 2 days to 92 months following successful transplantation (May 1992). Clearly these patients have outcomes equal to other heart transplant patients not requiring circulatory support before transplant.

LONG-TERM GOALS OF THE NOVACOR LVAS

Current clinical trials are establishing the efficacy of long-term support for patients who are not transplant candidates. The eventual goal is to utilize a completely implant-

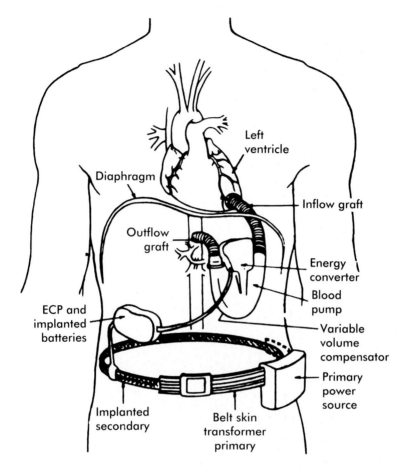

Fig. 8-5. A completely implantable version of the Novacor LVAS. Current practice is to anastomose the outflow graft to the ascending aorta. The original concept for the "permanent" means of support was for outflow return to the abdominal aorta. *ECP,* electronic control and power unit. (Courtesy Novacor Division, Baxter Healthcare Corporation, Oakland, California.)

able version of this device as a means of "permanent" support. Fig. 8-5 illustrates the implantable pump with a miniaturized implantable controller. A battery is housed in the implanted controller that ideally will be capable of supplying power for up to 1 hour without an external power source. During this time a patient could be free to shower or engage in other activities without wearing an external power pack. External power will be delivered to the implantable controller through the skin via transformer coils that encircle the waist in subcutaneous tissue. A second set of transformer coils is located in a belt that would be worn by the patient. The belt would also contain a pri-

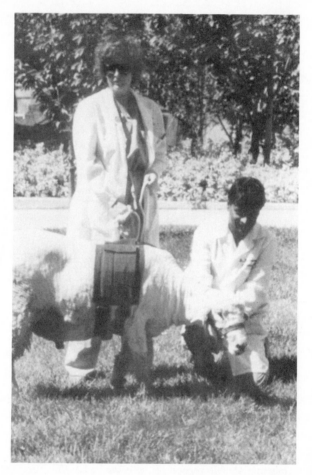

Fig. 8-6. A sheep with a totally implanted LVAS. Stored power to the implanted LVAS is delivered through the skin from a battery contained in the external belt worn by the animal.

mary stored power source that could be charged as needed from standard AC power outlets. Successful employment of this concept has already been achieved in animal studies. Fig. 8-6 shows a sheep with a totally implanted pump. The animal is wearing a belt that is supplying power to the LVAS. There are many potential candidates for this type of long-term support who exceed the age limit for heart transplantation, have other contraindications to transplant, or for whom a donor cannot be found.

CONCLUSION

Major progress has been made in the development and clinical application of the Novacor LVAS for long-term support. The majority of these patients survive to transplant in good condition. When they present for transplant, they are not dependent on inotropic support, they have recovered nutritionally, and their functional status has improved to a point that allows active exercise. The Novacor LVAS has played a major role in salvaging this small group of very terminal individuals. In the next decade we may see this application extend to individuals who do not receive transplants and choose to live with the extended support of this device in its completely implantable form.

ACKNOWLEDGMENT

The authors with to acknowledge peer, M. Porter Ph.D, for supplying data from the Novacor Division of Baxter Healthcare Corporation and Mary Hill for the preparation of this manuscript.

REFERENCES

1. Novacor Division: *Clinical data,* Oakland, California, 1992, Baxter Healthcare Corporation.
2. Portner PM, Oyer PE, Jassawalla JS et al: An alternative in end-stage heart disease: long-term ventricular assistance, *Heart Transplantation* 3(1):47, 1983.
3. Reedy JE, Ruzevich SA, Swartz MT et al: Nursing care of a patient requiring prolonged mechanical circulatory support, *Progress in Cardiovascular Nursing* 4(1):1, 1989.
4. Pennington DG, Bernhard WF, Golding LR et al: Long-term follow-up of postcardiotomy patients with profound cardiogenic shock treated with ventricular assist devices, *Circulation* 72(suppl II):216, 1985.
5. Shinn JA: Novacor left ventricular assist system, *AACN Clinical Issues* 2(3):575, 1991.
6. Ruzevich SA, Swartz MT, Pennington DG: Nursing care of the patient with a pneumatic ventricular assist device, *Heart Lung,* 17:399, 1988.
7. Teplitz L: Patients with ventricular assist devices: nursing diagnosis. *DCCN* 9(2):82, 1990.
8. Schoen FJ, Palmer DC, Bernhard WF et al: Clinical temporary ventricular assist, *J Thorac Cardiovasc Surg* 92:1071, 1986.

CHAPTER 9

HeartMate ventricular assist system

Nancy Abou-Awdi and O. H. Frazier

INTRODUCTION

The HeartMate (Thermo Cardiosystems Inc., Woburn, Mass.), a pneumatically actuated left ventricular assist device (LVAD), has been under clinical investigation since 1986. Currently this LVAD is used in cardiac transplant candidates whose hemodynamic status deteriorates, placing them at risk for permanent end-organ damage and thus compromising their transplant candidacy status. The HeartMate, which provides adequate end-organ perfusion, can support the patient until a suitable donor is found, even when extended support (>30 days) is necessary. In our experience the medical status of most patients has improved to the extent that they are optimal transplant candidates.[1] We will describe the development of the HeartMate, system operation, patient management, and future directions.

HISTORY

In 1978 Norman et al.[2] successfully used a left ventricular assist device (LVAD) to support a patient with "stone heart" syndrome for 5 days until cardiac transplantation could be undertaken. Although the patient died after transplantation, the experience was encouraging because it demonstrated the ability of an LVAD to support a patient in biventricular failure. The LVAD used in that case (Fig. 9-1) was a precursor to the HeartMate LVAD (Fig. 9-2), which is currently undergoing clinical investigation. The original pump was elongated to facilitate implantation from the left ventricle to the abdominal aorta. Later the pump was rounded to improve fit in the left subdiaphragmatic position and to ease the anastomosis to the ascending aorta. The new design also required a less extensive implant operation.

The blood-contacting surfaces of the HeartMate are textured, a unique feature that promotes the formation of a biological lining within the pump, helping to reduce the risk of thromboembolic complications. Texturing of blood-contacting surfaces in the original pump was initially done by gluing polyester fibrils to the pump surface. Because the fibrils could potentially become dislodged and increase the risk of embo-

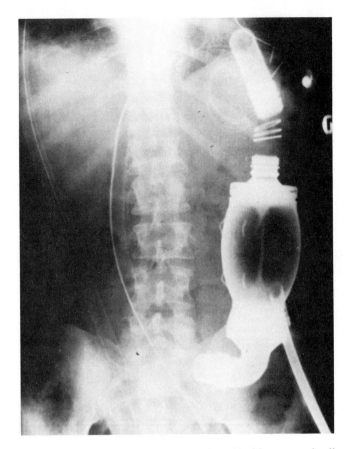

Fig. 9-1. X-ray film of implanted LVAD developed by Norman and colleagues.

lization, a process of integrally texturing blood-contacting surfaces was instituted to avoid this risk. Although minor alterations have been made to the pump, the basic design and simplicity of operation have remained unchanged.

THEORY OF OPERATION

The HeartMate consists of a pneumatically actuated, implantable blood pump and an external console/driver (Fig. 9-3). The blood pump is contained within a rigid titanium housing. A flexible diaphragm and pusher plate separate two chambers within the pump and isolate air from blood. A "stroke limiter" attached to the pusher plate prevents blood-contacting surfaces of the diaphragm from coming into contact with the opposing surface at the end of ejection. A stroke-volume sensor within the pump continuously reports pump volume to the console, the amount of which is displayed on the

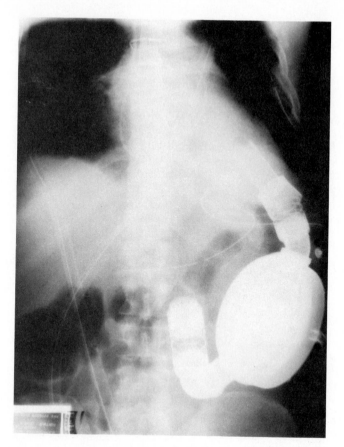

Fig. 9-2. X-ray film of implanted HeartMate.

console. At a maximum stroke volume of 83 ml, the pump is capable of providing outputs of up to 10 L/min. The pump diaphragm is fabricated of integrally textured polyurethane, and the metallic surfaces are sintered, a process whereby titanium microspheres are heated so that they fuse to the metallic surface. A thin coagulum forms between the blood and these textured surfaces, which is thought to reduce the incidence of excessive thrombus formation within the pump.[3,4] The Dacron inflow and outflow conduits each contain a 25 mm, one-way porcine xenograft valve (Medtronic Blood Systems, Irvine, Calif.) that produces unidirectional blood flow through the pump. The driveline, which extends inferiorly from the air chamber, provides communication between the pump and console by way of an interconnecting cable.

Affixed to a cart for easy maneuverability, the console/driver is a self-contained unit, powered by either a standard electrical outlet (AC) or an internal, rechargeable battery (DC). The console contains a pulsatile air pump with a pusher plate and diaphragm

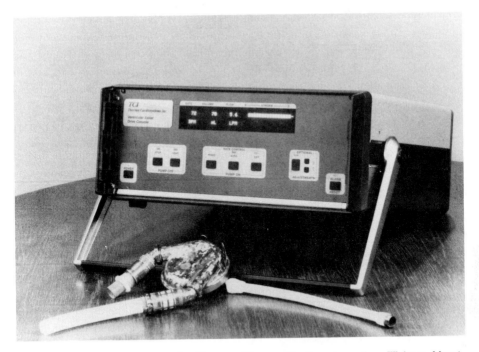

Fig. 9-3. Blood pump and console. (Courtesy Thermo Cardiosystems, Inc., Woburn, Mass.)

that function like bellows. Pump ejection is created when the bellows force compressed air through the driveline and into the air chamber of the implanted blood pump, operating the blood pump diaphragm and thus forcing blood to move through the outflow conduit. At the end of ejection, as the bellows relaxes, the pusher plate passively returns to its starting position.

The console may be operated in one of three modes: fixed rate, automatic, or external synchronous. For fixed-rate mode, the operator sets the console at the number of pulses, or beats per minute, to be delivered (range, 20 to 140 pulses per minute). The duration of ejection is also manually adjusted to maximize stroke volume. For automatic mode, a Hall-Effect sensor in the air chamber of the blood pump measures the excursion of the pusher plate and signals the console to adjust the median end-diastolic volume of the pump to 90% capacity (Fig. 9-4). In this mode the pump is maintained near maximum as variations occur in the patient's cardiac output. The external synchronous mode is triggered by an adequate signal from the patient's electrocardiographic QRS detector. In this mode, pump systole occurs synchronously with the electrical impulse from the patient's R wave.[5] Should the electrical power supply be interrupted, the pump can be operated manually with a hand crank that attaches to an access port.

The front panel of the console has a continuous digital display that shows pump

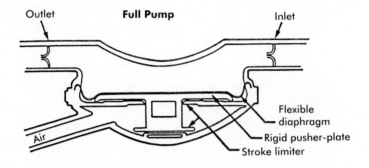

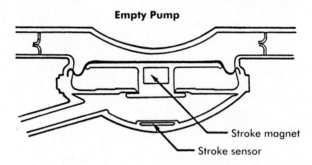

Fig. 9-4. Diagram of pump. (Courtesy Thermo Cardiosystems, Inc., Woburn, Mass.)

flow (L/min), pump rate (beats/min), and stroke volume (ml/min). Pump filling and ejection measurements are represented in a bar graph. Other panel controls include a power switch, a stop button (which must be compressed for 10 seconds to halt pump operation), and a vent button. The vent removes trapped air from the system and allows full excursion of the diaphragm and pusher plate. The venting cycle requires interruption of pumping for 8 seconds and then returns to full operation. An optional adjustment button allows the operator to change pump rate, duration of ejection, and alarm limits and to note the number of cycles completed by the console. A reset button allows an audible alarm to be temporarily disengaged.

PATIENT SELECTION

At present the investigational protocol for the HeartMate restricts use of the device to cardiac transplant candidates (see box on p. 121). The indication for implanting the LVAD is progressive cardiac deterioration despite maximal pharmacological and/or intraaortic balloon pump support. Experience has also shown the importance of instituting support before irreversible end-organ damage occurs. Thus indices reflecting renal and hepatic function are used to assess the need for support. Renal dysfunction is

---

INCLUSION CRITERIA FOR HEARTMATE CLINICAL TRIALS

Category I
Approved transplant candidate
Inotropic support
IABP support (if possible)
LAP or PCWP $\geq$ 20 mm Hg with:
   Systolic BP $\leq$ 80 mm Hg
       or
   Cardiac index $\leq$ 2.0 L/min/m^2

Category II
Approved transplant candidate
Inotropic support; IABP support (if placement possible)
Cardiac arrest
Systolic BP $\leq$ 60 mm Hg

BP, blood pressure; *IABP*, intraaortic balloon pump; *LAP*, left atrial pressure; *PCWP*, pulmonary capillary wedge pressure.

defined by a blood urea nitrogen level $>$ 40 mg/dl and/or a serum creatinine level $\geq$ 2 mg/dl, with urine output $<$ 0.5 cc/kg/hr despite treatment with diuretics. Hepatic dysfunction is defined by a total bilirubin concentration $>$ 2.5 mg/dl and/or a serum glutamic oxaloacetic transaminase concentration $>$ 500 IU/L.

Exclusion criteria for the device are numerous and include any condition that would adversely affect the outcome of cardiac transplantation (see box on p. 122). In addition, the size of the pump (11 x 4 cm; weight, 570 g) precludes its use in patients whose body surface area is less than 1.5 m^2.

INSERTION TECHNIQUE

The operation to implant the HeartMate begins with a median sternotomy.[6] The incision is extended to just above the umbilicus. Cardiopulmonary bypass is instituted with standard cannulation methods. The left ventricular apex is cored with a circular cutting knife, then a sewing ring is sutured to the opening. The pump is placed in the abdominal cavity, just below the left diaphragm. The inlet conduit is tunneled through an incision in the diaphragm and through the sewing ring into the left ventricle. The diaphragm is then closed around the conduit. The outflow conduit, a preclotted Dacron graft, is placed over the diaphragm and anastomosed to the ascending aorta. The pneumatic drive line exits the body through a stab wound in the left lateral abdominal wall, above the iliac crest (Fig. 9-5). Before initiating pump support, air is removed from the heart and the pump outflow graft by placing the patient in the Trendelenburg position, clamping the outflow graft, inserting a 19-gauge needle into the graft, then slowly hand-

---

EXCLUSION CRITERIA FOR HEARTMATE CLINICAL TRIALS

Body surface area $< 1.5 \text{ m}^2$

Age > 70 years

Detection of the following contraindications:

Chronic renal failure; renal dysfunction requiring hemodialysis within 1 month before surgery

Severe emphysema and/or severe chronic obstructive pulmonary disease: forced expiratory volume/sec $< 50\%$ of the predicted value; normal pH with $CO_2 > 55$ mm Hg

Unresolved pulmonary infarction: pulmonary angiograms with evidence of significant embolism within 2 weeks before surgery

Severe chronic pulmonary hypertension: fixed pulmonary hypertension with a PVR > 6 Wood units after a trial of PGE_1 and O_2

Severely depressed right heart function: right ventricular ejection fraction estimated at $<10\%$

Intractable ventricular tachycardia: ventricular tachycardia that is unresponsive to all conventional medical treatment

Severe hepatic disease: total bilirubin values > 10 mg% or biopsy-proven liver cirrhosis

Cerebral vascular disease: previous stroke with unresolved carotid bruit

History of stroke; TIAs or NIVs consistent with high-grade stenosis

Carotid arteriogram demonstrating ulcerated plaque or high-grade stenosis

Severe gastrointestinal malabsorption steatorrhea or need for pancreatic enzyme replacement

Active systemic infection: positive blood culture with clinical evidence of sepsis unresponsive to culture specific antibiotics within 72 hr before surgery

Severe blood dyscrasia; PT > 16.0; PTT > 45.0, platelet count $< 50,000$; clinical history of bleeding (values obtained off anticoagulation)

Cancer; unresolved malignancy

Diffuse, severe peripheral vascular disease; presence of limb or chest pain with absent distal pulses

Refractory anuria: urine output 20 cc/hr in the presence of adequate renal perfusion

BUN > 100 mg%

Creatinine > 5.0 mg%

Positive HIV test

Long-term high-dose steroid treatment; continuous use of steroids for a period of 6 months or more with a dose 10 mg/day

Prolonged (60 minutes) unsuccessful attempts to resuscitate the fibrillating heart

---

cranking the pump. Once the air has been removed, the LVAD is set to operate in the fixed-rate mode at 20 beats/min. When the surgeon is confident that the pump is receiving an adequate amount of blood from the left ventricle, cardiopulmonary bypass flows are gradually decreased, while the HeartMate pump rate and thus stroke volume are increased. After insertion of a mediastinal tube and chest tubes, the abdomen and chest are closed.

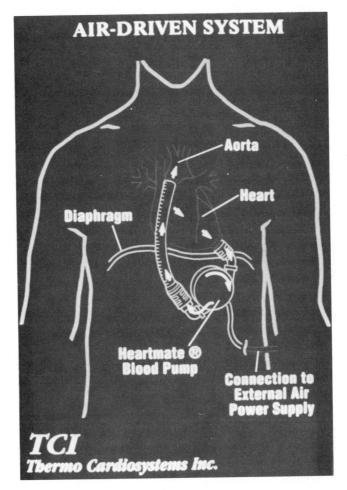

Fig. 9-5. Schematic of air-driven system. (Courtesy Thermo Cardiosystems, Inc., Woburn, Mass.)

POTENTIAL COMPLICATIONS

Patients are monitored for complications that might occur during LVAD support. These include infection, thromboemboli, bleeding, hemolysis, multiorgan failure, and device failure. Clinical experience, however, has shown the complications related to HeartMate support to be minimal. The biological lining that forms on the blood-contacting surfaces reduces the risk of thromboemboli and allows minimal anticoagulative therapy. Patients are generally maintained on aspirin and dipyridamole alone. The pulsatile flow created by the device does not cause undue trauma to the red blood cells, as evidenced by plasma free hemoglobin measurements within normal ranges in patients who are supported for more than 2 weeks. Despite implantation of the device, the risk of infections has been low. Most have occurred at the driveline site and have resolved after appropriate treatment. Finally, in our experience, no instances of mechanical failure have occurred.

During device support, patients are also monitored for preexisting conditions that could cause complications. End-organ function is continually assessed to determine the effectiveness of support. When support is instituted early, renal and hepatic function usually improve.

ANTICOAGULATION

Anticoagulative therapy is initiated after postoperative bleeding has been controlled. Low molecular weight dextran is infused at 10 ml/hr until patients are able to tolerate a regular diet, usually on postoperative day 7. At that time, aspirin (80 mg/day) and dipyridamole (75 mg, 3 times per day) are administered and continued through the remainder of LVAD support.

MORBIDITY AND MORTALITY

At present 14 sites are approved to use the HeartMate as a bridge to transplantation. A total of 43 patients have been supported by the device for durations of 1 day to 324 days, with the cumulative support time being 7.5 years. Mortality and morbidity have been low in patients receiving HeartMate support for more than 14 days. Hepatic and renal function are usually normalized after 30 days of support. The chief causes of death have been irreversible end-organ dysfunction and right heart failure requiring mechanical circulatory support. Right heart failure that does not require mechanical support can usually be reversed within 48 hours by treating the patient with pharmacological and ventilatory support.

Device-related complications have been minimal. Driveline infections have been found at the site of externalization, but they respond well to antibiotic therapy and have not altered patient outcomes. To date only one thromboembolic event has been documented and was attributed to a mechanial aortic valve, not the LVAD.

PATIENT TRANSPORT

The decision to transfer a patient from the critical care unit to the transplantation unit depends on numerous factors. The patient must be hemodynamically stable, must have adequate pulmonary function without mechanical ventilator support, must have resumed a regular diet, and must be ambulatory. As investigators gain confidence with the HeartMate, patients are being transferred from the critical care unit much earlier, usually within 7 to 10 days.

DATA COLLECTION

Clinical protocol requires documenting the patient's status before insertion, at insertion, during support, at transplant, and at specified intervals up to 1 year after transplant. Initially, hemodynamic status and pump parameters are recorded at 4-hour intervals and then once daily after the first week of support. Routine laboratory studies are conducted to assess hematology, coagulation, and blood chemistry. Arterial blood gases are also measured on a routine basis. Data are maintained in an individual patient study file and forwarded to the sponsor, as indicated in the investigational protocol.

PATIENT MANAGEMENT AND PSYCHOSOCIAL SUPPORT

A collaborative effort among nurses, cardiologists, surgeons, research personnel, physical therapists, dieticians, and the sponsor is necessary to ensure a positive outcome for patients receiving mechanical circulatory support with an investigational device. In addition to the surgical team, the research team must be present at the implant operation to set up the equipment, to monitor the device at initiation of support, and to document the procedure. Adequate pump flow depends on maintaining an adequate supply of blood to the pump. Inadequate volume status or the inability to circulate blood through the pulmonary circuit can decrease the amount of blood delivered to the pump. Inotropic support may be necessary to improve right ventricular function; sodium nitroprusside is indicated to decrease systemic vascular resistance; low doses of dopamine are indicated to improve renal function. Coagulopathies are a frequent problem in patients with end-stage cardiac disease. These conditions need to be identified and treated promptly. After hemodynamic stabilization is achieved, usually within 48 hours of implant, the patient is weaned from mechanical ventilator support. To address potential infections at the driveline site, the area is cleaned three times daily; at each time a thin film of 1% silver sulfadiazine is applied to the site. Table 9-1 contains primary nursing diagnoses and expected outcomes for patients on HeartMate support.

Early mobilization and adequate nutritional status are primary therapeutic objectives to prevent postoperative complications and to begin rehabilitation of the patient.[7] Rehabilitation actively begins when the patient is transferred from the critical care unit to a hospital room. Use of the HeartMate LVAD in bridge-to-cardiac transplantation procedures has afforded these patients an opportunity to dramatically improve their health status. Patients receiving extended support ($>$30 days) have been in New York Heart Association functional class I at the time of transplant.

After transfer to the transplant floor, these patients are encouraged to become increasingly independent in self-care and regular daily activities. Some have administered their own medications and changed their own dressings. Nursing goals during this period are aimed at improving the overall physical and mental status of the patients so that they are in optimal condition for cardiac transplantation. Rehabilitation programs include walking and riding stationary bicycles to improve muscle strength. Some patients have participated in more rigorous physical activities such as lifting weights and walking on an incline treadmill.

Psychosocial support is provided not only by the medical team, but also by family members and other patients. During LVAD support, patients are encouraged to attend support groups for transplant candidates. Their mental outlook is also improved by edu-

Table 9-1. Nursing care plan for patients on Heartmate support

Nursing diagnosis	Nursing interventions	Outcome
Alteration in cardiac output, decreased Related to bleeding	Monitor hemoglobin, hematocrit, and coagulation studies Assess blood loss every hour Administer blood products as ordered Be aware of blood component availability Monitor pump flow every hour and PRN	Controlled blood loss with continuing decreased pump flow > 3.5 L/min
Related to hypothermia	Use warming blankets as ordered	Temperature 98°-100°F
Related to increased pulmonary vascular resistance	Monitor central venous pressure (CVP) and pulmonary artery pressures Administer pulmonary vascular dilators as ordered	PVR decreased
Alteration in fluid volume deficit related to volume overload, retention, or shifts	Monitor volume status every hour Assess for edema Monitor CVP every hour	No edema Urine output > 20 cc/hr CVP 5-12 PCWP 12-16
Impaired gas exchange related to O_2 supply, blood flow, or alveolar capillary membrane changes	Assess breath sounds every hour and PRN Monitor chest x-ray and ABGs Sedate patient as ordered to decrease work of breathing O_2 consumption (do not overly sedate)	Breath sounds clear and equal bilaterally PO_2 > 80 pH 7.35-7.45 Svo_2 > 60%
High risk for infection related to surgical procedure, invasive lines, and preoperative status	Assess incision lines for redness, tenderness, or drainage Notify physician if invasive lines need to be changed or discontinued Monitor temperature every 4 hours and PRN Monitor WBCs Culture central line catheters when discontinued	Infection-free
Alteration in nutrition decreased related to preoperative status and size of implanted pump	Monitor oral intake accurately Encourage small, frequent, high caloric feedings Assess nutrition (dietician) Instruct patient and family regarding diet	Adequate nutritional intake
Mobility impaired, related to preimplant physical status and surgical pain	Initiate program of progressive mobilization (physical therapy) Educate patient	Increased mobilization and tolerance for physical activity

cating them about the LVAD. Patients and their families are taught how the LVAD works and what to do if the system fails. The more confidence the patient has in the device and in the hospital personnel, the more the patient is able to attain physical and psychological well-being.

A major challenge in caring for the HeartMate patients is alleviating their boredom. Restrictions of assist device support include not being able to leave the nursing unit unattended, which has necessitated creative alternatives to satisfy patients' need for independence. Allowing them to eat their meals in the hospital cafeteria provides time for socialization. Walking outside the hospital has also proved beneficial, as has participation in support group activities. Patients on HeartMate support are frequently the most willing to visit other patients or families within the hospital.

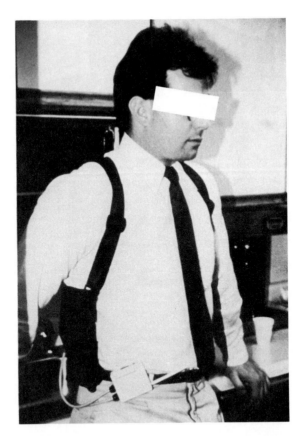

Fig. 9-6. Next generation of the HeartMate. (Courtesy Thermo Cardiosystems Inc., Woburn, Mass.)

DEVICE REMOVAL

The pump is removed at the time of transplantation. Cardiopulmonary bypass is instituted, and cardiac arrest is induced with cardioplegic solution. A femoral artery is cannulated for arterial return, which facilitates placing the cross-clamp on the aorta. The superior and inferior venae cavae are cannulated for venous return. After pump support has been discontinued, the outlet and inlet conduits are removed, the pneumatic drive tube is transected and removed, and the pump is dissected free. Orthotopic or heterotopic heart transplantation is then performed using standard methods. For a heterotopic transplant, however, the apex of the native heart must be repaired before the donor heart is placed.

CONCLUSION

The waiting period for patients requiring heart transplantation has increased because of a lack of donor organs. Implantation of the HeartMate allows the patient to regain a measure of good health during this time. Our experience has also shown the potential for providing long-term, mechanical circulatory support with a left ventricular assist device. These results are encouraging given that 30% to 40% of transplant candidates die while awaiting transplantation.[8]

Recent clinical trials of the electric HeartMate device have been initiated. This system is transcutaneously powered by two gel-cell, lead-acid batteries (Fig. 9-6). Although the system is not totally implantable, it leaves the patient untethered and allows a greater degree of mobility than can be achieved with any other device currently in use.

REFERENCES

1. Frazier OH, Duncan JM, Radovancevic B et al: Successful bridge to cardiac transplantation using a new left ventricular assist device, *J Heart Lung Transplant* (in press).
2. Norman JC, Brook MI, Cooley DA et al: Total support of the circulation of a patient with postcardiotomy stone-heart syndrome by a partial artificial heart (ALVAD) for 5 days followed by heart and kidney transplantation, *Lancet* 1:1125, 1978.
3. Dasse K, Chipman SD, Sherman CN et al: Clinical experience with textured blood contacting surfaces in ventricular assist devices, *Trans ASAIO* 19:418, 1987.
4. Nakatani T, Frazier OH, McGee MG et al: Extended support prior to cardiac transplant using a left ventricular assist device with textured blood contacting surfaces, presented at the Seventh World Congress of the International Society for Artificial Organs, Sapporo, Japan, October 1989.
5. *HeartMate left ventricular assist drive console operating manual,* Woburn, Mass., 1990, Thermo Cardiosystems Inc.
6. Frazier OH, Radovancevic B: Ventricular assist devices, *Cardiac Surgery: State of the Art Reviews* 4:335, 1990.
7. Abou-Awdi NL: Thermo Cardiosystems left ventricular assist device as a bridge to cardiac transplant, *AACN Clinical Issues Critical Care Nursing* 2:545, 1991.
8. UNOS Registry, 1990 Statistics, Richmond, Virginia, United States Department of Health and Human Services, Division of Transplantation, Research and Policy Department.

CHAPTER 10

ABIOMED BVS 5000 assist device

John F. Dixon, Charlotte D. Farris, and G. Kimble Jett

INTRODUCTION

Several different types of ventricular assist devices are currently available to provide temporary or long-term mechanical support. Centrifugal pumps provide nonpulsatile flow, are inexpensive, and require constant attention. Pneumatic pulsatile pumps provide pulsatile flow, are expensive, and are under strict Food and Drug Administration regulatory control.[1] Key design goals are to develop a system that is simple, reliable, and cost-effective. ABIOMED BVS 5000 combines advantages of other devices through lower cost, pulsatile flow, and minimal operator involvement.

THEORY OF OPERATION

ABIOMED BVS 5000 is an external pulsatile assist device designed for short-term univentricular or biventricular cardiac support (less than 2 weeks). It is composed of three parts: (1) transthoracic cannulas, (2) disposable external blood pumps, and (3) a microprocessor-controlled pneumatic drive console (Fig. 10-1). The physician inserts transthoracic cannulae into the right atrium and pulmonary artery for right support and left atrium and ascending aorta for left support. Inflow cannulae are wire reinforced polyvinyl chloride, size 46 French, and 40 cm long. Outflow cannulae are similar except that a precoated 14 mm Dacron graft is attached to the end, allowing anastomosis to the great vessel (pulmonary artery or aorta). Exterior surfaces incorporate a Dacron velour sleeve at the skin interface. Blood drains from the atria by gravity into two-chambered blood pumps externally located by the bedside. This passive filling avoids native atrial collapse, inflow cannula suction of air, and/or hemolysis.

Each single-use blood pump houses two Angioflex atrial and ventricular polyurethane bladders. These simulate native heart function, acting as a bypass for ventricular filling. Trileaflet valves are positioned between ventricular and atrial bladders, and between ventricular bladder and outflow cannula, thereby ensuring unidirectional blood flow. A compressed air driveline connects the console with the blood pump's ventricular chamber. Compressed air enters the blood pump ventricular chamber during

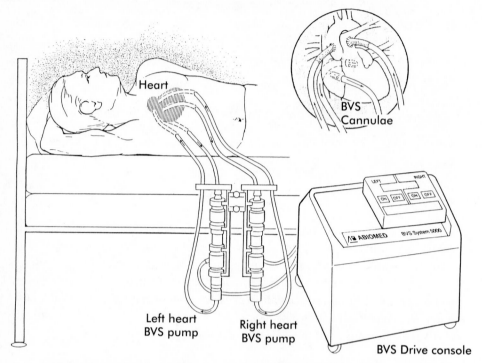

Fig. 10-1. ABIOMED BVS 5000. (Courtesy ABIOMED, Inc., Danvers, Mass.)

pump systole, causing bladder collapse, thus returning its blood volume to the patient. During diastole, air vents through the console to the atmosphere, allowing ventricular bladder filling. A single blood pump supports one side of the heart (Fig. 10-2).

Atrial bladders operate in a fill to empty mode. Inadequate atrial filling occurs if the external blood pump position is too high; prolonged filling may occur if the blood pump is positioned too low. Nurses visually inspect atrial filling, adjusting pump height if needed. Adequate hydration is mandatory for optimal pump flows. Filling pressures are checked before any height changes are made. Typical height is approximately 25 cm below the patient's atria. In some biventricular cases, it is necessary to adjust right and left blood pump heights independently. The system takes 2 minutes to equilibrate after each height change.

The BVS console is an automated, self-regulating, pulsatile support device controlled by a microprocessor. It automatically adjusts external blood pump beat rate and systolic/diastolic ratio. The BVS strives for an optimum stroke volume of 82 ml, pumping up to approximately 5 L/min if patient hydration is adequate. The microprocessor makes adjustments based on external system compressed air flow. The console senses bladder filling and returns blood to the patient whenever the ventricular chamber is full.

BVS 5000 Blood pump

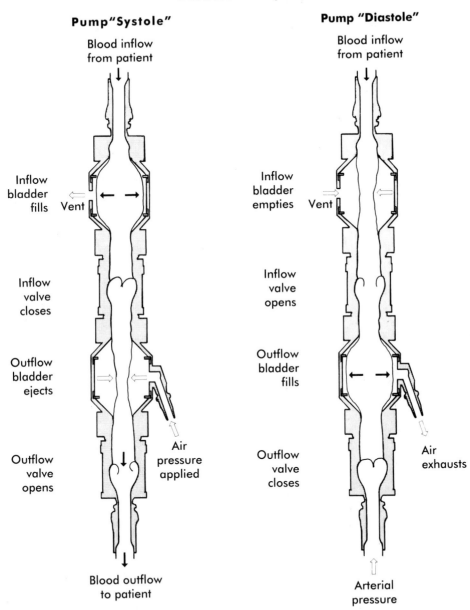

Fig. 10-2. External blood pump systole and diastole phase (cross-section). (Courtesy ABIOMED, Inc., Danvers, Mass.)

The BVS 5000 pumps independently of the heart, which simplifies its operation and minimizes the need for operator intervention. A single BVS console can operate and adjust one or two blood pumps. When using biventricular support, the console controls right and left blood pumps independently.

Care must be taken to ensure that right-sided flow does not exceed left-sided flow and thereby overload the pulmonary circulation with a resultant pulmonary edema. This can be controlled by using the wean control to reduce right-sided flow. An alphanumeric display shows external blood pump beat rate and L/min flow and alarm messages. Operator intervention is minimal because the console makes most necessary adjustments. Normal operation requires only turning on the console after connecting primed blood pumps. The only other control is for weaning, allowing flow rate reduction. This simplicity is an advantage compared with other devices that may require a perfusionist or continual adjustment and timing by a nurse.

PATIENT SELECTION

Currently, BVS research selection criteria involve two groups: postcardiotomy ventricular dysfunction patients and postacute myocardial infarction patients with cardiogenic shock. Cardiac surgical patients may fail to separate from cardiopulmonary bypass or develop postoperative cardiogenic shock. In both groups, patients must be refractory to standard pharmacological and mechanical interventions, including intraaortic balloon counterpulsation.

Patients excluded from this study include those with preexisting disease states (e.g., metastatic cancer, severe pulmonary disease), neurological compromise, and prolonged unsuccessful resuscitative measures.

INSERTION TECHNIQUES

Cannula insertion for the ABIOMED BVS 5000 is important for a successful intraoperative and postoperative result. Each cannula must be inserted in a fashion that allows unimpeded device filling and does not obstruct venous drainage. A small left atrium presents great difficulty for cannula insertion in the interatrial groove and may impair venous drainage from the superior vena cava. A left atrial dome approach between the superior vena cava and aorta, in this circumstance, has allowed easier cannula insertion and is less likely to impair vena caval drainage. Right atrial cannulation is best performed in the midatrial wall, with the cannula tip directed toward the inferior vena cava or tricuspid valve. Each cannula must be secured to the atrium to prevent inadvertent removal and subsequent air emboli. A double pledgetted purse-string suture with tourniquets applied over the sutures has been effective for cannula securing and for allowing easy removal once the patient is weaned from support. Cannula removal does not require cardiopulmonary bypass. Volume loading of the atrium being cannulated is important to prevent intracardiac introduction of air. The atrial cannula should be under fluid during initiation of ventricular support to prevent introduction of air into the inflow cannula. In addition, external blood pumps should be positioned level with the patient during initiation of support to prevent generation of negative atrial pressures. Attention to details of cannulation techniques will help ensure successful ventricular support.

POTENTIAL COMPLICATIONS

Complications may occur on insertion, during support, during removal, or after removal. These may be patient-related, device-related, or unknown. Patients are carefully assessed for embolic events. Early Jarvik devices had a high incidence of thromboemboli caused by a crevice at the atrial connector.[2] Anticoagulation minimizes this as does the BVS blood pump's smooth surface lining design and unique pump-cannula connectors designed to minimize such crevices.

Infection is a potential risk for patients with assist devices.[3] Not only are supported patients immunosuppressed,[4] but internally implanted pumps create a large dead space filled with a prosthetic device providing a good culture medium.[5,6] BVS patients are at an advantage compared with some patients using other devices because subcostal cannula externalization allows chest closure and external pump location. Sterile technique is closely followed, with all dressings and invasive lines being changed every 3 days. Postinsertion patients receive antibiotics for 72 hours minimum.

Other potential complications include renal failure, hemolysis, bleeding, reoperation, respiratory failure, blood pump failure, or console failure. In our experience, hemolysis has not been a problem with plasma free hemoglobin levels averaging < 10 mg/dl and with no appreciable decrease in platelets. Bleeding requiring reoperation has occurred in only one patient immediately postoperatively.

In our experience there has been no mechanical failure by any blood pump or console to date.

ANTICOAGULATION

Anticoagulation is begun for all patients during pump support to prevent pump system clot formation. The patient is anticoagulated only after postoperative hemostasis is obtained. All postcardiotomy patients have their heparin reversed with protamine sulfate in the operating room, and anticoagulation begins later postoperatively after hemostasis. Low dose heparin, dextran, or a combination of these provides patient anticoagulation. Activated clotting times (ACT) are maintained at 1.5 times control. These are measured using a bedside device. A maintenance infusion with periodic boluses based on ACT typically accomplishes this. During weaning or pump flow decreases, anticoagulation is increased to approximately twice baseline.

MORBIDITY AND MORTALITY

Baylor University Medical Center has had a very favorable experience with the ABIOMED BVS 5000. Results in our initial seven patients were outstanding. Complications were very low and usually patient-related. Only one patient bled excessively after device insertion, requiring reoperation. No thrombus was seen in these devices after explantation and there were no device-related neurological events or thromboembolism. Of our patients, 71% were weaned or transplanted. Three of these patients (43%) have survived and were discharged to home, comparing favorably with the National Registry survival rate of 23%.[7]

PATIENT TRANSPORT

During transport, battery power maintains console function for 1 hour when fully charged. External blood pumps remain on an intravenous pole mount or are placed on a bed mount. Care should be taken to avoid damage to the compressed air lines from the console to the blood pumps.

WEANING FROM THE DEVICE

The operator sets the weaning control from full flow to 0.5 L/min in 0.1 L/min increments. The BVS console then reduces flow by reducing pumping rate. To signal weaning mode, the console periodically beeps. An uninterrupted audible alarm sounds if flows go below 0.5 L/min. Assessments focus on maintenance of hemodynamic stability during weaning. Anticoagulation is increased during weaning. Right side weaning precedes left by approximately 30 minutes to reduce pulmonary strain in biventricular support cases.

After removal, external blood pumps and cannulae are carefully rinsed for return to the company. They are then photographed and samples are scanned, using an electron microscope.

DATA COLLECTION AND DOCUMENTATION

Because of classification as an investigational device, BVS 5000 data collection follows specific protocols. Vital signs (arterial pressures, filling pressures, blood pump flow and rate, intake and output) and laboratory tests (hematology, coagulation, blood chemistry, urinalysis, arterial blood gases) are recorded immediately before insertion, while on support, and 48 hours after removal. For patients on right heart support, thermodilution cardiac output (CO) is of questionable value as injectate may flow through the external blood pump. Data are recorded on designated forms.

ECG strips with arterial pressure tracings are obtained every 8 hours. The pump superimposes a pulsatile waveform on the patient's native arterial pressure tracing. This

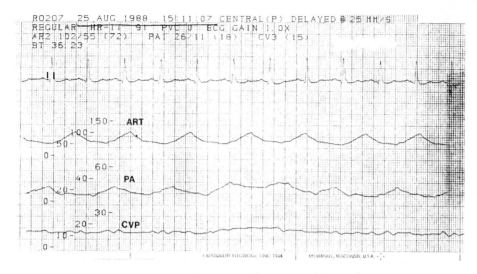

Fig. 10-3. Postinsertion pump effect on arterial waveform.

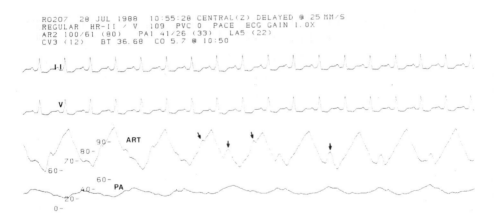

Fig. 10-4. Native recovery *(arrows)* interspersed with pump effects.

resembles a pyramid or upside down "V." Immediately after insertion, arterial tracings are predominantly pump artifact (Fig. 10-3). As the heart recovers, native contribution intersperses with pump waveforms (Fig. 10-4).

PATIENT/FAMILY PSYCHOSOCIAL ISSUES

Based on current patient selection criteria, this device provides a chance for a patient who is unresponsive to conventional pharmacological and intraaortic balloon pumping (IABP) therapies. As such, patient and family may view the device as the only option other than certain death. Because BVS support is investigational, questions may arise regarding quality of life issues and eventual outcomes. The initial family visit after insertion can be upsetting. An interdisciplinary approach involving the nurse, chaplain, and social worker aids the patient and family in creating a support network. Volunteers and guest relations representatives also are a valuable support resource. As the patient improves and is extubated, family anxieties tend to subside. In cases of failure to wean, the patient and/or a surrogate representative may decide between proposed options of cardiac transplantation or, if the patient is not a transplant candidate, withdrawing of BVS support and accepting the eventual outcome.

NURSING MANAGEMENT/CARE PLAN

Nurses are responsible for BVS management. This decreases demands on numbers of personnel required and eliminates perfusionist fees for the patient. Because the console is self-adjusting and operator intervention is minimal, this device is a minor part of total patient care.

Cardiac arrest and console failure are emergency situations requiring immediate intervention. During cardiac arrest, pump flows maximize, ensuring hemodynamic stability. Biventricular support patients in ventricular fibrillation may be awake with a 90 mm Hg arterial systolic pressure (Fig. 10-5). Thus no external cardiac compressions that could potentially cause cardiac damage because of in situ cannulas are needed. Dysrhythmias are treated using standard pharmacological measures, cardioversion, or

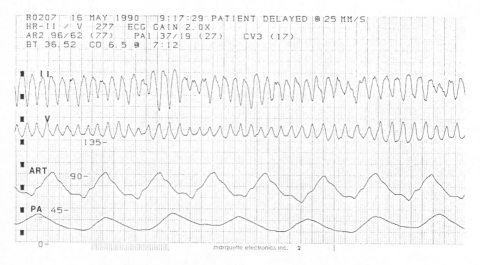

Fig. 10-5. Pump support during ventricular fibrillation.

########## ABIOMED BVS 5000 SYSTEM NURSING PROTOCOL ##########

Protocol Vitals *-Required:* BP (systolic, diastolic, mean), heart rate & rhythm, CVP/RAP, PAS, PAD, PAM, PAW/LAP, CO, CI, PVR, SVR, Pump Flow and Rate (for right and left sides)
-Pre-Insertion: immediately prior to insertion in O.R.
-Post-Insertion: immediately after BVS-on, then 4, 8, 16, and 24 hours after BVS-on
-On-Going: minimum q8h from 24 hours after BVS-on
-Post-Removal: immediately after BVS-off, then 8, 16, 24, 32, 40, and 48 hours after BVS-off
-also note any anticoagulants given (medication, dose, ACT), transfusions, and chest drainage as data becomes available

Protocol Labs *-Required:* PT, PTT, Fibrin Split Products, Fibrinogen, CBC, Platelet Count, Plasma Free Hemoglobin, SMA20, ABG, Urinalysis, and Anti-Thrombin III
-Pre-Insertion: send labs immediately prior to insertion in O.R.
-Post-Insertion: 12 hours after BVS-on, and then 24 hours after BVS-on
-On-Going: q24h from 24 hours after BVS-on
-Post-Removal: 12, 24, and 48 hours after BVS-off

Pre-Insertion Tasks and Assessments
-obtain Abiomed Data Log from central nurses' station cabinet
-send data collection forms to O.R. for pre-BVS and BVS-on (intraop) recordings
-arrange for private room if possible
-obtain insulating blanket to wrap cannulae, sheepskin for beneath cannulae, and eggcrate for bed
-have volume expanders (e.g., salt poor albumin, hetastarch, plasmanate) readily available
-obtain pulse oximeter and oximetric computer

Post-Insertion Assessments
-per standards of care for cardiac surgery
-vitals per Protocol Vitals
-labs per Protocol Labs

On-Going Assessments and Tasks
-per standards of care for cardiac surgery
-vitals per Protocol Vitals
-labs per Protocol Labs
-ECG rhythm strip *with* arterial pressure tracing q8h
-recalibrate SVO2 q24h
-dressing condition qshift
-dressing change q24h using strict sterile technique
-Activated Clotting Times (ACT) q1h or per physician order
-heparin sliding scale (plus possible dextran supplement) based on ACT per physician orders
-weigh patient only with a specific physician order
-tissue perfusion (skin color, temperature, capillary refill, peripheral pulses, edema, neuro status, urine output, pulmonary status)

Continued

_____ **ABIOMED BVS 5000 SYSTEM NURSING PROTOCOL—cont'd** _____

	-patient/family support and teaching -nutritional needs (enteral feeding, hyperalimentation, dietician consult) -keep pump plugged into electrical outlet at all times -do not lean or place any objects on control panel of pump -a brief extension of 1 beat q2minutes is normal (pump is recalibrating itself) -*atrial* bladder filling and emptying (*atrial* bladders should fill, hit walls of blood pumps, and immediately empty; position too high = inadequate filling, position too low = inadequate emptying) -after adjusting blood pump height, observe atrial bladder (upper chamber) filling for 2 minutes before adjusting again (if atrial bladder still does not adequately fill, patient may need volume) -instability of beat rate of pump may indicate blood pump placement incorrect in relation to patient -pump is ***never*** to be put on standby by anyone except by primary research physician
Weaning	-increase anticoagulation prior to commencement of weaning per physician order (typically ACT > 300 seconds) -assess hemodynamics 1 hour after each flow reduction -notify physician for decreasing arterial pressures, increasing LAP, or CI < 2.0 -if weaning from *biventricular* support, carefully assess for pulmonary intolerance (right pump weaning is begun 30 minutes prior to left pump to protect lungs) -pump periodically beeps to indicate the weaning mode is operational
Removal Equipment	-formaldehyde 1 gallon (obtained from Pathology Department, 5 Y-Wing) -removal kit (provided by physician)
Post-Removal Assessments and Tasks	-per standards of care for cardiac surgery -vitals per Protocol Vitals -labs per Protocol Labs -ECG rhythm strip *with* arterial pressure tracing q8h -signs and symptoms of bleeding -deterioration of hemodynamic status
Reportable Conditions to Physician	-alteration in neuro status -deterioration of vital signs and/or filling pressures -decreasing or no urinary output -ACT outside of prescribed parameters in spite of heparin/dextran -dysrhythmias refractory to treatment -signs and symptoms of bleeding -deterioration of oxygen status -flows < 2 L/min when not in weaning mode in spite of adjusting pump heights -intolerance to pump weaning [see Weaning]

——— **ABIOMED BVS 5000 SYSTEM NURSING PROTOCOL—cont'd** ———

Emergency Situations
-cardiac arrest (1-treat chemically and/or electrically per ACLS Standards, 2-notify physician) **[Do not perform CPR or deliver a precordial blow.]**
-console computer failure [see System Alarms-Emergency System On] (1-change out console, 2-notify O.R. Biomedical Services STAT, 3-notify physician)
-complete console failure (1-turn off console, 2-open back door of pump, 3-swing lever up to horizontal position, 4-pull out foot-plate by squeezing pedal closed, 5-completely depress the foot-plate and allow it to fully return to its original position, continue doing this until backup console is ready, 6-power up back-up console, 7-allow back-up console to run self-test, 8-initiate pumping on back-up console, 9-transfer drive lines from failed console to back-up console, 10-notify O.R. Biomedical Services STAT, 11-notify physician)

System Alarms Messages
-*Low Flow:* ($<$ 2 L/min) - check for obstruction of blood lines, blood pump too high relative to atrium, or hypovolemia
-*Low Pressure/Low Flow* - check for disconnection or leak in air line
-*High Pressure/Low Flow* - check for air line or blood pump lines kinked or occluded
-*Emergency System On* - microprocessor system failure, obtain back-up console
-*Battery On Low* - low batteries, less than 10 minutes of operation left, plug machine in or obtain back-up console (pump periodically emits a loud 4-beep signal as a reminder)
-*Battery Charging* - $<$ 80% capacity, message will disappear when fully charged
-*Battery On* - battery in use (pump periodically emits a 2 beep signal as a reminder)

Forms Used for Documentation
-*Nursing Assessment Checklist:* total systems assessment qshift
-*Vital Signs Flowsheet:* Page 1 - Vitals
-*Vital Signs Flowsheet:* Page 2 - Intake & Output, ACTs
-*Vital Signs Flowsheet:* Page 3 - Equipment: Abiomed Pump, sheepskin, eggcrate; Labs drawn
-*Nurses' Progress Notes:* notification of physician for problems [see Reportable Conditions], what problem, intervention, and response; patient/family teaching
-*Abiomed Data Log*

defibrillation. Preference is to correct dysrhythmias avoiding stasis of blood in the native heart and possible thrombus formation, but if the dysrhythmias are refractory, the pump will maintain adequate hemodynamics.

Three backup mechanisms exist for console failure. If AC power is lost, battery power automatically engages. An independent electronic system maintains uninterrupted fixed rate pumping if the microprocessor system fails. Operation by a foot-operated mechanical pump allows continued support for complete console failure while a backup console is readied. A backup console will automatically make adjustments regarding external blood pump beat rate and systolic/diastolic ratio after connection.

Nurses use the cardiac surgery care plan coupled with a nursing protocol[8] for this device (see box on pp. 137-139). The care plan is based on a nursing diagnosis format, allowing for individualization of interventions and outcomes. The nursing protocol is a single page, printed front and back, and addresses device specific issues: protocol vitals, protocol labs, preinsertion tasks and assessments, postinsertion assessments, ongoing assessments and tasks, weaning, removal equipment, postremoval assessments and tasks, conditions reportable to the physician, emergency situations, system alarms/messages, and forms used for documentation.

Because this device is preload dependent, maintenance of adequate hydration is pivotal. The greatest challenge usually appears immediately postoperatively. Chest drainage coupled with voluminous urine output secondary to increased renal perfusion can create a rapid fluid deficit. Bolus therapy with volume expanders (e.g., salt poor albumin, hetastarch, plasma protein fraction) are effective in maintaining adequate filling pressures. Anticoagulation also compounds risk for bleeding postoperatively, creating another potential volume loss.

Pulmonary vascular resistance (PVR) and systemic vascular resistance (SVR) elevations can potentially impede flow. Prostaglandin E1 (PGE1) infusion titrated through a jugular route is effective in controlling PVR.[9] To counteract possible peripheral vasodilatory effects of PGE1 and maintain a normal SVR, norepinephrine is infused through a left atrial line.

Development of hypoxia causes increases in PVR.[10] Arterial blood gases, saturation of arterial oxygen (Sao_2), and saturation of venous oxygen (Svo_2) are monitored and maintained within normal limits. Svo_2 decreases immediately postoperatively are often related to shivering and are effectively treated with pancuronium bromide and morphine sulfate.

Hypothermia contributes to increases in SVR.[11] Chest closure and the external blood pumps themselves account for minimal heat loss. The greatest source is the connecting tubing between patient and pump. Wrapping these with silver insulating blankets is effective in controlling this heat loss and maintenance of patient normothermia. External heating sources are not applied to the tubes or blood pumps because of possible thrombus formation and/or blood protein denaturation.

The abbreviated length of connecting tubing limits patient mobility and increases risk for potential pressure areas. Patients are on standard beds compared with open chest cases that return to the CVICU on an operating room table. Standard beds are an advantage, allowing repositioning in bed from side-to-side and changes in head elevation. The connecting tubing weight also can cause skin breakdown on the patient's abdomen. A sheepskin pad, woolside down, between the tubings and patient prevents this.

APPLICATION OF RESEARCH FINDINGS TO CLINICAL PRACTICE

Much has been learned from the initial clinical experiences with the BVS 5000. Right-sided pump flow should never exceed left-sided pump flow. If right-sided pump flow exceeds left sided, the pulmonary circulation can be overloaded leading to pulmonary congestion/edema. The wean control can be used to decrease right-sided flow in this instance. Native left output exceeds right pump output due to bronchial blood flow.

Patients on support can be extubated and have limited mobility. We have permitted patients on support to dangle their feet, but have yet to allow them out of bed. The upright position allows adequate drainage and function of the device. Only one nurse is required to care for the supported patient and manage the device.

CASE STUDY

A 33-year-old man went to his personal physician with complaints of low-grade fever, malaise, cough, and dyspnea and was placed on antibiotics. The next day he continued to experience mild dyspnea that worsened over the next 24 hours. He went to an emergency department in severe dyspnea and was diagnosed with fulminant pulmonary edema. He was intubated and placed on inotropic support. Continued deterioration (systolic BP 70s to 90s mm Hg, CO 2.8 to 3.4 L/min, oliguria) required transfer to another facility for intraaortic balloon therapy that day. The next day he was transferred to our CVICU for consideration for mechanical assistance or possible cardiac transplantation. Cardiac catheterization revealed PAW 35, CO 2.8 to 3.0 L/min, poor global left ventricular function, 5% ejection fraction, and normal coronary arteries. Endomyocardial biopsy showed lymphocytic infiltration consistent with myocarditis-like rejection seen in cardiac transplant patients. The patient was put on biventricular BVS support. Immunosuppressive therapy was discussed, but steroids because of BVS insertion and cyclosporin because of oliguria were contraindicated. It was decided to administer OKT3, a monoclonal antibody, 5 mg IVP for 8 days. After 5 days a transesophageal echo revealed a left ventricular ejection fraction of 25% to 30%. Repeat biopsy showed resolving lymphocytic infiltration with a predominantly intact myocardium.

By 8 days, his ejection fraction was 60%, weaning was accomplished, and the devices

Table 10-1.   ABIOMED BVS 5000 case study parameters

Parameter	Admission	Postinsertion (6° later)	Postremoval
BP	84/57	99/60	168/59
MAP	71	82	80
Rhythm	Complete heart block	Complete heart block	Sinus tachycardia
RR	20 (vent)	10 (vent)	10 (vent)
CVP	23	16	12
PAW	22	—	10
PAS/PAD	45/25	—	31/14
CO	2.8	6.0	6.9
CI	1.5	2.3	3.8
SVR	1427	866	741
Svo_2		—	73%
IABP	1:1 ratio	Removed	—
BUN	63	—	18
Creatinine	2.3	—	0.9
SGOT	720	—	16
SGPT	695	—	20
LDH	1140	—	217
CPK	330	—	61
Dopamine	17.5 μg/kg/min	3 μg/kg/min	—
Dobutamine	Titrating	Discontinued	—
Norepinephrine	Titrating	Discontinued	—

were removed (Table 10-1). The patient was discharged 1 week later. A year later a biopsy showed normal myocardium without interstitial scarring. He remains asymptomatic.

CONCLUSION

ABIOMED is currently applying for premarket approval for the BVS 5000 with the Food and Drug Administration. Such approval would allow access to the device by many institutions that would benefit many patients. This device is intended for temporary support. ABIOMED is also developing a total artificial heart to be used for permanent support.

REFERENCES

1. Smith RG, Cleavinger M: Current perspectives on the use of circulatory assist devices, *AACN Clinical Issues* 2:488, 1991.
2. Olsen DB, Unger F, Oster H et al: Thrombus generation within the artificial heart, *J Thorac Cardiovasc Surg* 70:248, 1975.
3. Hsu U, Griffith B, Dowling R et al: Infections in mortally ill cardiac transplant recipients, *J Thorac Cardiovasc Surg* 98:506, 1989.
4. Stelzer CT, Ward RA, Wellhousen SR et al: Alterations in select immunologic parameters following total artificial heart implantation, *Artif Organs* 11:52, 1987.

5. Gristina AG, Dubbins JJ, Giammora B et al: Biomaterial-centered sepsis and the total artificial heart: microbial adhesion vs. tissue integration, *JAMA* 259:870, 1988.
6. Griffith BP, Kormos RL, Hardesty RL et al: The artificial heart: infection-related morbidity and its effect on transplantation, *Ann Thorac Surg* 45:409, 1988.
7. Pae WE Jr: Temporary ventricular support: current indications and results, *ASAIO Trans* 33:4, 1987.
8. ABIOMED BVS 5000 nursing protocol, Dallas, Baylor University Medical Center.
9. D'Ambra M, LaRaia P, Philbin D et al: Prostaglandin E1: a new therapy for refractory right heart failure and pulmonary hypertension after mitral valve replacement, *J Thorac Cardiovasc Surg* 89:567, 1985.
10. Kersten L: *Comprehensive respiratory nursing,* Philadelphia, 1988, WB Saunders.
11. Biddle C: Hypothermia: implications for the critical care nurse, *Crit Care Nurse* 5:34, 1985.

CHAPTER 11

Bard cardiopulmonary support system

Terry K. Bavin and Sheldon E. Cohen

INTRODUCTION

A significant number of deaths in the United States are caused annually by cardiac arrest and sudden cardiac death.[1] Different mechanical support devices have been used to support standard cardiopulmonary resuscitation (CPR) for many years. The application of cardiopulmonary support used in open-heart procedures is one of those methods.[2] However, for several reasons, including difficulty of initiating the system, it was not readily accepted. A portable cardiopulmonary bypass support system (Cardiopulmonary Support [CPS] C.R. Bard, Billerica, Mass.) has recently been developed (Fig. 11-1). It allows cardiopulmonary support to be initiated easily and rapidly.

CPS supports the patient's cardiac and/or pulmonary function in the presence of a failing heart and/or lungs when conventional therapy has failed. This allows time for assessment of the patient and initiation of further therapeutic measures. Use of this CPS system has also been extended to supportive roles in patients who have significant cardiac or pulmonary dysfunction. An example of this is its role in coronary angioplasty (i.e., supported coronary angioplasty).[3]

The CPS system, as used today, is an outgrowth of extracorporeal pump oxygenated devices developed in the 1950s. Evolution of extracorporeal perfusion technology and materials, along with development of percutaneous techniques for femoral vessel cannulation, ushered the CPS system into modern day hospital practice.[4]

DESCRIPTION OF CPS

Cardiopulmonary Support is a femoral-femoral percutaneous portable cardiopulmonary bypass used as a temporary assist. Blood is removed from a cannula in the central venous circulation. This venous blood is pumped through a heat exchanger to maintain body temperature and a membrane oxygenator to provide O_2 and remove CO_2. Blood is then returned to the body via a femoral artery cannula.

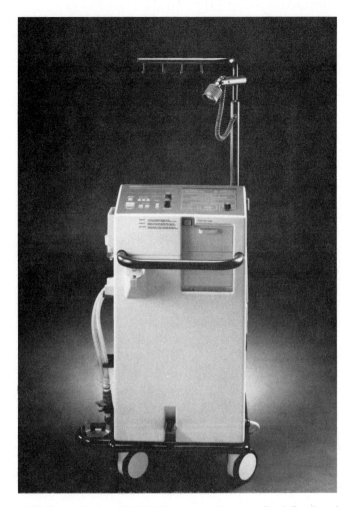

Fig. 11-1. Bard CPS ReAct System H-9000 Hardware. (Courtesy Bard Cardiopulmonary, Bille-rica, Mass.)

SYSTEM COMPONENTS

The Bard CPS perfusion circuit comes preassembled and ready to use (Fig. 11-2). CPS can be initiated within 15 minutes once all team members and equipment are assembled.[5] A Biomedicus pump head, which is magnetically coupled to the pump con-troller, receives blood and fluid from the patient via a venous line and rapid prime lines. Pump head rotating cones create a constrained vortex, aspirating blood from the venous end and producing positive pressure on the arterial side.

Blood flow and pressure are measured via a flow probe and pressure line. A sensor,

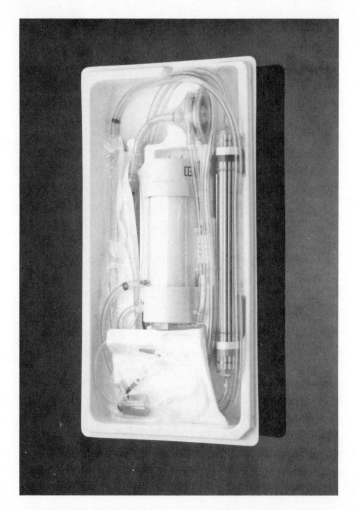

Fig. 11-2. Preassembled CPS circuit H-9400 (disposable circuit) including pump head, membrane oxygenator, heat exchanger, and rapid prime lines. (Courtesy Bard Cardiopulmonary, Billerica, Mass.)

located within the circuit, monitors temperature; the heat exchanger warms blood to maintain normothermia. The hollow fiber membrane oxygenator works by simple diffusion to supply O_2 and remove CO_2 from blood flowing through it. Blood is then returned through the arterial line to the body. Venous and arterial lines are anastomosed with a recirculation loop, which facilitates priming and air removal from the system during setup.

The CPS circuit interfaces with a cart. Hardware for this cart includes a Biomedicus-Medtronic pump controller (Eden Prairie, Minn.), which displays pump revolutions per minute (RPM) and pump flow (L/min). A battery pack is provided for portable operation. A normothermic water-based heat exchanger connects to the circuit and circulates warmed water around the blood to gently maintain body temperature.[6] The cart also houses an IV pole, in addition to brackets that secure both the O_2 tank and the membrane oxygenator.

HEMODYNAMICS OF CPS

Cardiopulmonary support is capable of supplying 100% of the cardiac output requirements up to 6 L/min, even in complete cardiac arrest situations. It is also capable of supplying 100% of the oxygen and ventilation requirements during arrest states. By aspirating blood from the right atrium, CPS unloads both right and left ventricles. This reduces CVP and PCWP to -5 to 5 mm Hg pressure. Reducing preload decreases the heart's work, leading to lower myocardial oxygen consumption.

PATIENT SELECTION

Use of emergency percutaneous cardiopulmonary support in patients with cardiopulmonary failure (or in extremis) unresponsive to advanced cardiac life support can temporarily give physicians the time needed to diagnose and correct reversible problems. Unless the patient is properly perfused and oxygenated, brain death or other vital organ dysfunction can occur. Although cardiopulmonary resuscitation (CPR) is a useful adjunct for short periods of time, it is able to support only 25% of the baseline cardiac output.[7]

Current reported criteria for emergent application of CPS include myocardial infarction, cardiac arrest, congestive heart failure, and cardiogenic shock.[8] Mechanical cardiac problems such as ventricular septal defect, mitral regurgitation, or cardiac tamponade may be fully supported until surgically corrected. Temporary life-threatening dysrhythmias resulting from drug overdose or electrolyte imbalance can be treated with CPS until the drug is metabolized or removed from the body. Reported cases of accidental hypothermia with cardiac arrest and intractable ventricular fibrillation have been successfully reversed with gentle rewarming by extracorporeal circulation.[9,10] Recovery from reversible respiratory failure has been proposed for use in smoke inhalation, near drowning, alveolar hyperproteinosis, pulmonary edema, and status asthmaticus.[11]

Beyond the emergent uses, CPS is being utilized in supported percutaneous transluminal coronary angioplasty. Inclusion criteria for the elective "Supported Angioplasty" Registry include (1) presence of severe or unstable angina; (2) at least one likely dilatable coronary stenosis; and (3) patients with a left ventricular ejection fraction $< 25\%$, and/or target vessel supplying half of the viable myocardium.[12]

Contraindications for the use of CPS include (1) untreatable terminal illness; (2) brain damage or death; (3) and aortic regurgitation. Aortic-iliac occlusive disease can preclude femoral catheter placement.

INSERTION TECHNIQUES

Cannulation can be accomplished by direct visualization of the vessels used or by the percutaneous method.[2,4] Vessels commonly used for this procedure are the femoral artery and vein. Alternative cannulation vessels are the internal jugular vein, right atrium, and ascending aorta.

Arterial and venous cannulae are prepackaged in a kit with necessary equipment for percutaneous insertion. A perfusionist assembles and primes the system during concomitant heparinization with 300 units/kg. The goal is to maintain an activated clotting time (ACT) greater than 400 seconds. During this time resuscitation or supportive measures are continued.

Once exposure of the femoral artery and vein is accomplished, cannula insertion can be performed by direct arteriotomy and venotomy, or by percutaneous technique. If good femoral pulses are obtained, percutaneous insertion can be attempted without direct visualization. If initially unsuccessful, direct visualization is necessary because time is of the essence.

Venous cannula tip placement should be in the right atrium to ensure maximal venous return and cardiac decompression. Once the cannulae are in place, CPS is initiated.

Surgical cutdown insertion requires closure of the incision around the CPS cannulae, followed with application of sterile dressings. Anchoring cannulae to the thigh prophylactically prevents movement, which could lead to vessel trauma and bleeding, disruption of flow, and/or kinking.

Heparinization is continued throughout the procedure to maintain an ACT greater than 400 seconds.

POTENTIAL COMPLICATIONS

Bleeding is a major potential complication associated with CPS due to platelet trauma from the pump head and membrane oxygenator. Heparinization to maintain the ACT greater than 400 seconds prolongs coagulation; hemorrhage can ensue. CPS requires extracorporeal blood circulation, which could leak, disconnect, or disrupt. Large cannulae, necessary for arterial and venous access, increase bleeding risk through injury to cannulation sites or by damage to catheters; this can lead to rapid loss of blood. One study reported blood loss requiring transfusion in 45 of 105 patients. A mean of 3.7 units of blood were required. Subsequent decannulation procedure changes have greatly reduced blood loss and need for blood transfusions.[13]

Embolic events to the brain, heart, mesenteric, kidneys or other vital organs are another potential complication. An embolic source may be from blood coagulating on foreign materials in the perfusion circuit. This can be related to inadequate blood flows or inadequate heparinization. Failure to remove CPS circuit air during priming or while connecting patient CPS catheters could be another embolic source. Open intravenous catheters or lines can allow air entry into the system due to low or negative CVP pressures. The incidence of total embolic events is less than 3%.[13]

Potential neurological complications include brain damage and/or death before CPS initiation, or cerebral vascular occlusive disease in conjunction with nonpulsatile blood flows (or low mean blood pressures). Factors contributing to bleeding may cause central nervous system hemorrhages. Transient femoral nerve injury from cannulation, cannula removal, and/or control of bleeding may cause weakness or sensory changes in the affected extremity (less than 2% incidence).[13]

Infection risks exist from poor surgical technique or poor preparation for insertion of the large arterial and venous cannula. Keeping the groin area free from bacteria can be particularly difficult. Therefore prophylactic antibiotics should be considered with the initiation of CPS.

Other potential complications include (1) renal failure, which can occur from inadequate circulatory support or prolonged shock states that happen before initiation of CPS; and (2) risk of skin breakdown while on the CPS system, which increases with the length of time the patient requires immobilization.

Problems such as inability to wean from CPS because of prolonged irreversible cardiac or respiratory failure will end in death without other long-term support access or treatments. Catastrophic illness may result in the patient or family being unable to cope with the situational crisis.

MORBIDITY AND MORTALITY

The majority of complications that occur have been previously discussed. Specific complications not mentioned before include vessel injury from cannulation and leg ischemia secondary to arterial cannulation.

During cannulation, vascular injury can occur, which may include intimal tear, dissection, and perforation. Perforation can cause retroperitoneal bleeding, which, if unrecognized, may result in death secondary to exsanguination.

Ischemic extremities have been described in 5% to 19% of patients who receive an intraaortic balloon (IAB) catheter.[14] CPS cannulae are considerably larger (18 to 20 French). Arterial occlusion can occur, leading to an ischemic injury when collateral circulation is lacking. This ischemia is tolerated only briefly; therefore a means of extremity circulatory support must be instituted via direct distal cannulation or crossover femoral-femoral bypass.

Defining CPS success is difficult. Is patient weaning from the system and/or transferring to another modality of cardiopulmonary support considered successful? Should it be considered successful only if the patient leaves the hospital? Various series report this in terms of long-term survival. Results with CPS range from 15% to 40% with most being between 15% to 25%.[13,15-17] In our series we have a 30% patient survival rate.[15]

Without CPS support, mortality "in extremis" has been reported as high as 100%.[17] Improved survival can therefore be achieved with cardiopulmonary support. At present, studies are being done to determine which categories of patients will benefit most from this intervention.

Postangioplasty vessel closure occurred in 4% of patients in CPS supported angioplasty (10 hrs to 4 days). Eight patients (7.6%) died during hospitalization (2 hours to 7 days) following the procedure. Four died following coronary artery closure and one each died from the following: abdominal hemorrhage, mesenteric artery thrombosis, femoral artery thrombosis, and during bypass surgery.[13]

Morbidity statistics from 105 patients undergoing elective CPS–supported angioplasty revealed femoral artery repair in four cases. The incidences of complication are as follows: one patient suffered femoral artery occlusion, three patients had femoral artery pseudoaneurysms, four patients had large hematomas, five patients experienced thrombophlebitis, eight patients developed cannula site infections, and transient femoral nerve injury occurred in two cases.[13]

PATIENT TRANSPORTATION

Because it is portable, CPS offers the ability to initiate support anywhere in a hospital. Once initial evaluation is completed, further diagnostic tests to better define the patient's problem may be necessary. Transportation for diagnostic studies (such as computerized tomography and nuclear medicine), or definitive treatments in the catheterization laboratory, or surgery require prior planning for a smooth transport. Each facility should define which personnel are needed and what equipment is required for monitoring to provide proper patient care during transport. Suggestions for a transport team include a perfusionist to operate the CPS system. Respiratory therapy staff may be necessary to provide for oxygenation and ventilation while on partial bypass. When available, our facility utilizes an anesthesiologist for patient airway management and ventilation, controlled sedation, and paralysis if necessary in restless and combative patients. The use of several nurses aids in transport by synchronizing gurney movement with the CPS cart, thereby protecting CPS cannula and lines. As an additional safety precaution, the physician who inserted the cannula should monitor transport.

ECG with arterial pressure display for monitoring the patient and a defibrillator are appropriate. Additional supplies include two full oxygen tanks, one for patient inspiration (via nasal cannula or mask) and the other for CPS membrane oxygenation. Additional fluids such as lactated ringers, normal saline or blood may be needed, as well as tubing clamps.

The CPS battery pack allows about 1 hour operation at 5 L/min dependent upon patient resistance. Attention to detail for interfacility transport is paramount, including space requirements for patient, equipment, and staff. Transport vehicle and/or aircraft must have a compatible AC power source to function with the CPS system. It is best to work through these details before the need to transport outside the facility arises.

NURSING MANAGEMENT

Nursing plays an important role in the care of patients requiring CPS. In some facilities, nurses are trained to set up and prime the system while the perfusionist is enroute to the hospital.[6] Although perfusionists are responsible for operating the CPS system in most medical centers, nursing care is essential to provide for the patient's needs.

Nursing diagnosis #1

Low cardiac output related to reduction in stroke volume as a result of mechanical, structural, or electrical problems requiring cardiopulmonary support.[18]

Assessing patient's adequacy of circulation on CPS is different from conventional patients. Since blood flow is nonpulsatile during CPS, pulses may be absent, even with excellent tissue perfusion. Blood pressure evaluation using the cuff method is therefore impractical; thus direct arterial pressure monitoring is highly desirable. Mean blood pressure (MAP) values above 60 mm Hg are required; upper limits of about 90 mm Hg are suggested. Skin color, warmth, capillary refill, and urine output are other parameters of perfusion that can be assessed.[18] During total bypass support, blood flow to the body is delivered entirely by the CPS system and can be measured from the pump controller. Blood flows of 2.2 to 2.4 L/min/M^2 are considered satisfactory. During supported PTCA, partial bypass support is used to supplement the patient's circulation. Blood flows are usually maintained at 2.0 to 3.5 L/min and increased if PCWP remains high or if blood pressure falls during the angioplasty.[19]

Arterial waveform analysis on total bypass with no cardiac contribution (such as in ventricular fibrillation) reveals a nearly flat arterial trace (Fig. 11-3, *A*). During partial bypass both the patient's intrinsic heart and the CPS system are contributing to patient perfusion.[18] The arterial waveform demonstrates weak to moderate pulse waveforms with diastole being flattened out while on partial bypass (Fig. 11-3, *B*).

As CPS is increased in patients exhibiting cardiac ejection, the right atrial pressure (RAP) and pulmonary artery pressure (PAP) decrease.[3] Lowered pulmonary artery and capillary wedge pressure (PCWP) measurements indicate the success of left ventricular unloading, which reduces cardiac work and improves subendocardial blood flow.

Low venous blood volume or inadequate venous return may cause a hazard known as "pump shutter," characterized by sudden falls in pump flow at a given RPM setting. The tubing shutters or shakes because of higher negative venous line pressures attained as the right atrium collapses, preventing flow to the catheter's lumen.[18]

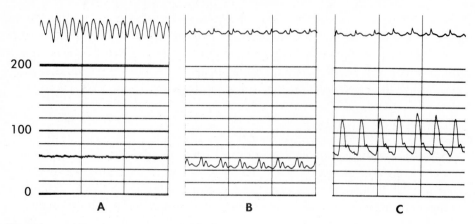

Fig. 11-3. A, Full bypass support in ventricular fibrillation. CPS at 4 L/min pump flow. **B,** Partial bypass support in normal sinus rhythm. CPS at 2.5 L/min pump flow. **C,** Arterial waveform after CPS support withdrawn following PTCA. Special thanks to David Debutts and Rick Hood for their assistance with this figure.

Systemic vascular resistance (SVR) can be calculated during full bypass support by the formula MAP/pump flow × 80, assuming that the RAP is zero. Unfortunately measurements taken in the right atrium are considered inaccurate because the CPS venous cannula aspirates blood from that site. Normal SVR is between 900 and 1100 dynes/sec/cm^{-5}. When pump flows are adequate and BP is low, vascular resistance needs to be increased. Drugs that increase SVR with little cardiac action (such as Neo-synephrine (phenylephrine hydrochloride) and Vasoxyl (methoxamine hydrochloride)) are preferred because the heart is often unloaded and unable to respond. In situations where the BP is high with normal pump flows, it is desirable to reduce BP with vasodilators, paying close attention to the potential need for IV fluids.

On partial bypass support the heart provides a portion of the cardiac output to the body. Measuring intrinsic cardiac output using standard thermodilution methods is considered inaccurate because of CPS system aspiration in the right atrium.[18] Mixed venous oxygen saturation (SvO$_2$) monitoring is helpful in determining overall tissue perfusion and oxygen delivery during partial bypass support.

Nursing diagnosis #2

Impaired gas exchange related to respiratory dysfunction not responding to standard ventilatory support and/or ventilation perfusion mismatch.

Evaluation of oxygenation is critical in CPS patients. Measurement of arterial blood gases (ABGs) is clinically useful in assessing alterations in pH due to metabolic or respiratory problems. Oxygenator membrane status can be assessed by looking postmembrane at difficulties causing gas diffusion, decreases in the Po$_2$ and increases in the Pco$_2$

levels. If this occurs, the membrane oxygenator may need replacement. Assessment of patient breathing during partial bypass support is critical. Blood ejected by the left ventricle goes first to the coronaries and brain. If the patient has a major mismatch of ventilation and perfusion, poorly oxygenated blood may go to vital organs.[18] Because the innominate artery is most proximal to the heart, pulse oximeter measurements from right hand fingers (with pulsatile blood flow) are the closest to the heart to detect this complication. ABGs from right radial artery lines are also useful to detect this situation. If Po_2 levels are low, supplemental oxygen by nasal cannula, mask, or even mechanical ventilation may be required.

Nursing diagnosis #3

High risk for injury to the patient related to bleeding, thrombus, or air embolus.

Assessing for and prevention of potential complications is also an important nursing function. Checking laboratory results for hemoglobin and hematocrit, platelets, and activated clotting times are important in evaluating causes of bleeding and when blood product replacement is indicated. Prevention of bleeding because of injury may require limb immobilization to protect the insertion site and cannula. Some patients are given sedation and are paralyzed with drugs to lessen patient movement.[18]

Embolic events may be as subtle as a change in bowel sounds for mesenteric infarcts or as gross as blown pupils for a brain-related catastrophe.

Nursing diagnosis #4

High risk for infection related to invasive line sites and depressed immune response of the patient.

Infection related to CPS may be observed at the cannula site and an increase in white blood cells (WBC) noted on complete blood counts (CBC).

Nursing diagnosis #5

Immobility due to CPS catheters in the groin and paralytic drugs or restraints to prevent injury to the patient.

Skin breakdown may be prevented with the use of special care air flotation beds. Some of these beds also provide kinetic therapy that may help prevent pulmonary complications.

DATA COLLECTION DOCUMENTATION

In our facility, no special forms are used to chart on patients. The perfusionist documents CPS-related information on the same record used for cardiopulmonary bypass: pump RPM, pump flow, O_2 sweep speeds, percent O_2 (if applicable), and blood temperature, along with some laboratory results (ABGs, CBCs, ACTs). Nursing documents vascular pressures, physical assessment findings, and any complications on the critical care record/nurses notes.

Our facility participates in the National Emergent CPS Registry (Jonathan Hill, MD registry director, Emanual Hospital and Medical Center, 2801 Gantenbein Ave., Portland, OR 97229), which is collecting data for patients treated on the system in extremis. Comprehensive information is compiled on each patient, including diagnosis, methods used applying CPS, complications, and outcome, along with other data.

There is also a National Registry for Elective Supported Angioplasty (Robert A. Vogel, MD registry director, Division of Cardiology, room N3W77, University of Maryland Hospital, 22 S. Green St., Baltimore, MD 21201). Initial data suggest that supported angioplasty can be used in high-risk patients with good short-term results.[13]

WEANING FROM CPS/DECANNULATION

After treating the problem that necessitated cardiopulmonary support, attention can be directed toward eventual recovery, sufficient to permit weaning. In uncomplicated angioplasty CPS patients, weaning may be as simple as slowly decreasing pump flows over several minutes and adjusting left ventricular preload to a PCWP value of 8 to 10 mm Hg or higher (dependent upon left ventricular function) and clamping the arterial and venous lines.[3] During this time blood pressure and PCWP are monitored and standard pharmacological support instituted. In complicated CPS cases, additional forms of cardiac and/or ventilatory support may be necessary, including intraaortic balloon pump support (IABP), ventricular assist device (VAD), or aggresive ventilatory support such as with long-term extracorporeal membrane oxygenation (ECMO). Following CPS support, ventricular assist devices may in some cases bridge patients to other interventions such as cardiac transplantation.

Following weaning, CPS femoral vessel cannulae are removed. Before decannulation ACT levels should be less than 240 seconds, either using protamine sulfate (for heparin reversal) or waiting for 5 to 6 hours for ACT values to decrease passively (for fear of early closure following PCTA). There are two methods for cannula removal. Our institution prefers surgical closure of vessel and groin insertion sites. Another method is by percutaneous removal using manual pressure over the insertion site for 30 minutes or longer, followed with clamp compressor for hemostasis. Careful assessment of peripheral pulses distal to the clamp and proper clamp placement to prevent femoral nerve injury are essential. After 90 minutes in the absence of bleeding, the clamp is gradually released 2 to 3 mm every 20 minutes.[19]

PATIENT AND FAMILY PSYCHOSOCIAL ISSUES

It is shocking to see a loved one critically ill, and dependent upon advanced medical technology such as CPS. Events leading to the situation can be sudden and unexpected, leaving the family emotionally unprepared. Patients may not have regained consciousness and may be unable to respond, making the potential loss all the more apparent. In emergencies, many of the patients may not be salvageable and will die.[13,15,16,17] To support the family and patient through the crisis, it is important to establish good lines of communication. Identify the key leader/spokesperson to pass information on to the family. Explanations should be appropriate for the family's educational background. Repeat explanations may be required. If a private conference room is available, family members may feel more free to discuss personal matters and display their emotions. Resources such as social workers, clergy, and psychologists can be beneficial.

In elective supported angioplasty patients, preprocedure teaching is needed, along with lots of reassurance. Fear and anxiety can be reduced by explaining the unknown. Medication for sedation and pain may make the experience less threatening and less unpleasant.

CASE STUDY

An 80-year-old man was admitted to the hospital with a diagnosis of aortic stenosis and congestive heart failure. He underwent aortic valvuloplasty to reduce the 50 mm Hg transvalvular gradient and to improve cardiac function. During valvuloplasty the patient complained of crushing chest pain; ST segments became elevated on the ECG. Catheterization revealed left main coronary artery occlusion. Rapid deterioration into ventricular fibrillation made the patient unresponsive to advanced cardiac life support (ACLS) measures. CPS took about 20 minutes to initiate from the onset of ventricular fibrillation. Within 10 minutes of initiating CPS, the patient converted spontaneously into normal sinus rhythm. He was quickly taken to surgery for an aortic valve replacement and saphenous vein coronary bypass graft past his left main occlusion. He required intraaortic balloon pump support and high-dose inotropic drug support for about 1 week. Although he had many problems, he was eventually able to walk out of the hospital and lived another 2 years.

CONCLUSION

Applications for the use of cardiopulmonary support in interventional cardiology are apt to increase in high-risk patients. CPS may eventually be used in coronary stents, laser treatments, and artherectomy patients.[13]

Improvements in perfusion circuits will allow support with little or no heparinization, permitting wider usage emergently, especially in trauma patients where the risk of bleeding is much greater. Reduction of bleeding complications following cannula removal could therefore be expected.

Results from additional studies will be required to predict the role of CPS in the future.

REFERENCES

1. Myerberg RJ, Castellanos A: Cardiovascular arrest and sudden cardiac death. In Braunwald E, ed: *Heart disease, a textbook of cardiovascular medicine, ed 3,* Philadelphia, 1988, WB Saunders.
2. Phillips SJ: Percutaneous cardiopulmonary bypass and innovations in clinical counterpulsation, *Crit Care Clin* 2:297, April 1986.
3. Shawl FA: Percutaneous cardiopulmonary support in high risk angioplasty, *Cardiol Clin* 7(4):865, 1989.
4. Phillips ST, Ballantine B, Sloving CP et al: Percutaneous initiation of cardiopulmonary bypass, *Ann Thorac Surg* 36:223, 1983.
5. Raithel SC, Swartz MT, Braun RR et al: Experience with an emergency resuscitation system, *Trans Am Soc Artif Intern Organs* XXXV:475, 1989.
6. Litzie K: Emergency femoro-femoral cardiopulmonary bypass, *Proc Am Acad Cardiovasc Perfus* 8:60, 1987.
7. Peters J, Ihle R: Mechanics of circulation during cardiopulmonary resuscitation: pathophysiology and techniques, *Intensive Care Med* 16:11, 1990.
8. Shawl FA, Domanski MJ, Hernandez TJ et al: Emergency percutaneous cardiopulmonary bypass support in cardiogenic shock from acute myocardial infarction, *Am J Cardiol* 64:967, 1989.
9. Husby P, Anderson KS, Owen-Falkenberg A et al: Case report, accidental hypothermia with cardiac arrest: complete recovery after prolonged resuscitation and rewarming by extracorporeal circulation, *Intensive Care Med,* 16:69, 1990.
10. Towne WD, Geiss WP, Yanes HO et al: Intractable ventricular fibrillation associated with profound accidental hypothermia-successful treatment with partial cardiopulmonary bypass, *N Engl J Med* 287(22):1135, 1972.
11. Overlie PA: Emergency use of portable cardiopulmonary bypass, *Cathet Cardiovasc Diagn* 20:27, 1990.
12. Shawl FA, Domanski MJ, Punja S et al: Percutaneous cardiopulmonary bypass support in high-risk patients undergoing percutaneous transluminal coronary angioplasty, *Am J Cardiol* 64:1258, 1989.
13. Vogel RA, Tommaso CL: Special feature: cardiopulmonary support; elective supported angioplasty: initial report of the National Registry, *Cathet Cardiovasc Diagn* 20:22, 1990.
14. Bolooki H: Complications of balloon pumping: diagnosis, procedures and treatment. In *Clinical Applications of Intra-Aortic Balloon Pump,* Mt Kisco, N.Y., 1984, Futura Publishing Company Inc.
15. Cohen S: Author's personal experience, unpublished data.
16. Mattox KL, Beall AC Sr: Resuscitation of the moribund patient using portable cardiopulmonary bypass, *Ann Thorac Surg* 22:436, 1976.
17. Reichman RT, Joyo CI, Dembitsky WP et al: Improved patient survival after cardiac arrest using a cardiopulmonary support system, *Ann Thorac Surg* 49:101, 1990.
18. Bavin TK: Nursing considerations for patients requiring cardiopulmonary support, *AACN Clinical Issues in Critical Care Nursing* 2(3):500, 1991.
19. Shawl FA, Domanski MJ, Wish MH et al: Percutaneous cardiopulmonary bypass support in the catheterization laboratory: technique and complications, *Am Heart J* 120(1):195, 1990.

CHAPTER 12

External counterpulsation

Mary Beth Farley Liska, Kristen E. Johnson, Marc R. Pritzker, Robert W. Emery, and **Stephanie Sevcik**

INTRODUCTION

The principle of diastolic counterpulsation was conceived in the late 1950s by Birtwell and Harken as a means of supporting dysfunctional hearts.[1] Originating from this concept the intraaortic balloon pump (IABP) was developed in the early 1960s by Moulopoulos to assist patients experiencing cardiogenic shock.[1] First successful IABP use was in 1967, when Kantrowitz used it in patients with cardiogenic shock, thus beginning the era of modern clinical intraaortic balloon pumping.[1] Despite rapid improvements in technology and understanding of physiologic principles governing balloon counterpulsation, this therapy remains invasive and expensive, necessitating specialized teams of support personnel and limiting its utilization to larger referral centers. Thus it is not surprising that over the last two decades considerable attention has focused on the potential for external use counterpulsation (ECP) devices to provide mechanical circulation assistance.

Advantages of this system over an IABP derive from its noninvasive nature and include (1) wider applicability of patient selection (women, children, and those with mild to moderate peripheral vascular disease), (2) potential use in a wider variety of hospitals, (3) potential cost efficiencies, and (4) generally, less or no monitoring in an intensive care unit, although patient hemodynamic instability may necessitate critical care nursing.[2,3] In our preliminary experience with ECP two trained nurses can initiate and implement effective diastolic counterpulsation in 10 minutes, a time considerably shorter and a process considerably less technically demanding than initiation of intraaortic balloon counterpulsation. With use of ECP it is possible to achieve approximately 60% of IABP support,[4] yet, unlike internal balloon counterpulsation, anticoagulation is not necessary because the device is not in direct contact with blood supply. However, ECP has been used in a limited number of patients receiving thrombolytic therapy without noted complications. No complications have been reported that could be directly attributed to use of external counterpulsation.[2]

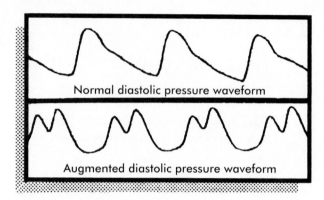

Fig. 12-1. Normal diastolic pressure waveform compared to a waveform augmented by an external counterpulsation device. (From Schwoebel J: *Sequential external counterpulsation system* [instruction manual], Santa Ana, Calif., 1989, Cardiomedics, Inc.)

PHYSIOLOGICAL EFFECTS

Diastolic augmentation through external sequential counterpulsation is achieved by using cuffs placed on patient's legs and inflated during diastole. This mechanically augments diastolic blood pressure, resulting in an increased volume of blood delivered to the coronary vasculature (Fig. 12-1). Immediately before systole, the cuffs are deflated, causing a reduction in aortic volume and pressure. Cuff inflation and deflation timing with an electrocardiograph (ECG) is crucial because accurate timing allows retrograde blood flow through the arterial system to the aortic valve. This flow, initiated by cuff inflation, may provide up to 225 mm Hg of pressure, generally equal to or greater than the systolic blood pressure at peak augmentation.[3] It is this increased pressure that augments blood flow to the coronary vasculature.

Systolic blood pressure is also affected because counterpulsation decreases afterload by reducing intraaortic volume when the device cuffs deflate. Oxygen demand is decreased by reducing myocardial workload and lowering intracardiac pressure, thus improving subendocardial perfusion. Consequently cardiac output may be increased 10% to 15%.[4,5] Increases in diastolic pressure generated by diastolic augmentation improves perfusion to the coronary arteries and thus may increase coronary collateral circulation.[3] Hemodynamic benefits of external counterpulsation can also extend to other organs (e.g., increased renal blood flow may have a positive effect on urine production).[1,3]

Device description and function

A control console, finger pulse pressure sensor (finger plethysmograph), ECG electrodes, and four leg cuffs comprise an external counterpulsation system (Fig. 12-2).

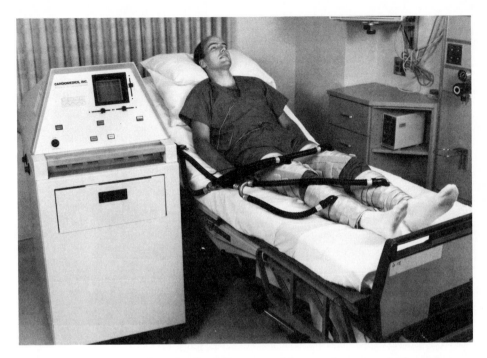

Fig. 12-2. Simulation of the Cardiomedics sequential external counterpulsation system.

Cuffs are available in various sizes for more accurate and comfortable fits. Flexible cuffs are placed on the calf and thigh of each leg. Air fills the calf cuffs first, thus compressing lower vessels. Blood is then displaced to the thigh; following a 20 msec delay the thigh cuffs inflate. This process forces blood back toward the heart. ECG data is relayed via electrodes to the system, where it is amplified and utilized in device timing and triggering. For monitoring purposes the patient's ECG and pulse wave (arterial waveform) are displayed on a strip chart recorder. Pressure and timing settings should be adjusted as necessary to provide greatest augmentation while maintaining patient comfort.[3] Weaning is initiated when the myocardium is able to function independently, maintaining adequate pressures and flow rates. Without data available to support a weaning protocol, decisions to wean and weaning schedules are the physician's responsibility.

SUPPORTING DATA

Amsterdam et al., in a randomized, prospective, cooperative study of 25 institutions, reported a mortality rate of 8.3% in patients who received 3 or more hours of ECP treatment during the early phase of acute myocardial infarction compared with a mortality rate of 17.5% in a control group.[2] Although this study was limited to 258 patients, its

_____ **CURRENT INDICATIONS FOR ECP** _____

Cardiogenic shock
Uncomplicated myocardial infarction
Unstable angina
Chronic stable angina
Hemodynamic decompensation
Postinfarction angina

From Schwoebel J: *Sequential external counterpulsation (SECP)* (inservice orientation), Santa Ana, Calif., 1989, Cardiomedics, Inc.

_____ **RECOMMENDED TREATMENTS** _____

Acute MI

Counterpulsation may be used in sessions lasting up to 4 hours with 10 minutes of rest after every hour. This should be followed by 1 hour of therapy every day until discharge. The duration of treatment and rest sessions should be ordered by the physician, taking into account the patient's tolerance and condition.

Cardiogenic shock

When using external counterpulsation for cardiogenic shock, the recommended protocol is the same as for patients with acute MIs. However, the patient may not be able to tolerate long rest periods. Therefore an attempt should be made to take a 2 to 5 minute break every hour.

Unstable angina

Counterpulsation for 2 hours with a 10 minute break after 1 hour until discharge is recommended for patients with unstable angina. The patient should have resting chest pain and alterations of the T-wave without elevations of the cardiac enzymes or evidence of an acute MI.

From Schwoebel J: *Multicenter post market randomized study of sequential external counterpulsation (SECP)*, Santa Ana, Calif., 1989, Cardiomedics, Inc.

mortality results are particularly interesting when compared to mortality results achieved in recent trials with thrombolytic therapy.[2] In a study by Soroff et al. using ECP to treat cardiogenic shock associated with acute myocardial infarction (MI) and unstable angina pectoris a survival rate of 45% (9/20) was found, compared with the usual survival rate of 10% to 20%.[6]

INDICATIONS FOR USAGE

Current acceptable indications for ECP device usage are noted in the upper box. These indications were derived from a series of clinical studies carried out between

CONTRAINDICATIONS FOR USING ECP

Peripheral vascular disease and deep vein thrombosis
Aortic valve insufficiency
Patients with DDD or atrial pacemakers (devices trigger off the QRS)
Amputated lower limbs
Chronic atrial fibrillation or uncontrolled arrhythmias
Left or right bundle branch blocks
Left ventricular hypertrophy
Pulmonary disease

From Schwoebel J: *Sequential external counterpulsation system* (instruction manual) and *Sequential external counterpulsation (SECP)* (inservice orientation), Santa Ana, Calif., 1989, Cardiomedics, Inc.

NURSING CONSIDERATIONS

Use of the device may cause increased urine production. Therefore it is important to have the patient urinate before initiating treatment.[3]
The head of the patient's bed may be elevated to 45 degrees, but the supine position is preferred.[3]
Use lead II for electrodes (upright deflection).[3]
Device should face same way as feet because of short hose length, and for ease of observation.[5]
Finger plethysmograph[3]
  The plethysmograph should be on an index or middle finger.
  Do not expose to fluorescent lights.
  Discourage patient movement.
  The amplitude of the pulse waveform will self-adjust.

1975 and 1990. Preliminary published and unpublished experience suggest ECP device usage is safe in patients with congestive heart failure and septic shock, although formal FDA approval of these indications is pending.[7,8] One manufacturer recommends treatment regimes for an acute myocardial infarction, cardiogenic shock, and unstable angina (see the lower box on p. 160). Contraindications to the use of an external counterpulsation device are listed in the upper box on this page.

Patient care

During ECP two primary complaints of patients and staff were lower limb discomfort[2] and, at our center, noise from the corresponding console.[9] Patients also voiced feelings of confinement while undergoing therapy.[2] These complaints are not

---

CUFF APPLICATION

Application of the cuffs is facilitated by two nurses, one to adjust the straps, the other to support the leg.

Cover skin before applying cuffs (with towel, pajamas, gauze, etc.).

Use the largest comfortable cuff; it should fit snugly.

Open the cuffs completely before applying.

   Apply thigh cuffs first. They should rest within ¼ inch of the crotch and not overlap the kneecap.

   Secure cuff snugly with velcro, adjusting distal strap last.

   The top of the calf cuff should fit just below the kneecap, and the bottom should be 3 in. above the ankle.

Attach air hoses after all cuffs are applied.

The system should be kept clean and dry.

Replace the paper, electrodes, and cuffs as needed. (The inner bladder of the cuffs usually lasts about 3 months.)

From Schwoebel J: *Sequential external counterpulsation system* (instruction manual), Santa Ana, Calif., 1989, Cardiomedics, Inc.

unlike those of patients who have experienced other circulatory assist devices. See the boxes on pp. 161 and 162 for nursing considerations and application of the cuffs.

Three primary nursing diagnoses for patients treated with ECP are decreased cardiac output, immobility, and lack of knowledge. Improvements in cardiac output should be noted shortly after initiation of ECP as diastolic augmentation increases. A Swan-Ganz heart catheter may be used for measuring and documenting cardiac outputs; however, an alternative noninvasive indicator of improved perfusion is increased urine production.

Cuff displacement resulting from patient movement can alter the degree of diastolic augmentation, thus influencing device efficacy. Therefore maintaining patient immobility during device operation is an important aspect of patient care.

Through explanations and teaching, nurses are often able to increase patient knowledge regarding their illness and treatment,[3] and eliminate many anxieties and concerns associated with hospitalization. Familiarity with a situation or object may contribute to the elimination of a frightening or anxious experience. Promotion of patient autonomy and self-worth is especially important when one is bedridden and care dependent. A care plan consisting of these three nursing diagnoses, with their expected outcomes and interventions, is provided in Table 12-1.

Safety

The Cardiomedics External Sequential Counterpulsation System (Cardiomedics, Inc., Santa Ana, Calif.) has important safety features that are listed in the box on p. 165.

Table 12-1.   Nursing care plan for the ECP patient

Nursing diagnosis	Expected outcome	Interventions
Decreased cardiac output related to cardiac dysfunction	Adequate cardiac output is maintained by (1) adequate diastolic augmentation, (2) Swan-Ganz catheter pressures within normal limits, (3) normal vital signs (BP, HR), (4) adequate urine output, (5) lack of arrhythmias, (6) normal CNS, (7) normal neurological function	Monitor timing of cuff inflation and deflation closely and adjust as necessary Adjust filling pressures per protocol and physician request Monitor BP and HR frequently; use an arterial line or automated cuff if necessary Monitor Swan-Ganz catheter readings frequently, if available. Also consider adjunct treatment with vasopressors and volume replacement, if necessary Maintain urine output at > 30 cc/1hr; use of diuretics and K^+ monitoring should be per physician and/or nurse discretion and hospital protocol Monitor patient for dysrhythmias Monitor CNS by assessing: (1)nailbed capillary refill, (2) color of skin and mucous membranes, (3) skin temperature Assess patient sensorium routinely, along with frequent reorientation
Increased anxiety related to knowledge deficit regarding disease process and alternative treatments	Patient, family, and significant others (SOs) will be knowledgeable about the disease and treatment, thus decreasing their anxiety	Nursing staff will discuss disease process with patient, their family, and SOs Nursing staff will teach the patient, their family, and SOs (1) the concept of external counterpulsation, (2) the device console, (3) the purpose and application of the cuffs, and (4) expected outcomes of the treatment The nursing staff will encourage questions from those involved regarding the disease and treatments The nurses will medicate the patient per physician's orders to decrease anxiety and promote relaxation

Continued

Table 12-1.   Nursing care plan for the ECP patient—cont'd

Nursing diagnosis	Expected outcome	Interventions
		The staff will offer relaxation techniques to the patient (e.g., music, imagery, dimmed lighting)
		Nurses will allow the patient to make decisions pertaining to their care when appropriate to promote autonomy and self-worth
		The staff will encourage family members and SOs to participate in the patient's care
Immobility due to treatment by external counterpulsation.	The patient will resume activity level experienced before hospitalization with knowledge of limitations	The nurse will teach the patient about the concept of counterpulsation and purpose of the device and cuffs
		The patient will accurately discuss the purpose of their treatment
		Slight changes in position are permitted
		Activity levels should be dictated by the physician
		The nursing staff will provide PROM and encourage AROM by the patient between ECP treatments
		The patient will be made aware of limitations to activity and voice symptoms and feelings to staff

Abrupt changes will disable the system and cause the device console recorder to print out error messages during failures, treatment delays, and changes in duration times and pressure settings. The system, however, is limiting because the patient's heart rate must be between 40 bpm and 120 bpm for the system to be operational. Outside of these limits, counterpulsation is automatically disabled by the device.[3] Nursing personnel should verify message accuracy, while reassessing the patient's condition, and then initiate treatment according to individual hospital protocols.[3]

POTENTIAL USAGE

Use of external counterpulsation may be beneficial as an interim treatment for patients requiring medical or surgical intervention. The noninvasive nature of external

_____ **SAFETY FEATURES** _____

Pressure within the cuffs is gradually increased.

The device is electrically isolated from the patient and is electrically grounded.

Patient arrhythmias will disable the counterpulsation as will an abrupt increase or decrease in the heart rate, <40 or >120 bpm.

A manual control allows the controller to suspend pulsation and release built up pressures to end treatments.

A loss of power will disable the system and deflate cuffs.

Through its internal circuitry, the system is prevented from applying the counterpulsation during systole.

From Schwoebel J: *Sequential external counterpulsation system* (instruction manual), Santa Ana, Calif., 1989, Cardiomedics, Inc.

counterpulsation makes it potentially useful in a variety of settings where conventional intraaortic balloon pumping has been either unavailable or difficult to apply.

ECP may provide favorable hemodynamic effects without the associated complications of IABP (e.g., noncardiac surgery in cardiovascular patients is known to carry a significant mortality that peaks on the third postoperative day). In high-risk patients, prophylactic use of an IABP has been limited by the significant procedures associated with morbidity, especially in women, small patients, patients with peripheral vascular disease, and patients requiring prolonged dwell times for anticoagulation.[11,12]

ECP may offset the risk of abrupt large vessel closure and hemodynamic instability induced by balloon inflation. Although prophylactic intraaortic balloon insertion or establishment of temporary extracorporeal circulation are generally declining in usage in favor of a surgical standby approach, ECP may allow the maintainence of satisfactory hemodynamics during balloon inflation or abrupt vessel closure.

ECP, because of its noninvasive nature and ease of use, may find a role in primary and secondary hospitals during initial treatment of acute or unstable patients. Currently, most forms of mechanical circulatory assistance are limited to secondary and tertiary care centers because of cost and specialized expertise required. However, the majority of acute or unstable patients present themselves to primary and secondary hospitals that do not have support systems to initiate mechanical circulatory assistance.

An ECP device adapted to aeromedical and medical ground transport special needs may provide an adjunctive therapeutic option. Because most primary and secondary centers are unable to initiate intraaortic balloon pumping, emergency transfer of acute or unstable cardiac patients to tertiary centers for angioplasty and thrombolytic therapy has become increasingly frequent. Unstable patients are managed currently with pharmacological therapies before and during transfer.

Patients with decompensated congestive heart failure may profit from sequential

ECP. Preliminary experience reported by Uretsky and Murali,[7] notes a trend toward reduction in pulmonary capillary wedge pressure and maintenance of satisfactory arterial pressures. At present, experience is too limited to predict which patients may respond favorably.

External counterpulsation may have a role in the treatment of chronic angina pectoris. In China, where a similar device has been utilized, patients treated for 1 hour a day for 12 days showed a tendency toward reduction in anginal frequency and improvement in exercise capacity.[13]

CONCLUSION

Sequential external counterpulsation appears to be a valuable adjunct to treatment of acute cardiac dysfunction. The true potential of this therapy remains to be explored by further usage. Advantages include ease of usage and application, and lower direct and indirect costs in comparison to invasive forms of mechanical circulatory assistance. These advantages also combine to extend its potential use to primary and secondary hospitals where mechanical circulatory assistance has traditionally not been available.

Further studies are underway to define its appropriate place in the field of current therapeutic choices for treatment of acute ischemic syndromes, as well as to extend its indications for treatment of heart failure, septic shock, and chronic angina pectoris.

REFERENCES

1. Bolooki H: *Clinical application of intra-aortic balloon pump*, ed 2, Mount Kisco, N.Y., 1984, Futura Publishing Company, Inc.
2. Amsterdam EA et al: Clinical assessment of external pressure circulatory assistance in acute myocardial infarction. Report of a cooperative clinical trial, *Am J Cardiol* 45:349, 1980.
3. Schwoebel J: *Sequential external counterpulsation system* (instruction manual), Santa Ana, Calif., 1989, Cardiomedics, Inc.
4. Schwoebel J: *Sequential external counterpulsation (SECP)* (inservice orientation), Santa Ana, Calif., 1989, Cardiomedics, Inc.
5. Sevcik S: Personal notes: Burke P: *Presentation on cardiomedics external sequential counterpulsation system*, Minneapolis, Minn., May 2-3, 1991.
6. Soroff HS et al: External counterpulsation, management of cardiogenic shock after myocardial infarction, *JAMA* 229(11):1441, 1974.
7. Murali S et al: Use of sequential external counterpulsation (SECP) for the treatment of chronic severe congestive heart failure, *Clin Res* 39(2):402A, 1991 (abstract).
8. Gunter JP Jr et al: Synchronized external systolic augmentation (SESA) improves hemodynamics in septic shock, *Am Rev Respir Dis* 143(4):A-86, April 1991 (abstract).
9. Rathbun V: *Letter to Gloria Metcalf*. Personal files of Vicki Rathbun, Minneapolis Cardiology Associates, Minneapolis, Minn., September 4, 1990.
10. Schwoebel J: *Multicenter post market randomized study of sequential external counterpulsation (SECP)*, Santa Ana, California, 1989, Cardiomedics, Inc.
11. Gottlieb SO et al: Identification of patients at high risk for complications of intraaortic balloon counterpulsation: a multivariate risk factor analysis, *Am J Cardiol* 53(8):1135, 1989.
12. Pedersen WR et al: Vascular complications in patients undergoing preoperative prophylactic intraaortic balloon counterpulsation, *Chest* 100:1145, Nov 1991 (abstract).
13. Zheng ZS et al: Sequential external counterpulsation (SECP) in China, *Trans Am Soc Artif Intern Organs* 29:599, 1983.

CHAPTER 13

Total artificial heart

Lawrence E. Barker and William C. DeVries

INTRODUCTION

In 1969 the total artificial heart (TAH) made an initial transition from the animal laboratory to clinical environment when Dr. Denton Cooley implanted an artificial heart developed by Dr. Domingo Liotta.[1] The device was implanted for 64 hours as a bridge to transplant. In 1981 Dr. William DeVries implanted the first permanent TAH in Dr. Barney Clark at the University of Utah in Salt Lake City. This was the first human application of the Jarvik-7-100. This particular device was the result of animal experimentation by Willem Kolff, MD, Cliff Kwan-Gett, MD, Robert Jarvik, MD, William DeVries, MD, Donald Olsen, DVM and numerous engineers and technicians.[2] Dr. Clark lived for 112 days after implant.

Three successive permanent implants were performed in Louisville, Kentucky by Dr. DeVries after moving his TAH program to Humana Hospital Audubon. One patient, William Schroeder, survived for 620 days. The third, Murray Haydon, survived 488 days. Half of these initial TAH patients suffered from device-related complications of bleeding, infection, device fit, and thromboembolic events.[3] It became apparent to researchers that the early TAH configuration was not suitable for long-term support; however, for short-term support as a bridge to transplant it appeared to have an immediate future. As a result, Symbion, Inc., manufacturer of the Jarvik TAH, trained numerous transplant centers in the United States, Canada, and Europe to implant their TAH as a bridge to transplant. Dr. DeVries' program at Humana was the only U.S. permanent TAH implant program approved by the Food and Drug Administration (FDA).

In 1985 the first Symbion J-7-100 TAH implantation bridge to transplant was performed by Dr. Jack Copeland at the University of Arizona. This patient was supported on the device for 9 days and was successfully transplanted and discharged home. In the last 6 years, more than 170 patients have been bridged utilizing the Symbion J-7 TAH with over 70% of these patients being successfully transplanted. Thromboembolic events have been significantly reduced with better understanding of anticoagulation requirements. Infection continues to be the greatest potential complication.[4] Problems with proper device positioning in the patient's chest were significantly reduced with development of the Symbion J-7-70. This TAH was identical in construction and function to the J-7-100, with the exception of smaller ventricles to facilitate easier placement. Although a number of other total artificial hearts are being developed and researched worldwide, the Symbion J-7 TAH has been used most often as a bridge to transplant.

TAH DESIGN

The basic TAH pneumatic design consists of a flexible diaphragm inside semirigid ventricles composed of polyurethane polymer (Biomer) molded with Dacron polyester mesh. The diaphragm is composed of four Biomer layers each 0.18 mm in thickness; graphite powder is placed between layers to prevent creasing of the diaphragms, which could lead to possible rupture. Air is pulsed to the ventricles through internal drivelines, causing diaphragm inflation and subsequent blood ejection. The diaphragms collapse with diastolic filling.

Medtronic-Hall tilting pyrolitic carbon discs with titanium valve rings and struts are utilized as inflow and outflow valves. The ring and strut are machined from a single section of titanium to eliminate the need for welds, which can be prone to failure. The valves are seated in polycarbonate rings to comprise a fitting that joins the atrial cuffs and great vessel grafts to the ventricles.

THEORY OF OPERATION

Symbion J-7-70 and J-7-100 are pneumatically driven devices. A difference exists in the ventricle capacity, which is 70 cc vs. 100 cc (Fig. 13-1). The J-7-70 is used most often because of its smaller size, which facilitates easier chest placement. Surgical device implantation involves excising the native ventricles through a median sternotomy along the atrioventricular groove.[5] Atrial cuffs are sutured to the remnant atria; Dacron grafts are sutured to the aorta and pulmonary artery. Internal drivelines are tunneled through subcutaneous tissue, exiting in the left periumbilical area. They are then passed through velour-covered Silastic percutaneous leads as they exit the patient's body. Exiting drivelines are subsequently attached to 7 feet of external driveline (Fig. 13-2), which are then connected to the Circulatory Support System (CSS) console (Fig. 13-3). The CSS is a semiportable unit, supplying pneumatic drive for the TAH. Compressed air is supplied from an independent air source via outlets in selected OR suites and patient rooms. The CSS also contains two high-pressure air tanks for backup and for patient transport. Each CSS contains two TAH controllers; one serves as primary controller and the other is a backup (Fig. 13-4). Adjustments for heart rate, systolic duration, left and right drive pressure, and a battery backup in the event of electrical power failure are contained within the controller. An alarm panel, with audible and visual alarms, alerts staff to alarm conditions such as loss of air, low cardiac output, and left/right output imbalance (Fig. 13-5).

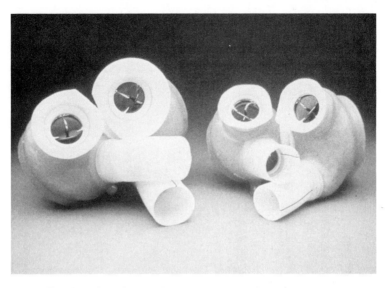

Fig. 13-1. Symbion J-7-70 and J-7-100 Total Artificial Hearts.

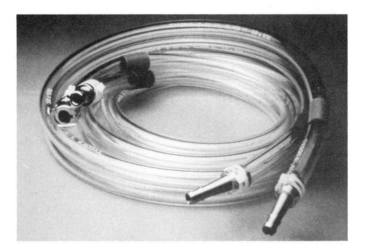

Fig. 13-2. External drivelines.

The CSS uses a COMPAQ dual drive PC that utilizes Cardiac Output Monitoring and Diagnostic Unit (COMDU) software to monitor TAH function. Two primary waveforms are monitored to assess ventricular filling and blood ejection from the ventricles. The first waveform is the COMDU diastolic flow curve (Fig. 13-6). This waveform is generated by air passing through two CSS Fleisch pneumotachometers. For each milliliter of blood entering the ventricles, 1 ml of air is forced through the pneumotach-

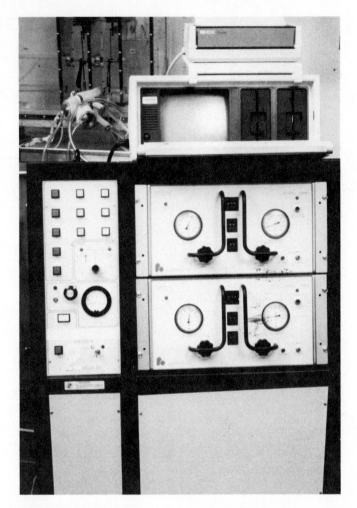

Fig. 13-3. Symbion Circulatory Support System.

ometers. The computer digitally converts an analog signal, which is displayed on the computer screen as airflow waveforms, to determine ventricular filling in liters per minute. The computer integrates area under the flow curve to determine filling volumes in milliliters, which is then multiplied by the heart rate to derive the cardiac output. This is done simultaneously for left and right ventricles. Device ejection is monitored by CSS pressure transducers, which generate drive pressure waveforms that are also displayed on the computer screen (Fig. 13-7). There are a number of features on the drive pressure waveform that must be observed to ensure proper ejection. The initial steep

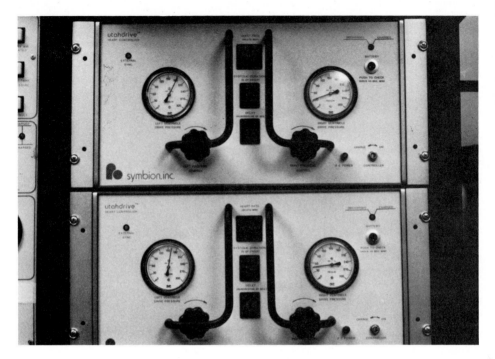

Fig. 13-4. Primary controller and backup controller.

upward portion of the waveform is time, during which air pressure increases to equal the diastolic pressure. As pressure becomes greater than end diastolic pressure, blood is ejected. This ejection phase is seen as the lesser sloped portion of the waveform. As diastole begins, a sudden downward slope occurs. The ejection point indicates full diaphragm excursion and full ejection of blood. The systolic/diastolic ratio of each cardiac cycle is regulated through the controller, utilizing a percent systole control.

TAH operation is based on a principle of "partial fill" and "full ejection."[6] Partial or incomplete filling allows the device to operate on the Starling Curve and requires much less drive parameter manipulation (Fig. 13-8). This can be seen in the following example, where there is a fixed rate but variable filling volume:

HR	Filling volume (cc)	CO (L/min)
100	55	5.5
100	65	6.5

Full ejection is the other TAH operating principle, which ensures that all blood entering the TAH is completely ejected during systole, allowing proper filling in diastole. Maintaining these two operating parameters makes the TAH very easy to manage and requires fewer drive system changes. Full ejection requires that the patient have adequate circulating volume and good vascular tone and integrity.

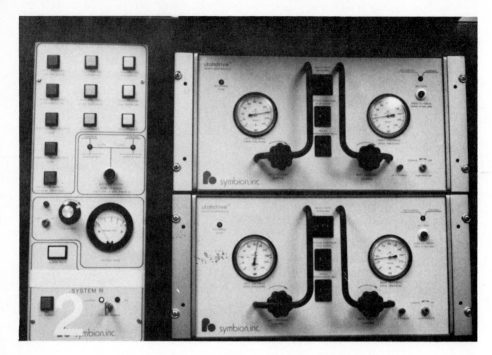

Fig. 13-5. Primary controller, backup controller, and alarm panel.

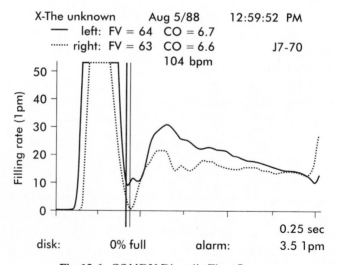

Fig. 13-6. COMDU Diastolic Flow Curve.

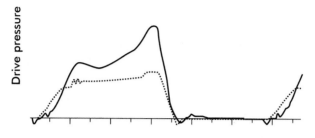

Aug 5/88   1:11:01 PM
—   left: FV = 63   CO = 6.7
······ right: FV = 62   CO = 6.5   J7-70
105 bpm

Fig. 13-7. Drive pressure waveform.

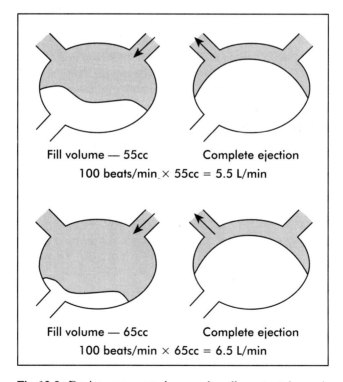

Fill volume — 55cc   Complete ejection
100 beats/min × 55cc = 5.5 L/min

Fill volume — 65cc   Complete ejection
100 beats/min × 65cc = 6.5 L/min

Fig. 13-8. Device response to increased cardiac output demand.

PATIENT SELECTION

The TAH is presently intended solely as a bridge-to-cardiac transplant; all patients considered for this device must meet each institution's transplant protocol. These absolute medical guidelines differ from institution to institution. TAH implantation can potentially reestablish renal perfusion and reverse acute renal failure secondary to low output syndrome. The most significant contraindication to implantation of the TAH is active infection. Mortality rates of implant patients with active infections are nearly 60%.[7] Other less invasive means of mechanical support, such as the biopump, rollerpump, or pneumatic ventricular assist devices should be considered in patients with documented infections.

POSTOPERATIVE DRIVE SYSTEM MANAGEMENT

Following excision of the native ventricles and TAH implantation, driver function is initiated. After air is aspirated from the left ventricular de-airing port and the external drivelines are attached to the controller, the left ventricular drive pressure (LDP) is set at 90 mm Hg, percent systole at 40, and heart rate at 40. The right ventricle is then aspirated, and right ventricular drive pressure (RDP) is set at 40 mm Hg. LDP is slowly increased to overcome the pressure generated by the cardiopulmonary bypass circuit. Extracorporeal flow is slowly reduced, and the heart rate, percent systole, and ventricular drive pressures are increased to maintain complete ejection. Adjustments in heart rate, percent systole, and left/right drive pressures are made, based on patients clinical assessment and monitoring of drive pressure and COMDU waveforms and data.

COMDU-recorded outputs that are above average suggest hypovolemia. Diuretic therapy and/or fluid restriction is the treatment of choice. Temporary increases in device heart rate can facilitate moving this excess volume. Left ventricular filling and cardiac output may also be controlled by decreasing the RDP to reduce the amount of blood going through the pulmonary bed to the left ventricle. Hypovolemia can exist if left/right complete ejection is present with lower than desired filling volumes. Volume replacement is the treatment of choice in this scenario. Ventricular filling and cardiac output can be increased by using vacuum applied to the console exhaust ports. A vacuum of 10 to 15 mm Hg reduces ventricular filling resistance and facilitates filling in hypovolemic states. Increasing diastolic filling time by reducing the percent systole can also increase ventricular filling and cardiac outputs. These temporary adjustments should be made until the underlying clinical problem (i.e., hypervolemia or hypovolemia) can be treated.

Systemic hypertension is recognized by loss of an ejection point on the drive pressure waveform, indicating incomplete ejection of left ventricle blood volume. This will lead to a significant decrease in cardiac output. Rapid and early filling will be displayed on the COMDU tracing. Increasing percent systole and/or drive pressure in an attempt to decrease left atrial pressure will reduce the possibility of pulmonary edema with persistent hypertension. The patient should be treated with antihypertensives to correct this problem. Pulmonary hypertension with resultant decrease in left cardiac output can be overcome by increasing RDP until pharmacological therapy can be introduced.

Because of the hemolytic nature of the TAH, care should be taken to reduce the degree of hemolysis as much as possible, thus avoiding frequent transfusions of blood.[8] This can be accomplished by keeping the dP/dt (the first derivative of pressure over time) as low as possible. The dP/dt is used to describe the natural ventricles[1] contractility and rate of change in pressure in circulatory assist devices. The TAH dP/dt is measured from the drivelines and is a determining factor in the rate at which blood is ejected. By decreasing heart rate, drive pressures can be lowered secondary to increased diastolic filling time. This can be further enhanced by adjusting the percent systole. Making these adjustments will lower the dP/dt and subsequently reduce the degree of hemolysis.

POTENTIAL COMPLICATIONS

Three complications have been observed in the TAH recipient population. The first is bleeding often observed in or around atrial cuff suture lines and great vessel grafts, especially the posterior side of the aortic graft. Bleeding can quickly lead to a tamponade, which could seriously affect device filling. Bleeding is manifested on the COMDU

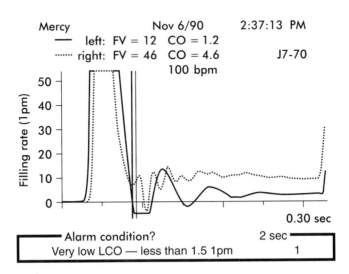

Fig. 13-9. Note lower filling volumes and cardiac output of left ventricle, indicating possible left atrial tamponade.

flow curve waveform as lower filling volumes, decreased filling rates, and possible left/right imbalance alarms (Fig. 13-9).

Infection is always a possibility because the periumbilical driveline exit interrupts the skin. Infectious organisms may develop in the mediastinal "dead space area" surrounding the TAH. The nonvascular TAH housing limits infection management by conventional modalities, often requiring a continuous irrigation solution with antibiotics flowing in the mediastinum to overcome potential life-threatening infections. Active infections involving the TAH often result in very high mortality.[7]

ANTICOAGULATION

Thromboembolism has become less of a complication presently than it was with the permanent implants because of a much better understanding of the anticoagulation requirements in these patients. There is a narrow margin between over-anticoagulation, with the risk of excessive bleeding, and undercoagulation, which may cause an embolic event. Anticoagulation is usually maintained by heparin infusion maintaining the PTT at 1.5 times to 2.0 times control. Persantine is administered to prevent platelet aggregation. For longer term support the patient can be switched to Coumadin. Patient volume status should also be monitored closely to prevent increases in blood viscosity. Platelets also require frequent measurement because there appears to be a correlation between platelets and an increase in embolic events.

Mechanical failures with this TAH have been rare. In Dr. Barney Clark a ventricular valve strut fractured, allowing the tilting disk to lodge in the left ventricle. Dr. Clark was returned to surgery to have the left ventricle replaced. Drive parameters were adjusted to successfully manage this particular failure. The valves were subsequently replaced with Medtronic-Hall valves without recurrence.[2,5] There have been reported cases of diaphragms sticking to ventricular housings, but this was corrected by the manufacturer without further incidents. This is a testament to the durable nature of the Symbion TAH.

PATIENT TRANSPORT

In most cases a minimum of four persons is required for patient transport. One person should be on each side of the driver with one hand on the bed rail and one hand on the console. A distance of 10 to 12 inches between the foot of the bed and the back of the console should be maintained. Careful attention should be given to the drivelines so that they are not pulled taut, kinked, or compressed. The other transporters guide the head of the bed and IV poles.

External air tanks and extension cords should be available if a long stay is anticipated where wall air is not available and power outlets are not in the vicinity. This will avoid using the reserve tanks and batteries. Before transporting the patient, the primary and reserve air tanks should be checked to make sure they are fully pressurized (4000 to 4500 psi). Each of the three battery test buttons should be pressed and held for 10 seconds to ensure the batteries are fully charged.

The console usually leaves the room first and is moved into the new area first. The air lines are connected to the external tanks, and AC power cords are connected to wall outlets. During transport, COMDU waveforms should be monitored to ensure that activities are not interfering with proper filling or ejection of the ventricles.

WEANING FROM THE TAH

When a suitable donor has been found for the TAH patient, the patient is returned to the surgery suite. After being placed on cardiopulmonary bypass, flow is reduced through the TAH until the patient is being supported totally by the CPB circuit. At this time the TAH is removed and the remnant atria, aorta, and pulmonary artery are prepared for implantation of the donor heart. The TAH is gently rinsed with saline and inspected closely for thrombus formation and any defects. The TAH is placed in a formaldehyde/formalin solution to be returned to the manufacturer for closer inspection.

NURSING MANAGEMENT

Assessment of the TAH patient is similar to other open heart patients with exceptions:

1. There are no ECG rhythms to monitor as both native ventricles are excised. P-waves may be observed since recipient atria are left in situ.
2. TAH prosthetic components may make lung auscultation difficult.
3. Swan-Ganz catheters cannot be used in this setting secondary to the mechanical

Table 13-1.   Nursing diagnosis of the TAH patient

Diagnoses	Related to
Alteration in cardiac output	Difficult positioning of TAH during surgery, impeding good filling of device, decreased circulating volume
Impairment of skin integrity	Exiting of drivelines from periumbilical area
Alteration in tissue perfusion	Decreased cardiac output, hypovolemia, and hypotension
High risk for infection	Exiting of drivelines from periumbilical area, nonbiologic surfaces inside device, invasive lines
Alteration in comfort	Exiting of drivelines from left periumbilical area
Impaired physical mobility	Drivelines and large console, need for air source
Disturbance in self-concept, body image	Excision of native ventricles and implantation of TAH, attachment to console via drivelines

Table 13-2. Circulatory support system flowsheet

SYSTEMS CHECKS°

1. Batteries: Primary driver
   Backup driver
   System power/alarm
2. Alarms: (audible and visual)
3. Key in backup driver
4. Air supply (wall, primary, reserve)
5. Backup driver set
6. Check paper in printers
7. % Full of data disk
8. Data and plot storage intervals check

Date	Time	System checks °	PSI		Drive pressures		Heart rate	% Systole	Delay	Vacuum	LCO/RCO	Sync mode	Comments	Initials
			Primary	Reserve / Wall pressure	Left	Right								

Systems checks "q" shift

valves in the TAH. Swan-Ganz catheters make these valves significantly more regurgitant when used with the TAH. Left atrial pressure, right atrial pressure, and pulmonary artery pressure lines can be inserted but are not recommended. The insertion sites of these lines can become areas of bleeding when removed before TAH explantation, especially when the patient is anticoagulated.

4. Filling pressures and volume status can be determined by observing the COMDU filling waveforms, which will indicate a high, normal, or low rate of filling (in liters per minute).
5. Driveline exit sites must be observed closely for evidence of infection.
6. Strict aseptic technique should be used for dressing changes.
7. Cardiac transplant isolation procedures should be implemented.
8. Indwelling catheters should be removed as soon as possible.
9. Early mobilization is recommended to increase physical recovery and psychological well-being.
10. Sudden positional changes should be avoided because these patients seem to be more prone to postural hypotension.
11. Avoid kinking or stressing drivelines.

Nursing diagnoses are outlined in Table 13-1. Circulatory Support System documentation is shown in Table 13-2.

PATIENT/FAMILY PSYCHOSOCIAL ISSUES

Many patients and families are intimidated by the "high tech" nature of the device and monitoring equipment. This requires nursing staff to encourage the patient and family to verbalize their concerns and questions relating to the TAH and support equipment. Nursing staff should use strategies to promote emotional and psychological adaptation for the patient and family. Interventions include answering questions in clear simple terms, providing explanations for procedures and equipment, and updating the patient's condition. Encouraging frequent family visits may alleviate anxiety. Primary nursing with continuity of care can establish a comfortable relationship between staff, patient, and family.

CONCLUSION

The Symbion TAH at present is not used for permanent implantation. Totally implantable hearts may be necessary to obtain success with long-term support. Devices requiring external power sources may not be acceptable secondary to infection and lack of mobility. As a bridge to transplant, the TAH has proven very effective. However, even with short-term support, the bridge to transplant patient is susceptible to infection. Future research should be directed toward the totally implantable artificial heart to meet the demands of an increasing recipient population and a declining donor pool.

REFERENCES

1. Cooley DA, Liotta D, Hallman GL et al: First human implantation of cardiac prothesis for staged total replacement of the heart, *Trans Am Soc Artif Intern Organs* 15:252, 1969.
2. DeVries WC, Anderson JL, Joyce LD et al: Initial human application of the Utah total artificial heart, *N Engl J Med* 310:273, 1984.
3. DeVries, WC: The permanent artificial heart, *JAMA* 259:849, 1988.
4. Joyce LD et al: Results of the first 100 patients who received Symbion total artificial hearts as a bridge to cardiac transplantation, *Circulation* 80(III):192, 1989.
5. DeVries WC, Joyce LD: The artificial heart, *Clin Symp* 35:(6), 1983.
6. Mays B, Williams M, Barker L et al: Diagnostic monitoring and drive system management of patients with total artificial heart, *Heart and Lung* 15:466, September 1986.
7. Kunin CM, Dobbins JJ, Melo JC et al: Infectious complications in four long-term recipients of the Jarvik-7 artificial heart, *JAMA* 259:860, 1988.
8. Levinson MM et al: Indexes of hemolysis in human recipients of the Jarvik-7 total artificial heart: a cooperative report of fifteen patients. *J Heart Transplant* 5:236, 1986.

CHAPTER 14

Total artificial heart development at the University of Utah

The Utah-100 and electrohydraulic cardiac replacement devices

R. Keith White, George M. Pantalos, and **Don B. Olsen**

INTRODUCTION

Of the 2.5 million patients with chronic heart failure, more than 600,000 deaths occur annually in the United States secondary to the complications of coronary atherosclerosis.[1] In 1987 approximately 300,000 coronary revascularization procedures and 1400 cardiac transplants were performed in this country to treat the sequelae of coronary occlusion and other primary myocardial diseases.[2,3] Cardiac transplantation could theoretically benefit approximately 15,000 patients; however, a limitation of available donor organs usually restricts this mode of therapy to less than 2000 patients per year in this nation.[4] The National Institutes of Health and the Heart Failure Study Group estimate that cardiac assist or replacement devices could treat between 35,000 and 165,000 patients per year in the United States alone and several thousand more worldwide. Research and development at several centers throughout the world are ongoing to produce models that will minimize the devastating complications previously associated with earlier cardiac replacement devices. Although the current trend may seem to be directed primarily toward cardiac assistance as a bridge to transplantation and for the patient with postcardiotomy shock, devices that totally replace the diseased native heart and provide a comfortable existence for at least 2 years are undergoing intense testing in the animal model in four major research centers in the United States. Cardiac assistance and replacement should not be thought of as two disparate ideologies in the realm of cardiovascular support but rather as two methods by which the patient may eventually achieve independence. At this institution we are currently in the advanced stages of development of both a pneumatic total artificial heart (Utah-100) and an electrohydraulic total artificial heart (EHTAH) that may be implanted for temporary or chronic circulatory support.

PATIENT SELECTION FOR TAH IMPLANTATION

The decision to implant a device for cardiac assistance or replacement is usually made when all medical and most other surgical alternatives have been exhausted. The patient typically has not been able to maintain an acceptable cardiac output or systemic perfusion pressure either while being weaned from cardiopulmonary bypass (after surgical treatment of acquired or congenital heart disease) or while waiting for a suitable heart for orthotopic transplantation. Rigid guidelines have not been presented that currently define the best candidates for total cardiac replacement; however, data from large groups of patients with end-stage cardiac disease that have been implanted with either ventricular assist devices (VAD) or the TAH as a bridge to transplantation reveal that failure to implant the device before multisystem organ dysfunction worsens the final outcome. Those with postcardiotomy heart failure, who are often elderly or undergoing "redo" procedures, are accounting for an increasingly larger proportion of patients requiring temporary VAD or TAH assistance. Maximal inotropic support consisting of sympathomimetic drugs such as dopamine, dobutamine, epinephrine, or others such as the phosphodiesterase inhibitors (amrinone, enoximone) along with afterload reducing agents have usually been administered before or in conjunction with insertion of the intraaortic balloon pump (IABP). Augmentation of the cardiac output occurs in most instances with these conventional methods; however, if the heart failure persists (in the absence of surgically correctable lesions such as pericardial tamponade, ventricular septal rupture, valvular dysfunction) and no hope for myocardial recovery exists, TAH implantation should be contemplated if the patient meets all the requirements for cardiac transplantation. Great need for such a TAH exists since the only device that was approved by the Food and Drug Administration (FDA) for total cardiac replacement as a bridge to transplantation is no longer available for implantation.

Cardiogenic shock that is refractory to treatment with the previously mentioned pharmaceutical agents and the IABP is currently the most reported indication for ventricular support or replacement, and only recently have specific cardiovascular parameters been discussed especially for this reason (see box on p. 183). The decision to proceed to total cardiac replacement with the TAH, instead of employing uni- or biventricular assist devices is often difficult.[5] TAH implantation should be employed when there is severe biventricular failure that is resistant to all pharmacological adjuncts and IABP therapy, while avoiding certain complications as outlined by Griffith[6]: (1) presence of active infection, (2) previous median sternotomy, (3) age > 60 years, (4) evidence of preformed antibodies to human lymphocyte antigen (percent reactive antibody > 20), (5) established acute tubular necrosis, (6) unresponsive or comatose patient, and (7) small size or weight of the patient.

At this institution a worldwide registry of TAH recipients is updated routinely; its recent report is summarized in Table 14-1. Of the different devices, 11 have been implanted in 225 patients, and except for 5 patients who received the device for attempted long-term support, all of the remaining patients were implanted with the

```
_____ CRITERIA FOR CARDIOGENIC SHOCK _____

Cardiac index < 2.0 L/m²/min
Systemic vascular resistance > 2100 dynes/sec/cm⁵
Atrial pressure > 20 mm HG
Urine output < 20 cc/hr with:
    Optimal preload
    Maximal drug therapy
    Corrected metabolism
    Intraaortic balloon pump
```

Within the box, the equations render as:

$$\text{Cardiac index} < 2.0 \text{ L/m}^2/\text{min}$$
$$\text{Systemic vascular resistance} > 2100 \text{ dynes/sec/cm}^5$$
$$\text{Atrial pressure} > 20 \text{ mm HG}$$
$$\text{Urine output} < 20 \text{ cc/hr with:}$$

Table 14-1.   Human orthotopic total artificial heart implantations (April 1969 to March 1991)

Device	Patients	Transplanted (TX)	Alive	% TX	% TX/living
Liota	1	1	0	100	0
Akutso	1	1	0	100	0
Jarvik-7	44	26	11	59	35
Jarvik-7-70	146	107	46	73	43
Penn State	2	1	0	50	0
Phoenix	1	1	0	100	0
Berlin	6	2	0	33	0
Unger	6	5	1	83	20
BRNO	3	0	0	0	0
Poisk	13	0	0	0	0
Small Vienna	2	2	1	100	50
TOTAL					
11 devices	225	146	59	65	40

TAH as a bridge to transplantation. All devices were pneumatically driven and consisted of two implantable pumps with elastomer blood sacs housed within a biocompatible rigid casting. Pulsatile flow was delivered to the pulmonary and systemic circulations by contracting blood diaphragms within the TAH, which were powered by compressed air delivered by transcutaneous low compliance lines. Of the patients implanted with the Jarvik-7-70 TAH, 73% eventually proceeded to orthotopic cardiac transplantation with a 43% survival rate. These patients would have otherwise died because of the immediate unavailability of a donor heart.

REQUIREMENTS FOR THE CARDIAC PROSTHESIS

Advancements in surface-tissue interaction, implantation, and durability of the artificial ventricle are by no means complete; however, new steps toward achieving the total implantation of a cardiac replacement device and support system that will, it is hoped, allow the device to be employed for long-term use are underway. Since Kolff's first model of the TAH in 1959, experience from previous attempts at permanent cardiac replacement and 20 years of use of the TAH as a temporary bridge to transplantation have shown that certain requirements must be fulfilled by the future totally implantable models.[8,10]

The device must be totally implantable in the future, must fit into the chest with a minimum of dead space, and should not disturb adjoining mediastinal structures. Implantation and removal must be relatively easy, especially if the device requires emergent replacement or if implantation of a donor heart is required. The prosthesis must be reliable for at least 2 years and must be physiologically responsive. An acceptable quality of life must be afforded the patient and should include autonomy from the hospital. Medical intervention should be infrequent and the device should be equipped with diagnostics and controllers for normal range of function. The system should be relatively affordable, with recipient and attendee training easily taught and learned. Soft failures of the device should not endanger the life of the recipient and diagnostics should alert the patient of the problem.

The electric-powered TAH that is currently being developed at four research centers in the United States, under the auspices of the National Institutes of Health, has been engineered to satisfy many of the above requirements. Unfortunately, all foreign material implanted into the body, especially with blood-contacting surfaces, will harbor the possible consequences of sepsis and thromboembolism. It is hoped total implantability of the device (without percutaneous drive lines) will minimize the infectious complications, as it has for other medical hardware (e.g., arteriovenous fistulas for hemodialysis access and pacemakers). Coating the blood-contacting surfaces with different biocompatible materials that impede the formation of clot and pseudoneointima has been an ongoing enigma in research for several decades and may in the future minimize the complications of peripheral thromboembolization.

THE UNIVERSITY OF UTAH'S ELECTROHYDRAULIC TAH
Systems development

Since 1988, at the University of Utah Artificial Heart Research Laboratory, an electrohydraulic total artificial heart (EHTAH) has been conceptualized, fabricated, and is currently undergoing intense in vivo testing. The current design began with the initial iteration, the EHTAH 10 series, which was employed for in vitro mock circulation testing and acute animal implantation for evaluation of energy converters, pressure transducers, and methods to achieve right and left heart balance in the TAH. The EHTAH 40 model will be a totally implantable TAH, complete with a transcutaneous energy transmission system (TET), and is scheduled for completion by 1993. The EHTAH system is based on three subsystems interconnected in structure and function: (1) blood

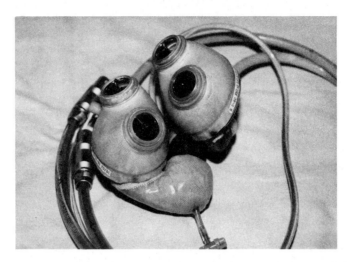

Fig. 14-1. University of Utah electrohydraulic total artificial heart model 20.

pump subsystem, (2) energy converter subsystem, and (3) the power, control, communication, and monitoring (PCCM) subsystem. Chronic in vivo animal implantation experiments have been conducted with the EHTAH 20 system (Fig. 14-1), which is a partially implantable model; production of prototypes for the next iteration is currently underway.

Blood pump design

Seamless polyurethane (Biomer, Ethicon, Inc., Somerville, NJ) is employed for the ventricular housing; this and the multilayered flexible diaphragms have a record of excellent results in both durability and performance. The ellipsoid right and left ventricles have a static stroke volume of approximately 70 ml and are somewhat smaller than the earlier models to reduce dead space from the housing, to allow the placement of pressure transducers on the ventricular base, and to simplify implantation. Inflow and outflow connectors for arterial grafts and atrial cuffs house Medtronic-Hall pyrolytic carbon-suspended disk valves (Medtronic, Minneapolis, Minn.). Screw-type connectors are employed to attach the ventricles to the atrial cuffs.

It has been well established that the net output from the right side of the TAH exceeds that of the left, and several mechanisms have been described to define this flow discrepancy.[11,12] Volume-displacement chambers, regurgitant pulmonic valves, and disproportionately sized left and right ventricles have been used to establish balance between the two ventricles, with equivocal results.[13,14] We have reported on excellent in vitro and in vivo results with the use of an interatrial shunt (IAS) created between the atrial cuffs of the TAH to maintain ventricular flow balance over a wide range of preload and afterload conditions.[15–17] This shunt has been modified in the EHTAH 20 by machine forming a 3 ml to 5 ml circular defect in the artificial interatrial septum of the atrial cuffs, thus obviating the need for a tubular conduit.

Energy converter design

A single energy converter, which is a three phase Hall-effect brushless, direct-current motor with fixed stators and a bladed rotor fixed to the motor shaft as an axial flow pump, is interposed between the two pumping chambers. Pure monomer reagent grade decamethyltetrasiloxane oil of low viscosity acts as the hydraulic fluid and actuates the diaphragm of the ventricle. Reversal of the motor changes the direction of the hydraulic fluid and initiates a different phase of the cardiac cycle in each of the ventricles. The maximum cardiac output of our current energy converters has been approximately 7.7 L/min.

PCCM design

The physiological control of the EHTAH 20 is based on a previously developed system at this institution for a volumetric and rate-coupled prosthesis. A full-stroke volume, variable heart rate control algorithm that has been extensively tested in vitro and in animals is employed.[18,19] Two pressure transducers located on the hydraulic fluid side of each ventricular base provide sensory information for a closed loop feedback system.[20] These transducers will serve as an indicator of full ejection of blood from the respective ventricle. At the end of systole, the diaphragm is distended and the hydaulic pressure in the ventricular base rises rapidly. The control system responds to a predetermined pressure level and after being reached signals full ejection; diastole is then initiated. The transducers will also serve as an indicator of desired heart rate. During the diastole of each ventricle, the mean filling pressure is monitored and compared with a preset value. If the mean pressure is greater or less than the preset value, the motor speed is increased or diminished by a fixed amount of 200 RPM. The pressure at end diastole is maintained at −6 mm HG, which has been found to augment ventricular filling. This control produces a Starling response as the TAH responds to varying amounts of venous return by altering its cardiac output accordingly.[16,21,22] The physiological controller also is supported by internal and external controllers. The internal controller software monitors the input of the pressure waveforms and data sent from the external controller with its output directed to the energy converter. The external controller is currently an IBM PC–compatible laptop computer that sends and receives information to and from the internal controller. Parameters that can be modified vary, depending on the internal controller setting (automatic or manual).

The TET, telemetry, and battery design are currently undergoing development and production. The peak efficiency of the TET system is approximately 85%, with peak power capability of 25 watts. The telemetry system can operate at 4800 baud; however, at this point it is very sensitive to noise. The internal battery delivers 10 watts for about 1 hour at 12 volts nominal and the external battery delivers 21 watts for approximately 3.5 hours at 12 volts nominal.

In vivo animal implantation results

At this time, seven animal implants have been performed employing the EHTAH 20 model, with a survival of 1 to 9 days. Valuable data have been gathered on size constraints of the prosthesis, right-to-left ventricular flow balance, and blood flow characteristics. Cardiac output was severely limited from the device in the early experiments secondary to thoracic cavity volume to implant size mismatch. Impingement of the device on the pliable vena cavae of the calf restricted venous inflow into the atria and thus limited cardiac output. Animals with mass greater than 90 kg allowed easier implantation of the TAH without crowding vital mediastinal structures and resulted in an 115% increase in the cardiac output.

Ventricular flow imbalance noted in the bovine model is due to a variable anatomic left-to-left shunt, resulting from bronchial blood flow (BBF) returning to the left atrium.[23] The IAS that is earlier described performed well and adequately maintained interventricular flow balance and physiologic pressure gradients between the right and left atria. Since the BBF is extremely variable in this species (2% to 25%), its volume, compared with the cardiac output, must be formulated intraoperatively, and the atrial cuffs containing the correctly sized IAS should be implanted to ensure good balance.[24,25] No thrombosis or obstruction of the IAS has been documented, and no intraventricular clot has been noted. The EHTAH 30 model will be a more streamlined version of the 20 system to alleviate the size constraints of the device without sacrificing cardiac output.

THE UTAH-100 PNEUMATIC TAH

Systems development

The Utah-100 TAH has been under development and testing at the Artificial Heart Research Laboratory for over 8 years and is currently under evaluation by the FDA for an investigational device exemption to be used as a mechanical bridge to transplantation. There has been one previously approved human implantation of a permanent TAH at the University of Utah, in 1982, and since that time this institution has designed, developed, and fabricated an elliptical TAH with a 100 stroke volume that would more easily fit into the thoracic cavity of a recipient than the Jarvik-7 TAH.[26] Although experience with centrifugal blood pumps for patients who require circulatory support postcardiotomy and before transplantation has been gained over the last decade at the University of Utah, no total artificial heart has been used, and currently a TAH is not available for this indication. The Utah-100 with its relatively small size and larger stroke volume, and its rigorous reliability and performance testing, may in the future fill this void.

Device description

The Utah-100 is designed to have a dynamic stroke volume of approximately 100 ml. Each ventricle has a modified cylindrical shape that is 9.5 cm long, 6.5 cm wide,

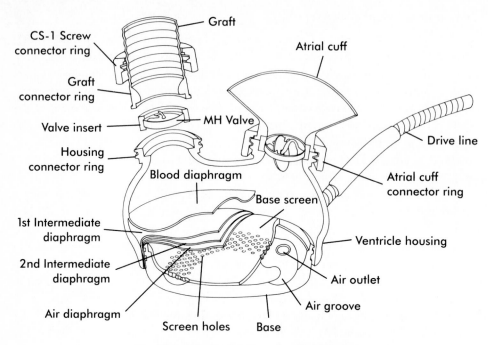

Fig. 14-2. The Utah-100 total artificial heart.

and 5.5 cm high (Fig. 14-2). The cylindrical shape is chosen to improve the fit inside the cardiac cavity that remains when the natural ventricles have been removed. Ports accommodating the Medtronic-Hall tilting disk inflow and outflow prosthetic valves are located on the top of the blood chamber housing. A size 27 mm mitral valve is employed in the inflow position and a size 25 mm aortic valve is used in the outflow position.

A precision machined connector is incorporated in the inflow and outflow port to permit easy and reliable connection of the atrial sewing cuffs and outflow grafts to the TAH. Since thrombus formation near the native tissue-connector interface has been a problem in the past, a connector system has been produced that has a continuous, smooth surface contour that eliminates gaps and has reduced the incidence of thrombus formation (verified by direct observation of retrieved artificial ventricles after animal implantation).[27] These connectors can also be rotated during implantation, which allows for greater maneuverability of the cuffs during suturing and connection. Likewise, if it becomes necessary to replace a ventricle or valve, this task does not require placement of any additional sutures.

The pumping mechanism of the Utah-100 is a multilayer flexing diaphragm system made of solution cast Biomer. The blood-contacting surface is cast into the chamber housing to provide a continuous surface without thrombogenic seams as blood flows into the ventricle. Three other diaphragms (two intermediate and one air-contacting diaphragm) are separately solution-casted and incorporated into the blood chamber housing at the time of ventricle assembly. Between each diaphragm is a thin layer of powered graphite lubricant.

A rigid base is attached to the circumference of the blood chamber housing assembly where the pneumatic driveline exits. Machined to the base is a screen system that allows for rapid exhaust of air from beneath the diaphragm system as blood enters the ventricle. This screen acts to prevent blockage of the driveline that allows an unimpeded exhaust of air to promote ventricular filling and also to limit the lower excursion point of the diaphragm during filling.

An inverted conical sewing cuff made of solution-casted Biomer is trimmed and sewn to the native atrial remnant. Woven Dacron vascular graft material (30 mm) is employed as the pulmonary artery and aortic outflow conduits.

Heart controller and monitor

The System II Utah Drive console is used to control and monitor the Utah-100 TAH and consists of a primary and backup Utah Heart Drive controller. Each controller has an independently set pressurization control to inflate the left and right ventricle of the artificial heart at a rate of approximately 2500 mm Hg/sec. Heart rate and percent systole are set by thumb switches. Each controller is equipped with a set of batteries that can provide up to 90 hours of function; the console is similarly suited to provide up to 45 minutes of diagnostic unit function in the event of a power loss.

The output of the artificial heart is determined with the cardiac output monitor and diagnostic unit (COMDU) that displays the filling wave form of each ventricle during diastole. A computer calculates the volume of blood that has entered the ventricle, makes a correction for valve regurgitant losses, multiplies the stroke volume by the heart rate, and gives a determination of the cardiac output.[28] The computer displays this information every third heart beat and summarizes the last 2 hours of cardiac function on a separate screen. The console also contains a panel of warning lights that indicate inadequate right and left driveline pressures, low or imbalanced cardiac outputs, and inadequate pressure sources. A vacuum pump is also integrated into the console to make it possible to augment filling of the prosthetic ventricles by applying diastolic vacuum through the drivelines when desired.

Utah-100 in vitro and animal performance testing

Pumping function and durability of the Utah-100 heart has been determined during several years of in vitro testing by placing the devices, along with the clinical console, on mock circulation test beds. Ventricular function curves from this extensive testing revealed that this TAH showed a Starling response to increased atrial filling pressures and that there was acceptable agreement between the COMDU and turbine flow cardiac output values. Durability data on Utah-100 ventricles were obtained from mock

Table 14-2.   UTAH 100 total artificial heart animal implantation record

Experiment number	Animal name	Species	TAH design	Implant wt (kg)	Days survived	Reason for termination
PH86C012	Domingo	Calf	UTAH 100	85	18	Died
PH86S002	Kellog	Sheep	UTAH 100	80	331	Died
PH86C029	Christian	Sheep	UTAH 100	55	106	Elective
PH86C039	Daniel	Calf	UTAH 100	70	94	Elective
PH86C049	Lucio	Calf	UTAH 100	62	1	Died
PH86C086	Phillippe	Calf	UTAH 100	73	109	Elective
PH86C098	Denton	Calf	UTAH 100	77	202	Elective
PH87C022	Norman	Calf	UTAH 100	82	19	Died
PH87C016	Sandy	Calf	UTAH 100	125	11	Elective
PH87C038	Hilda	Calf	UTAH 100	86	22	Elective
PH87C047	Tammy Fae	Calf	UTAH 100	85	26	Elective
PH87C067	Macbeth	Calf	UTAH 100	86	121	Elective
PH87S001	Wallace	Sheep	UTAH 100	102	22	Died
PH88C006	Pokey	Calf	UTAH 100	93	9	Died
PH88C007	Regulus	Calf	UTAH 100	98	97	Elective
PH88S001	Sparky	Sheep	UTAH 100	131	21	Elective
PH88C017	'57 Chevy	Calf	UTAH 100	62	6	Died
PH88C026	Screw Loose	Calf	UTAH 100	85	50	Died
PH88C027	Dave's Hernia	Calf	UTAH 100	88	25	Died
PH89C002	Alchemist	Calf	UTAH 100	78	17	Died
PH89C012	Coquette	Calf	UTAH 100	70	<1	Died
PH89C013	Easy	Calf	UTAH 100	54	143	Died
PH89C022	Cold Fusion	Calf	UTAH 100	95	<1	Died
PH89C021	Deuterium	Calf	UTAH 100	92	60	Elective
PH89C022	Paladium Rod	Calf	UTAH 100	93	145	Elective

Cumulative animal experience with final animal version = 1657 animal days (4.5 years)
Mean duration = 66 ± 79 days   Range = <1 day to 331 days
10 animals ≥ 60 days with final clinical version

PH89C026	Uno	Calf	UTAH 100	80	127	Died
PH89C029	Shabash	Calf	UTAH 100	92	183	Elective
PH89C033	Bilbo	Calf	UTAH 100	78	317	Elective
PH89C034	Shakespeare	Calf	UTAH 100	78	65	Died
PH90C015	Longfellow	Calf	UTAH 100	80	21	Elective
PH90C019	Yoho	Calf	UTAH 100	66	39	Elective

Cumulative animal experience with final animal version = 2409 animal days (6.6 years)
Mean duration = 78 ± 87 days   Range = <1 day to 331 days
14 animals ≥ 60 days with final clinical version

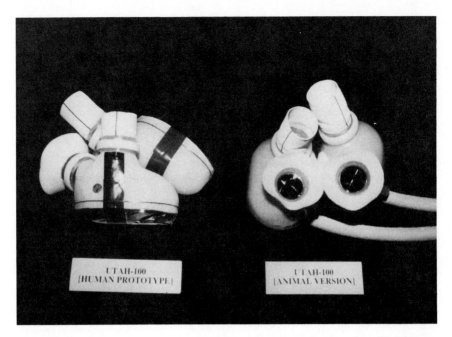

Fig. 14-3. Human and animal versions of the pneumatic Utah-100 total artificial heart.

circulation testing and by chronic animal implants. A minimum time to failure of nearly 1 year or more was achieved for all ventricles tested that failed.

Calves and adult sheep were used for a total of 31 implantations with the final animal version of the Utah-100 TAH. These animals were selected based on their appropriate size, cardiac output requirements, and anatomic similarity to adult humans, along with their ability to withstand open-heart surgery with long-term recovery for device evaluation. As can be shown (Table 14-2), several years of experience with animal implants has been afforded this device. The in vivo durability testing revealed that 2409 animal days (6.6 years) of pumping were performed with the Utah-100 TAH without evidence of catastrophic mechanical failure of the valves or pumping diaphragms.

Five cadaveric and 13 transplant intraoperative human fit trials have also been performed to test the human version of the Utah-100 because differences in orientation of the atria and great vessels do exist between the two species (Fig. 14-3). These trials reveal that both Utah-100 ventricles can fit comfortably into the pericardial space of humans as small as approximately 60 kg without compression of vital structures.

CONCLUSION

No clinical version of a total artificial heart is currently available for use as a bridge to transplantation or for chronic use. Research and development continues in major centers to produce a device that can be reliably employed as a totally implantable cardiac prosthesis to support the recipient comfortably for years. Likewise, a device more suited for short-term implantation that can sustain adequate perfusion after severe biventricular failure is also needed. Continued progress in both previously described devices may someday alleviate these needs.

REFERENCES

1. Spencer FC, Sabiston DL, eds: *Bypass grafting for coronary artery disease.* In Spencer FC, Sabiston DL, eds: *Surgery of the chest,* Philadelphia, 1990, WB Saunders Company.
2. Califf RM, Harrell FE, Lee KL: The evolution of medical and surgical therapy for coronary artery disease, *Ann Thorac Surg* 37:412, 1984.
3. Gay WA, O'Connell JB: *Cardiac transplantation.* In Spencer FC, Sabiston CL, eds: *Surgery of the chest,* Philadelphia, 1990, WB Saunders Company.
4. Evans RM, Maier AM: Outcome of patients referred for cardiac transplantation, *J Am Coll Cardiol* 8:1312, 1986.
5. Pennington GD, Joyce LD, Pae WE et al: Patient selection, *Ann Thorac Surg* 47:77, 1989.
6. Griffith BP: Interim use of the Jarvik-7 artificial heart: lessons learned at Presbyterian-University Hospital of Pittsburgh, *Ann Thorac Surg* 47:158, 1989.
7. Olsen DB: Registry and tabulations of orthotopic total artificial hearts in man. Personal communication.
8. Kolff WJ, Akutsu T, Dryess B: Artificial hearts in the chest and the use of polyurethane for making hearts, valves, and aortas, *Trans Am Soc Artif Intern Organs* 5:298, 1959.
9. Ghosh PK: *Precedents and perspectives.* In Unger F, ed: *Assisted circulation 3,* Berlin, 1989, Springer-Verlag.
10. Hahn C: Replacement of the heart, *Heart Transplant* 4:494, 1985.
11. Nabel HJ, Schmitz KP, Urbaszek W et al: Relationship between design and control of the artificial heart for protection of the right/left imbalance, *Intern J Artif Organs* 13:51, 1990.
12. Olsen DB, Butler M, Morgan D et al: Factors influencing right to left ventricular filling volumes, *Am Soc Artif Intern Organs* 15:10, 1986 (abstract).
13. Weiss WJ, Rosenberg G, Snyder AJ et al: In vivo performance of a transcutaneous energy transmission system with the Penn State motor driven ventricular assist device, *Trans Am Soc Artif Intern Organs* 35:284, 1989.
14. Jarvik RK: The total artificial heart, *Sci Am* 244:66, 1981.
15. Crump KR, Khanwilkar PS, Long JW et al: In vitro analysis of an atrial shunt in balancing an electrohydraulic total artificial heart, *Am Soc Artif Inter Organs* 20:7, 1990 (abstract).
16. Olsen DB, Long JW: Simplified right to left balance for the implanted artificial heart. In Tetsuyo A, ed: *Artificial Heart,* Tokyo, 1990, Springer-Verlag.
17. Olsen DB, White RK, Long JW et al: Right-left ventricular output balance in the totally implantable artificial heart, *Intern J of Artif Organs* 14:359, 1991.
18. Lioi AP, Olsen DB: *Physiologic control of the electric total artificial heart,* Final Report NIH Grant No.2r01-HL-24388, Devices and Technology Branch, National Heart, Lung, and Blood Institute of the National Institutes of Health.
19. Jarvik RK, Isaacson MS, Nielsen DB: Toward a portable human total artificial heart utilizing a miniature electrohydraulic energy converter, *J Artif Organs* 3:320, 1979.
20. Khanwilkar PS, Crump KR, Bearnson GB et al: Development of the physiologic control scheme for an electrohydraulic total artificial heart. Proceedings of the Annual International Conference of the IEEE. *Engineering in Medicine and Biology Society* 11:149, 1989.
21. Lioi AP, Orth JL, Crump KR et al: In vitro development of automatic control for the actively filled electrohydraulic heart, *Artif Organs* 12:152, 1988.
22. Guyton AC, Jones CE, Coleman TC: Circulatory physiology. In Guyton AC, ed: *Cardiac output and its regulation,* Philadelphia, 1973, WB Saunders.

23. Nakajura M, Fujimasa I, Imachi K: Left and right cardiac output differences in the artificial heart under right output in the physiologic range, *Jpn J Artif Organs* 13:146, 1984.
24. White RK, Bliss RS, Everett SD et al: Comparison of microsphere and intraoperative quantitation of bronchial blood flow, *Trans Am Soc of Artif Int Organs* 37:M507, 1991.
25. Kinoshita Y, Hansen C, Khanwilkar PS et al: Determination of atrial shunt size to balance the electro-hydraulic total artificial heart, *Trans Am Soc of Artif Inter Organs* 37:M264, 1991.
26. Taenaka Y, Olsen DB, Murray KD et al: *Development of an elliptical total artificial heart for smaller-sized recipients.* In Nosé Y, Kjellstrand C, Ivanovich P (eds): *Progress in artificial organs—1985,* Cleveland, 1986, ISAO Press.
27. Holfert JW, Riebman JB, Dew PA et al: A new connector system for total artificial hearts—preliminary results, *Am Soc Artif Int Organs* 10:151, 1987.
28. Willshaw P, Nielsen SD, Nanas J et al: A cardiac output monitor and diagnostic unit for pneumatically driven artificial hearts, *Artif Organs* 8:215, 1984.
29. Murray KD, Olsen DB: The use of calves and sheep as total artificial heart recipients, *Am Soc Artif Int Organs* 8:128, 1985.

CHAPTER 15

Clinical application of ventricular assist devices in Japan

Kazuhiko Atsumi, Iwao Fujimasa, Kou Imachi,
and **Yukiyasu Sezai**

INTRODUCTION

In 1959 research and development on the total artificial heart (TAH) was started in the University of Tokyo. Many kinds of blood pumps, driving mechanisms, sensors, and control systems have been constructed and tested in the mock circulatory models and also in the animal experiments. Since 1970 pneumatic units with sac type blood pumps have been used as the most convenient system for TAH animal experiments. After many years' experience using various animals, such as dogs, calves, and sheep, the goat has been selected as the most appropriate one and has been used in most of our animal experiments since 1971. In 1984 the longest survival (344 days) of a TAH goat was obtained in our laboratory by use of the pneumatic unit.

In 1980 the sac-type blood pump was modified and the pneumatic driving unit was miniaturized, and both were used for clinical cases of left and/or right ventricular assist devices (VAD).

In the National Cardiovascular Center (NCVC), the VAD system of diaphragm-type blood pump with pneumatic driving unit was developed and used clinically in 1984. The diaphragm-type of blood pump of Tomas Technical Laboratory was developed and applied clinically. The Pierce–Danathy blood pump was also used in clinical cases.

These VAD systems are pulsatile type; nonpulsatile pumps have also been used in clinical cases in Japan.

Japanese clinical experiences utilizing the pulsatile VAD are discussed in this chapter.

CLINICAL APPLICATION OF CARDIAC VENTRICULAR ASSIST DEVICES (VAD)

The first clinical case of VAD

In June 1980 the first clinical case of VAD using a pulsatile pump was performed at Mitsui Hospital in cooperation with our laboratory at the University of Tokyo. The patient suffered from cardiogenic shock caused by myocardial infarction after double-valve replacement surgery; cardiac assist was carried out for the patient by venoarterial pumping (VAP) and intraaortic balloon pumping (IABP). In spite of the cardiac assist, the circulatory condition of the patient did not improve, and biventricular assist was attempted and carried out. A diagram of the biventricular cannulation is shown in Fig. 15-1. The blood pumps are connected from the left atrium to the ascending aorta in the left heart bypass and from the right atrium to the pulmonary artery in the right heart bypass.

The ventricular assist bypass and the IABP were weaned instantly. After 3 hours of biventricular assist, the right ventricular assist device (RVAD) was weaned, and the patient's circulation was maintained by the left ventricular assist device (LVAD) only.

However, the shock condition of the patient gradually deteriorated and LVAD was stopped after 40 hours of pumping.

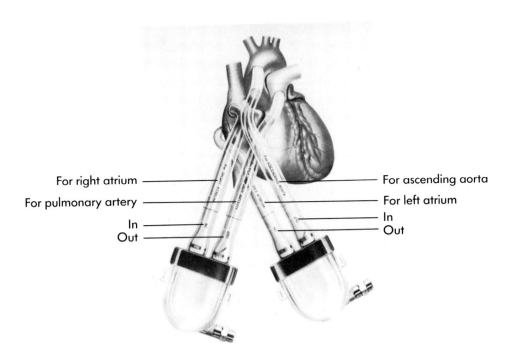

Fig. 15-1. Diagram of biventricular cannulation of VAD (Tokyo University).

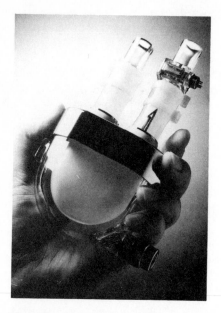

Fig. 15-2. Sac type of blood pump for clinical use (Tokyo University).

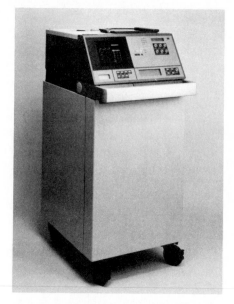

Fig. 15-3. Pneumatic driving unit (Tokyo University).

Clinical VAD system

From clinical experience and animal experiments a newly designed VAD system for clinical use was constructed in our laboratory, in cooperation with Aisin Seiki Company (driving and monitoring unit) and Nippon Zeon Company (blood pump). The VAD system was applied in a clinical case of cardiotomy in 1982.

Blood pump

The blood pump is the sac type, driven by air pressure with 40 ml sac volume. The pump is made from medical-grade PVC coated with Cardiothane, with two Björk–Shiley valves incorporated; the maximum output is 4.0 L/min (Fig. 15-2). An electromagnetic flow probe is mounted on the outlet canula of the blood pump to measure the blood flow. These blood pumps, inlet and outlet cannulae, and accessories are packed and sterilized with ethylene oxide.

Driving and control unit

The driving and control unit is the air-driven type. It is 540 mm wide, 698 mm deep, and 1208 mm high (Fig. 15-3). The air compressor and vacuum pump are incorporated inside the unit. In general the power for the driving and control unit is supplied by AC

Table 15-1. Performance of pneumatic driving unit (Corart 103)

Parameter	Specification
Pneumatic flow	Max. 18 L/min
Pneumatic pressure	−150 to +300 mm Hg
Pulse rate	Max 250/min
Systolic duration	29% to 90%
Synchronized delay	0 to 900 msec
Mask	¼, ½ to ⅛
Power supply	AC 100 V, 50 to 60 Hz, 0.7 kV
	Backup battery DC 48 V
Monitoring	External analogue signal (5 channels)
	Driving pressure
	Battery voltage
	Power voltage source
Synchronized trigger signal	ECG, BP, Other external signals (3 channels)
Helium gas cylinder	300 mm Hg regulated
Alarm	Buzzer, TV display, external signals

electric sources. When it is necessary to transfer the system from the surgical operation room to the intensive care unit (ICU), the power can be changed automatically to a DC battery.

The air pressures of the compressor and the vacuum pump are regulated by valves that are regulated by a controller, and the data is displayed on the front of the driving unit. The control and monitoring units are based on microprocessors.

In this system, electrocardiogram (ECG) synchronization is possible, and it is automatically returned to the internal pulse mode when severe tachycardia or bradycardia has occurred.

The standard specifications—pulse rate, systolic duration, air pressure, air flow, synchronizing delay, masking, and power supply—are shown in Table 15-1. These specifications can be altered using the microprocessing software.

Support van

Although the driving and monitoring unit is reliable, to ensure complete reliability for clinical cases, a backup system with a support van has been constructed and applied in practical use. The van can carry the blood pumps and driving system anytime and anywhere when an emergency arises (Fig. 15-4). The monitoring and communication systems installed in the van can be connected with the sensors in the operating room and support the VAD operation.

Other clinical (pulsatile) VAD systems in Japan

Several clinical VAD systems were developed or imported besides our system. In the National Cardiovascular Center (NCVC), a blood pump and pneumatic drive unit

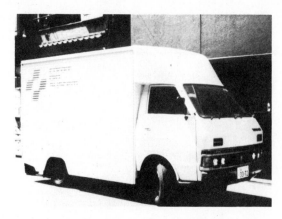

Fig. 15-4. Support van for VAD backup system to carry VAD hardware in case of emergency.

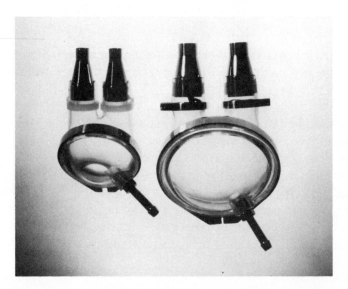

Fig. 15-5. Diaphragm blood pump for clinical use (National Cardiovascular Center).

were developed in cooperation with the Toyobo Company and first used clinically in 1984. The blood pump is a diaphragm-type made of segmented polyurethane (TM-3); two Björk–Shiley valves are incorporated in it. The pneumatic driving unit is 600 × 520 × 1500 mm in size and 250 kg in weight. An automatic control to keep the left atrial pressure or total cardiac output as a constant value is available in this system (Fig. 15-5, Fig. 15-6).

A diaphragm-type blood pump made of segmented polyurethane and incorporating

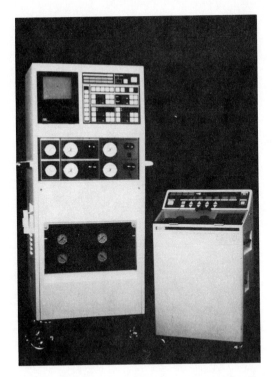

Fig. 15-6. Pneumatic driving unit for clinical use (National Cardiovascular Center).

two Hall valves was developed at Tomasu Technical Laboratory. A sac-type blood pump and pneumatic driving unit were developed at Tohoku University (Fig. 15-7, Fig. 15-8). A Pierce–Donachy blood pump and a pneumatic drive unit made by Thoratec Laboratory were imported and used clinically.

Clinical cases of (pulsatile) VAD in Japan

The clinical application of a ventricular assist device was not frequently performed in Japan until 1983; however, since 1984 the clinical cases have been increasing year by year as shown in Fig. 15-9.

In 1984 the registry committee of VAD was organized in Japan. Dr. T. Horiuchi (Tohoku University) and Dr. Y. Sezai (Nihon University) were appointed as chairman and vice-chairman respectively and Dr. K. Atsumi was appointed as the consultant. Since 1988 Dr. Y. Sezai was appointed as chairman and Dr. T. Fujita (National Cardiovascular Center) was appointed as vice-chairman.

In February 1989 the 177 clinical cases of VAD (115 [65%] males and 62 [35%] females) were registered (Table 15-2).

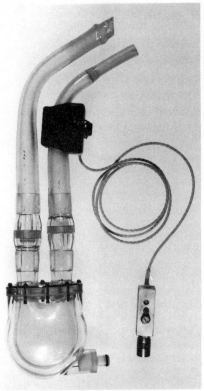

Fig. 15-7. Sac type of blood pump for clinical use (Tohoku University).

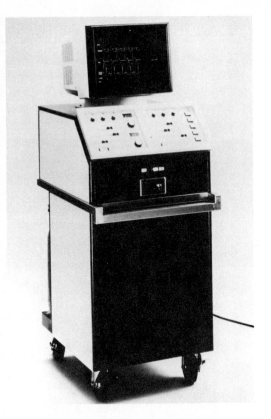

Fig. 15-8. Pneumatic driving unit for clinical use (Tohoku University).

Table 15.2   Clinical results of VAD patients classified by sex

	Clinical cases (%)	Weaned cases (%)	Discharged cases (%)
Male	115 (65.0)	59 (51.3)	21 (18.3)
Female	62 (35.0)	33 (53.2)	14 (22.6)
Total	177 (100.0)	92 (52.0)	35 (19.8)

Ages

The ages of the VAD patients in Japan are classified in Fig. 15-10. The largest number of VAD recipients is 60 to 70 years of age, followed by those 50 to 60 years old. Twenty-three patients are over 70 years old, an impressive number indeed.

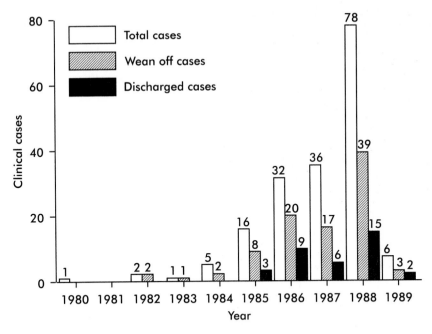

Fig. 15-9. Number of clinical cases of VAD by years.

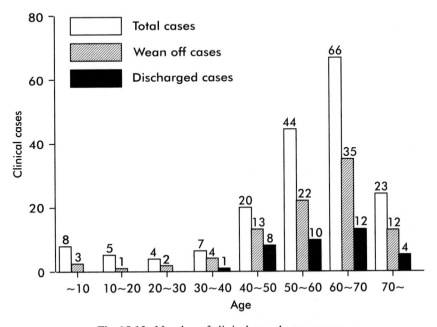

Fig. 15-10. Number of clinical cases by age-group.

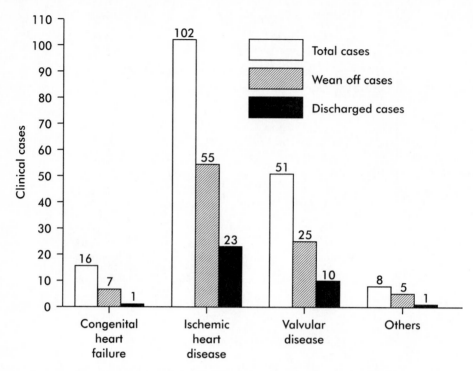

Fig. 15-11. Original heart disease and clinical results in VAD patients.

Table 15-3.   Clinical results classified by VAD modes

Mode	Clinical cases	Weaned cases (%)	Discharged cases (%)
RVAD	17	11 (64.7)	7 (41.2)
LVAD	148	80 (54.1)	28 (18.9)
BVAD	12	1 (8.3)	0 (0)
Total	177	92 (52.0)	35 (19.8)

Heart diseases in VAD patients

Among the 177 cases of VAD, 102 ischemic heart diseases (IHD), 51 heart valve replacements (VD), 16 congenital heart diseases (CHD) and 8 nonsurgical diseases are registered as shown in Fig. 15-11. Most of the patients of VAD come from IHD and valve patients.

In the valve group the number of female patients is greater than that of male patients; however, in the IHD group the relation is reversed. In the IHD group, 55 (53.9%) cases were weaned and 23 (22.5%) cases were discharged. However, in the VD group, 25 (49.0%) cases were weaned and 10 (19.6%) cases were discharged.

Causes of VAD application

Among the 85 cases of VAD, 58 cases (68.2%) are the patients who could not be weaned from extracorporeal circulation, and 23 cases (27.1%) are the low cardiac output patients who suffered from acute myocardial infarctions or postcardiac surgery. The four cases (4.7%) of the nonsurgical operation group were included.

Modes of VAD

In the total 177 cases, 92 (52.0%) were weaned and 35 (19.8%) were discharged.

The modes of VAD are divided into three types: (1) left ventricular assist device (LVAD), right ventricular assist device (RVAD), and biventricular assist device (BVAD). In Japan, among the 177 VAD cases, 148 (83.6%) are registered as LVAD (L), 17 (9.6%) are registered as RVAD (R), and 12 (4.5%) are registered as BVAD (R + L).

The modes of VAD and their clinical results are shown in Table 15-3. In the 17 cases of RVAD, 11 (64.7%) were weaned and 7 (41.2%) were discharged. In the 148 cases

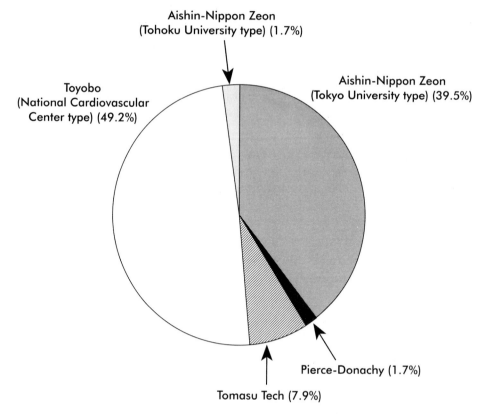

Fig. 15-12. Blood pumps used in VAD patients.

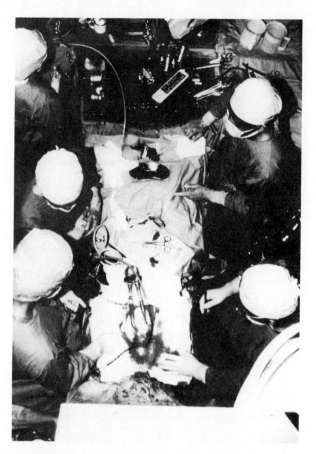

Fig. 15-13. Sac type of blood pump (Tokyo University) was connected to a patient who was in cardiogenic shock after double-valve replacement (Nihon University).

of LVAD, 80 (54.1%) were weaned and 28 (18.9%) cases were discharged. However, in the 12 cases of BVAD, only one (8.3%) was weaned and none were discharged.

In comparison with international VAD application, the use of RVAD is large in Japan, and the poor result of BVAD is the same as that of other countries.

Blood pumps used in VAD

The 5 types of blood pumps (pulsatile) used in the 177 cases include (1) the 87 (49.2%) NCVC (National Cardiovascular Center) type, (2) the 70 (39.5%) UT (University of Tokyo) type, (3) the 14 (7.9%) TM (Thomas) type, (4) the 3 (1.7%) UTH (University of Tohoku) type, and (5) the 3 (1.7%) PD (Pierce–Donachy) type (Fig. 15-12). The Japanese-made blood pumps were used in most of the clinical cases of VAD in Japan (Figs. 15-13 and 15-14).

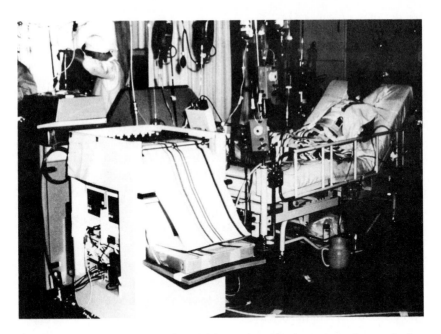

Fig. 15-14. Patient with LVAD. The driving and monitoring unit can be seen in front.

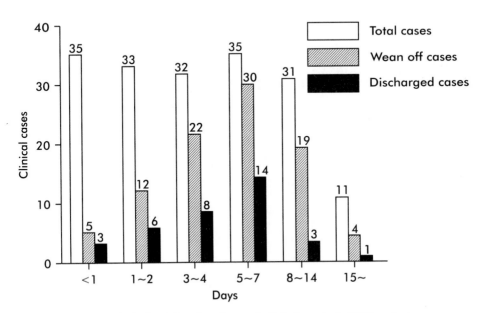

Fig. 15-15. Assisted duration time and clinical results in VAD patients.

Assisted duration time of VAD

The assisted duration time of the VAD patients is shown in Fig. 15-15.

The duration time is from 1 hour to 70 days and most of the cases are less than 14 days. The duration times are different between the weaning cases and the nonweaning cases.

In the group of medium duration time, from 3 days to 14 days, there are 71 (72.4%) weaning cases and 25 (19.4%) discharge cases among the 98 cases. The results are considered to be fairly good. However, in the group of short duration time, less than 3 days, there are 17 (25.0%) weaning cases and 9 (13.2%) discharge cases among the 68 cases.

In the group of long duration time, over 14 days, there are 4 (36.3%) weaning cases and 1 (9.1%) discharge case among the 11 cases. These results reveal that VAD patients of short- and long-term duration cases are difficult to wean and discharge.

Extracorporeal circulation time and clinical results

Among the 60 cases, 14 (23.3%) cases were discharged. However, among the 37 cases of the group of more than 6 hours of extracorporeal circulation time, only 3 (8.1%) were discharged (Fig. 15-16). The group of less than 6 hours of extracorporeal circulation time are counted in the 60 cases.

When the extracorporeal circulation time is over 6 hours for VAD application, it is difficult to cure the patients. It is suggested that VAD application should be decided before 6 hours' extracorporeal circulation.

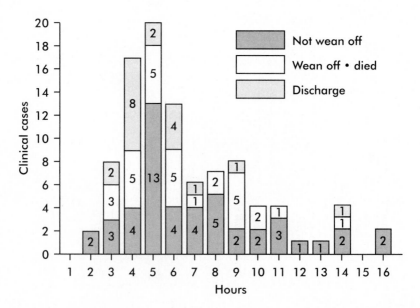

Fig. 15-16. Extracorporeal circulation time and clinical results in 97 VAD patients.

Table 15-4.   Use of anticoagulants and thrombus formation in blood pumps

Anticoagulant	Clinical cases	Thrombus formation
Heparin	45	4
Heparin + Foy	8	2
Foy	12	3
Others	4	1
None or no recording	46	12

Table 15-5.   Clinical complications in VAD use

Complications	Clinical cases (%)
Renal insufficiency	46 (40.0)
Bleeding	33 (28.7)
MOF	32 (27.8)
Infection	27 (23.5)
Peripheral circulatory insufficiency	24 (20.9)
Thrombus and emboli	23 (20.0)
Right heart insufficiency (LVAD)	12 (10.4)
Respiratory insufficiency	9 (7.8)
DIC	6 (5.2)
IABP-related (85 VAD cases)	4 (3.5)

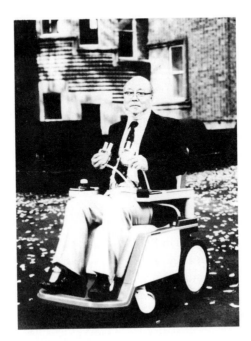

Fig. 15-17. Sac type of blood pumps and movable driving unit—an electric wheelchair (Tokyo University).

Use of anticoagulants and thrombus formation in blood pumps

In general, before VAD pumping, heparin was administrated to the blood pump to protect clotting. However, anticoagulants were introduced only in cases of long-term use or expected cases of clotting tendency (e.g., high viscosity, multiple valve replacement, and left atrial thrombus). The relationship between the use of anticoagulants and thrombus formation in the blood pump is shown in Table 15-4. 10% to 20% of thrombus formations were detected in the blood pumps; however, the rare complication cases of severe emboli could be detected in the clinical VAD cases.

Complications and causes of death in VAD

The major complications in VAD are shown in Table 15-5. The most frequent complication is renal insufficiency, followed by bleeding, multiple organ failure (MOF), and infections. These complications are the causes of death in VAD patients.

Movable VAD system

The movable VAD system was constructed by Tokyo University, cooperating with the Aisin Company.

The sac-type blood pump is the same as those developed for clinical use.

The pneumatic driving unit is a movable electric wheelchair. Positive and negative air pressure generators, the control unit of three microprocessors, the sensors, and the miniaturized monitoring TV system, and the batteries for energy sources are incorporated in the system (Fig. 15-17).

CONCLUSION

Of the 177 clinical cases of pulsatile VAD experienced in Japan from 1980 to 1988, 92 (52.0%) were weaned and 35 (19.8%) were discharged. Of the original heart diseases using VAD, the most frequent was ischemic heart disease, 102 (57.6%); valvular disease was 51 (28.8%); congenital heart disease was 16 (9%); and the others were 8 (4.5%). For the VAD systems, Japanese-made units were those most applied; there were a few Pierce–Donachy pumps used. For the VAD mode, LVAD was the most frequently applied, 148 (83.6%) cases. RVAD was used in 17 (9.6%) cases; BVAD was used in 12 (6.7%) cases. The wean rate and discharge ratio were 80 (54.1%) and 28 (18.9%) in LVAD, 11 (64.7%) and 7 (41.2%) in RVAD, and 1 (8.3%) and 0 (0%) in BVAD respectively. BVAD showed the world result. The clinical results were closely related to the extracorporeal circulation time before VAD application. In the cases of time less than 6 hours, good results were obtained. The assist duration time of VAD was also related to the discharge ratio of the patients. The cases of time within 1 day or longer than 2 weeks showed the worse results. Despite anticoagulant use during VAD pumping, thrombus formations were detected 10% to 20% of the time in the clinical cases. The major complication was renal insufficiency, followed by bleeding, MOF, and infection. These complications became the causes of death in the VAD patients.

CHAPTER 16

Cardiac circulatory support at the Moscow Institute of Transplantology

V. I. Shumakov

INTRODUCTION

Various methods of mechanical circulatory support are being utilized in Russian tertiary surgical centers; from Vilnius in the west to Blagoveshensk in the east; and from Murmansk in the north to Tashkent in the south. A summary of circulatory assist experience in the Russian Federation (RF) is provided in Table 16-1.

Intraaortic balloon counterpulsation (IABC) was initially used in May 1989 to stabilize a patient in cardiogenic shock as a complication of myocardial infarction. Furthermore, arterial–venous extracorporeal bypass of one or both ventricles and a noninvasive method of assisted circulation (external counterpulsation) are also employed in Soviet cardiovascular clinical practice.

At the Scientific Research Institute of Transplantology and Artificial Organs (SRITAO), a ventricular assist device (VAD) is currently being used successfully in cases of irreversible cardiomyopathy. Only two medical centers, the Scientific Surgical Center of the Academy of Medical Sciences of the USSR and the Scientific Research Institute of Transplantology and Artificial Organs of the Public Health Ministry, have initiated extensive assisted circulation research and incorporated almost all the above listed methods.

Every 5 years, study findings and issues surrounding mechanical support are discussed at a Specialized All-Union Symposium. Conferees are specialists in transplantology and artificial organs.

RUSSIAN VENTRICULAR ASSIST DEVICES (VADS)

Since 1990 RF synthesis of hemocompatible polymers, with excellent physical and chemical properties, has led to successful development of artificial ventricles. These

Table 16-1.   Summary of RF IABP experience

Center	Number of patients	Myocardial infarction secondary to cardiogenic shock	Complications after EC	Prophylaxis
Cardiovascular Surgery Institute Bakulev, Moscow	272	200/40°	72/55°	
Cardiovascular Surgery Institute Bakulev, Moscow	34			34/25°
Research Institute of Transplantology and Artificial Organs, Moscow	129	87/11°	42/9°	
Center of Cardiovascular Surgery, Minsk	61	12/9°	24/16°	25/26°
Center of Cardiosurgery, Donetsk	32			
All-Union Scientific Center of Surgery	50		36/13°	4/3°
Center of Cardiosurgery, Tallin	89	31/29°		57/52°
University Cardiovascular Surgery Center, Vilnius	202		163/86°	49/23°

EC, extracorporeal circulation; *CS,* coronary shock.
°survivors.

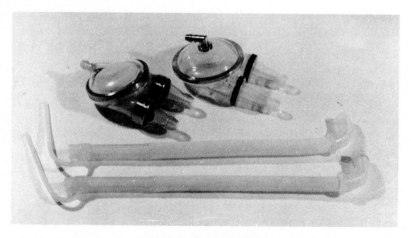

Fig. 16-1. Yasen-17 VAD.

polymers, made on a base of polyurethane, are biologically inert, non-antigen producing, and do not exert a thrombogenic influence on blood components.

Successful results have been achieved with the engineering, design, and clinical
application of Russian VADs. There are two models: (1) Yasen-17 and (2) Modul, manufactured by two different Moscow enterprises. The Yasen-17 (Fig. 16-1) is a sac diaphragm-type VAD with a filling capacity of 110 cc and stroke volume of 50 cc. The
blood-contacting components are produced by immersing a mold into a solution of sil-
urem. The diaphragm is manufactured from compressed silicon rubber, a material that
facilitates ejection of a predetermined stroke volume. Both housing and pneumatic lid
are made of polycarbonate by means of mechanical pneumatic formation; the connecting pipe is also made of polycarbonate. Connective elements (collapsible hoop,
spinned hoop, and screws of a connecting pipe) are made of titanium. Disk valves
(Amix) with an internal control diameter of 22 mm, manufactured in the RF, are used
in this model. The main advantage of the Yasen-17 is the capability to replace the blood-
contacting components after explant and therefore to reuse the device.

The Modul VAD (Fig. 16-2) is a kind of membrane blood pump. Its outer housing
is made of limid polyvinylchloride. Its blood-contacting surface has a high degree of
purity ($>\Delta 10$). The membrane is made of polyurethane. Modul is equipped with two

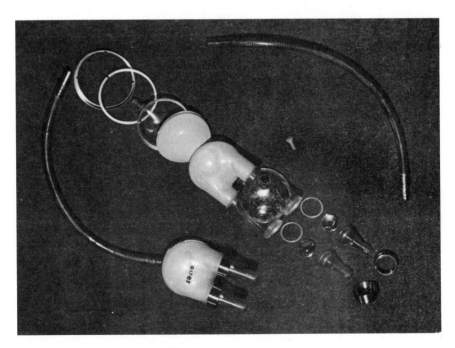

Fig. 16-2. Modul VAD.

disk inlet and outlet valves made of uglesital, an analog of pyrolyte. Inlet and outlet Modul-connecting tubing is designed to attain laminar blood flow, thus avoiding stagnation.

Modul's filling capacity is 120 cc, with a stroke volume of approximately 90 cc. The pump is characterized by a high sensitivity to blood inflow. It can be easily stripped and sterilized by ethylene oxide.

USE OF OTHER FORMS OF MECHANICAL ASSIST IN THE RF

An armamentarium of different types of apparatus for mechanical circulatory assistance have been utilized with good results in the RF.

Datascope and AVCO-manufactured consoles and balloons are utilized for IABC. Another type of balloon pump, the Unit Sinus VK2 (Fig. 16-3) is also used. Its drive

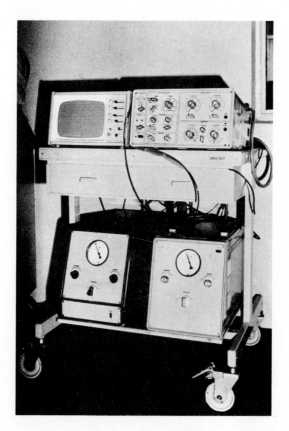

Fig. 16-3. Sinus VK2.

unit is pneumatic. It has two identical canals, each equipped with a cardiosynchronizer that can trigger from an R wave. The electrocardiogram, schemes of formation for delay, and duration of pressure pulses, power amplification, and electropneumatic transformation all function in absolute periods of time. A generator functions as a backup power source and provides an internal trigger in the event that the R wave signal is lost. It employs a solenoid engine with little inertia.

The Sinus-VK2 has been used recently for IABC and as a VAD. The Sinus VK2 is an autonomous pneumatic driver, containing two small canals with a control system.[1] This pneumatic system is charged from a small two-chamber compressor. Positive pressure changes from 0 to 400 mm Hg.

Diastolic pressure can be changed from +30 to -50 mm Hg. The controller accurately tracks pneumatic impulses from 10 to 160 a minute, synchronizing from the ECG. Its weight is about 30 kg.

Disadvantages of the Sinus VK2 include (1) high speed, (2) inefficiency associated with a preliminary processing of information, (3) manual intervention required for car-

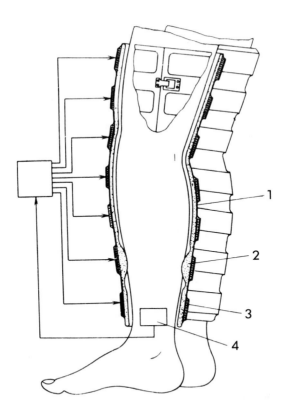

Fig. 16-4. Ferromagnetic external counterpulsation system; *1*, external sheath; *2*, magnetic field; *3*, solenoid; *4*, ECG.

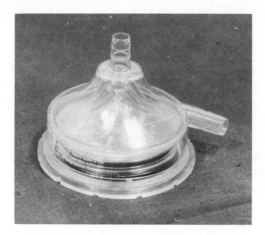

Fig. 16-5. GOFR centrifugal VAD.

diosynchronization, arrhythmias, and phasic synchronization based on analysis of heart rhythm, (4) prevention of false start during rapid changing of ECG and electrical systole, (5) control of pressure impulses, their slope and front form, depending on heart rate, and (6) automatic disconnection during drive unit disorders.

The Sinus-AH pneumatic drive unit has been used during implantation of a total artificial heart. There is a pneumatic scheme on every canal, including pressure receiver and vacuum, servomechanism, sensory element, and expenditure of air. The drive unit is supplied with a pressure of $+0.5$ atmospheres at the pneumostation outlet and a vacuum pressure of -0.5 atmospheres. Maximal flow rate is about 10 L/min; its weight is about 15 kg.

Two systems have been developed using a pneumatic and hydrodrive unit for external counterpulsation. Technical characteristics of the latter are higher and more accurate than those of the former. A ferromagnetic fluid external counterpulsation system (Fig. 16-4) is now undergoing evaluation. The obvious advantage of this system is that the drive unit is less cumbersome.

The centrifugal GOFR Pump (Fig. 16-5) has been developed at SRITAO. It has two discs or rotating cone surfaces that transport blood with minimal turbulence and cavitation. With the same speed of rotation, the efficiency of the GOFR Pump is greater than that of the Biopump.

CLINICAL EXPERIENCE
Intraaortic balloon counterpulsation

Indications for IABC are summarized in the box on p. 215. Both surgical cutdown and percutaneous techniques are used. Instituting percutaneous insertion has increased usage of IABC and lowered the complication rate from 30.5% to 9.5%.[2]

```
 _____ INDICATIONS FOR USE OF IABC IN RF _____

   Coronary disease
      Shock associated with myocardial infarction
      Transmural myocardial infarction
      Left main coronary disease
      Unstable angina
      Complications associated with coronary angioplasty
   Low output syndrome following extracorporeal circulation
   Septic and traumatic shock
   As a bridge to cardiac transplantation
   Ventricular rupture
```

Table 16-2.   Left ventricular assist experience

Center	Number of patients	Kind of pump		
		Membrane	Roller	Centrifugal
Scientific Research Institute of Transplantology and Artificial Organs, Moscow	21	8	6	7
Medical Institute, Blagoveshensk	37	7	36	
All-Union Scientific Center of Surgery, Moscow	43	4	39	
Institute of Cardiovascular Surgery, Kiev	36	5	31	

Left heart bypass

A summary of left VAD support is listed in Table 16-2. These figures represent approximately 2% of all extracorporeal, circulation-supported, surgical cases performed. In most cases, left VAD inflow cannulation is via the left atrium and outflow is via the ascending aorta. Research undertaken by the All-Union Scientific Center of Surgery has demonstrated very successful outcomes with left VAD support. The algorithm in Fig. 16-6 illustrates the decision-making process employed when managing myocardial pump failure following withdrawal of cardiopulmonary bypass.

If a membrane VAD is utilized for left ventricular bypass, IABC is considered to be unnecessary because of unjustified waste of time. When we use roller and centrifugal pumps, the obvious advantage is pulsatile blood flow. With successful left ventricular

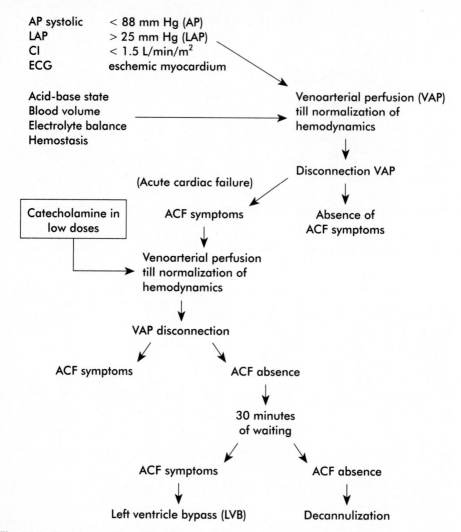

Fig. 16-6. Decision-making algorithm used when withdrawing patients from extracorporeal support.

Table 16-3. Demographics of complications observed°

Type	Number of patients (total)	Complication abolished	Complication as a reason of death
Failure	13 (35.1%)	10 (29%)	3 (8%)
Bleeding	6 (16.2%)	3 (8.1%)	3 (8.1%)
Air embolism	1 (2.7%)	—	1 (2.7%)

°Data from Medical Institute in Blagoveshensk.

assist, the patient's hemodynamic normalizes, encephalopathy disappears, the level of catecholamine support decreases, and renal perfusion improves. We have isolated three phases of left ventricular support.

The initial phase is concerned with recovery of normal blood circulation without using high doses of catecholamines, elimination of pulmonary edema, afterload reduction, improvement of coronary perfusion, and decreasing myocardial ischemia. Controlled pulmonary ventilation is very important during this initial phase of VAD support. Prevention of right ventricular dysfunction is also critically important. Positive end-expiratory pressures as great as 17 to 20 cm water with 100% oxygen therapy have been used in shock lung. High levels of positive end-expiratory pressure are not tolerated because this lowers left ventricular filling volume and lowers VAD output.

The second phase consists of VAD support maintenance. The third phase consists of pump disconnection after the myocardium has demonstrated its recovery with a cardiac index >2.5 L/min/m^2.

COMPLICATIONS

Complications associated with left VAD include right ventricular failure, surgical and nonsurgical bleeding, air embolism (rare), thromboembolism, infection, and right ventricular failure. Demographic characteristics of complications observed in our program are listed in Table 16-3.

Right ventricular failure

Right ventricular failure limits blood flow to the left atrium and therefore left VAD outflow, which sometimes has to be lowered to 1 to 3 L/min, and even discontinued. Clinical symptoms of right ventricular failure include a central venous pressure >200 cm H$_2$O, decreased left atrial and VAD filling, which necessitates decreasing VAD flow. Arterial pressure decreases, and cardiac output and left atrial pressures remain low. Right ventricular hypokinesis can be visually observed in the operating room.

Right ventricular structure changes have been observed via myocardial biopsy performed during left VAD support. Characteristics included swelling of the myocardium with partial crists reduction and matrix homogenization of mitochondria.[1] Glycogen content was considerably lowered in the cell sarcoplasma. Contractile proteins were less affected by right ventricular failure. A schematic suggestive of the pathogenesis of right ventricular failure seen in LVAD patients is illustrated in Fig. 16-7.

Bleeding

Bleeding occurred in 6.2% of all left VAD cases. Known causes are extracorporeal circulation and heparinization. Bleeding is not immediately obvious in left VAD patients. Table 16-4 illustrates a typical hemodynamic profile associated with a LVAD patient who is bleeding.

In general, mechanisms of RVF development during LVB vary. These mechanisms are illustrated below.

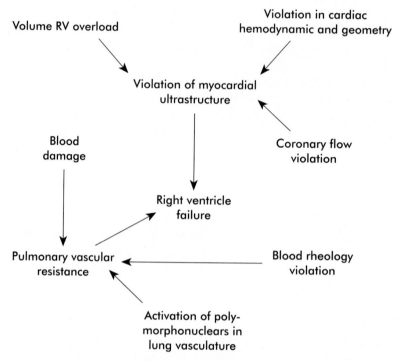

Fig. 16-7. Schematic of possible pathogenesis of right ventricular failure in left VAD patients.

Table 16-4. Typical hemodynamic profile of a bleeding LVAD patient

Indices	LVB	Bleeding	P
Pa mean	92.3 ± 1.6	64.2 ± 3.1	0.01
CVP mm H$_2$O	118.3 ± 4.2	60.1 ± 3.7	0.001
LAP mm Hg	10.1 ± 0.6	9.1 ± 0.4	0.05
Pump flow rate L/min	4.1 ± 0.3	2.2 ± 0.5	0.05

Air embolism

Although rare, air embolism is nevertheless considered to be one of the most dangerous complications.[4,7] Even the slightest amount of air that enters the return arterial circulation can result in serious neurological sequelae. During VAD operation, aspiration of the nonhermetic connective points in the negative pressure phase is essential. Potential for air aspiration is less when using a roller pump device because of the short duration of the negative phase. We also do not allow left atrial pressure to fall below 1 to 2 mm Hg as a prophylaxis against air embolism. It is noteworthy that left atrial pressure predictably falls during the initial minutes of left VAD support because of left atrial blood decompression. VAD flow acceleration must therefore increase slowly to prevent this sudden drop in left atrial pressure.

Thrombosis and thromboembolism

Thrombus formation has been noted within the interior VAD, but it has not been associated with thromboembolism. We have used VAD support for >5 days; flow during the last 24 hour period was less than 1 L per minute.

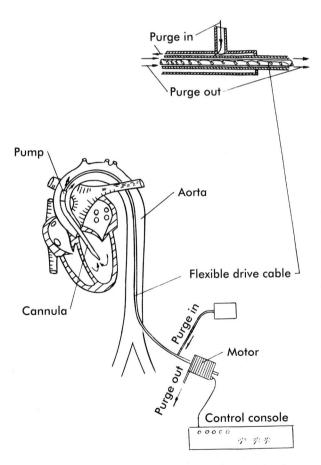

Fig. 16-8. Multifunctional pumping system (MPS) high speed circulatory assist device.

Infections

The presence of large foreign body plastic surfaces in the thorax predisposes to infections. Two left VAD-support patients in our series developed infections and died, despite aggressive treatment with antibiotics, immunocorrection, application of hemoabsorption, and use of xenospleen. One patient implanted with the Poisk M artificial heart developed a purulent mediastinitis, which was the cause of his death on the tenth postoperative day of his two-stage heart transplantation.

HIGH SPEED TECHNOLOGY FOR CIRCULATORY SUPPORT

Current technology is able to design devices with high reliability and performance. Advantages are obvious: (1) minimum weight and dimensions, and (2) simplicity and reliability in exploitation. An example of this high speed technology used for circulatory support is the Multifunctional Pumping System (MPS) (Fig. 16-8). Clinical indications include (1) temporary circulatory support for heart failure associated with myocardial infarction, and (2) as an implanted device, partially or fully supporting the heart (Fig. 16-9).

The MPS high-speed circulatory assist device comprises a micropump assembly, a block of medicaments and lubricant dosages, and a drive and control block. The pump assembly consists of a micropump, inflow cannula, and a flexible drive cable.

For temporary circulatory support, the micropump XAT5-7.5 is used; its diameter

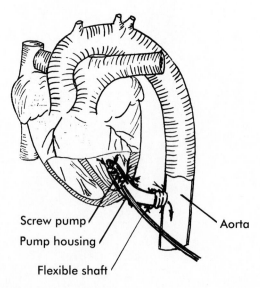

Fig. 16-9. Implantable high speed circulatory assist device.

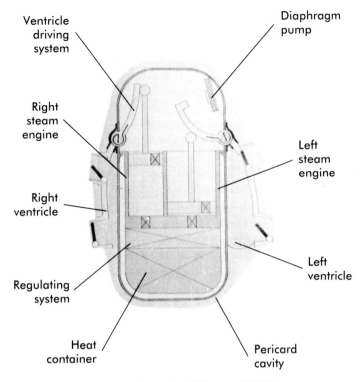

Ventricle driving system

Diaphragm pump

Right steam engine

Left steam engine

Right ventricle

Left ventricle

Regulating system

Heat container

Pericard cavity

Fig. 16-10. Schematic of Micron artificial heart.

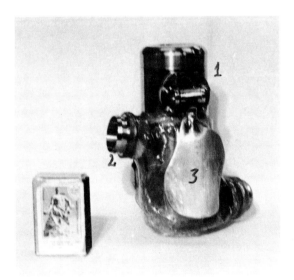

Fig. 16-11. Micron-M compared in size with a match box; *1*, heart engine; *2*, pump; *3*, pusher.

is 5 to 7.5 mm. It can pump 0.5 to 51 L/min of blood. This micropump is manufactured from titan with a high surface quality. Hemolysis is limited to 40 mg/%. XAT5-7.5 insertion is via the femoral artery, advanced through the aortic valve into the left ventricle. It rotates up to 30,000 rpm. Advantages include simple and rapid implantation through the femoral artery, significant left ventricular unloading, and pump sizing from 5.0 to 7.5 mm.

ARTIFICIAL HEART USED AS A BRIDGE TO TRANSPLANTATION

Three categories of patients have been bridged to transplantation with an artificial heart: (1) those awaiting transplantation who suddenly develop severe failure; (2) patients who cannot be weaned from extracorporeal circulation; and (3) irreversible rejection following transplantation. Of the artificial heart implants using the Poisk IOM, 13 have been performed at SRITAO, the duration of support ranging from 3 to 10 days.

AUTONOMIC IMPLANTABLE SYSTEM

Since 1976 Soviet researchers have been developing an implantable artificial heart, the Micron (Fig. 16-10), as well as a system of assisted circulation with Micron-M, a thermomechanical drive unit working on the principle of a steam machine (Fig. 16-11). Development of these models was centered on creating a physiological drive unit with direct host *back connection.* No electrical control is needed because the system is totally mechanically operated. Mock circulation testing of these systems has occurred. Animal model testing of the Micron-M was planned to begin at the end of 1991, with human trials planned for 1995.

PATIENT MANAGEMENT

Some Russian medical centers (e.g., SRYTO and the All-Union Institute of Surgery) utilize a family of VADs. In these centers mechanical assist research laboratories have been established, consisting of physicians, physiologists, engineers, and ancillary personnel. These laboratories develop pumps and drive systems, and perform mock circulation testing. Russian equipment is used, with the exception of the U.S. Datascope balloon pump and, occasionally, a U.S. manufactured centrifugal Biopump.

Researchers employed by the laboratory comprise a VAD support team. Each member is trained in medicine or biomedical engineering and is responsible for all types of circulatory support. Cardiovascular surgeons work with the VAD team for pump implantation.

Protocols have been established that include indications,[3] VAD operation manuals, anticoagulation, hemodynamic monitoring, and prophylactic antibiotic therapy. The

VAD team manages the patient while he or she is on circulatory support. Ancillary support services (e.g., assisted ventilation) are provided by physicians and nurses from the clinical department of the institute's care unit. Our ICU physicians and nurses are not certified in VAD patient management. Therefore all patient problems and decisions regarding VAD management are assumed by the specially trained VAD support team.

REFERENCES

1. Шумаков ВИ, Махатадзе ШМ, Толпекин ВЕ: Аппараты и методы вспомогательного кровообращения. Тбилиси, 1990.
2. Petrovsky B, Kniazev M, Konstantinov V: Three clinical methods of circulatory assistance, *Artif Organs* 11:9, 1987.
3. Ведерникова ЛА: Лечение острой сердечной недостаточности способом левожелудочкового обхода после операций с искусственным кровообращением, Дисс. канд. мед. наук, Благовещенск, 1984.

CHAPTER 17

Optimizing hemodynamics and assessing myocardial recovery

H. David Short III and **George P. Noon**

INTRODUCTION

Successful use of mechanical circulatory support beyond intraaortic balloon pumping requires considerable clinical judgment for selection of appropriate patients. Early institution of support, management of hemodynamics, and avoidance of complications are important in achieving myocardial recovery and a successful clinical outcome. After a discussion of appropriate patient selection as well as device selection in patients who have reversible myocardial injury, this chapter will discuss maintenance of hemodynamics on mechanical support and methods to assess ventricular recovery to aid in the timing of device removal.

INITIATION OF SUPPORT
Patient selection

Patients who are reasonable candidates for temporary mechanical circulatory support generally fall into a few categories. Most surgeons consider that patients unable to be weaned from cardiopulmonary bypass after conventional cardiac surgery make up the majority. These may be patients undergoing emergency surgery following cardiac catheterization laboratory catastrophes, such as cardiac arrest during catheterization, failed angioplasty, or cardiac perforation. They may also be patients who have had elective cardiac surgery with prolonged cardiopulmonary bypass or suboptimal myocardial protection. These patients should have had acceptable ventricular function preoperatively to anticipate any possibility of myocardial recovery and successful resuscitation using mechanical circulatory support. Patients with shock following myocardial infarction might also be considered for temporary, mechanical, circulatory support. This complication of myocardial infarction has a high mortality rate and is usually associated with extensive myocardial damage.[4] Newer methods of clinical management, including thrombolytic therapy and early revascularization with coronary angioplasty or surgery, may limit the size of infarction. Since reversal of severe "stunning" has been documented in patients with acute myocardial insults,[2] these patients may also be candidates for mechanical circulatory support. In both postcardiotomy patients and postinfarction patients, if transplantation is not an option, careful patient selection is necessary for there to be any hope of weaning them from the device. In patients with marginal ventricular function before the superimposed acute insult or with extensive infarction, use of ventricular assist devices, although heroic, is usually futile.

In the transplant population, several other clinical settings may require the use of temporary, mechanical, circulatory support. In severe acute rejection, single or biventricular support may be required to tide the patient over until rejection can be controlled or until it is evident that recovery is unlikely, at which time retransplantation might be considered. Immediately after orthotopic transplantation, right ventricular dysfunction is not uncommon in patients with labile pulmonary vascular resistance. With elevated pulmonary artery pressures, right ventricular dysfunction in the graft may cause severe hemodynamic disturbances and temporary right ventricular support may be required to sustain the patient in the early posttransplant period. A final example occurs in patients with Novacor ventricular assist systems for left ventricular support as a bridge to transplant. Right ventricular failure has been successfully managed in our institution with temporary right ventricular assistance using a BioMedicus pump, which can be used until right ventricular recovery and then removed, leaving the patient with only left ventricular support as a long-term bridge.

Devices

Devices that have been used as temporary support fall into several broad categories. Extracorporeal membrane oxygenation (partial cardiopulmonary bypass) has been used occasionally for patients with severe acute rejection to immediately resuscitate the patient, to assess multiple organ failure, or to evaluate cardiac function when hemodynamic deterioration is rapid and the clinical cause is not immediately apparent. Long-term extracorporeal membrane oxygenation has not generally been successful in most clinical settings. Patients requiring prolonged support will need other devices, after initial stabilization with femoral-femoral bypass. Extracorporeal pulsatile pumps were first used in our hospital over 20 years ago for temporary ventricular support.[3] Since then a number of similar devices have been used in both the single and biventricular configurations for a variety of clinical indications. However, the most experience has been with continuous flow pumps. The BioMedicus pump is generally available in most cardiac centers and can easily be used for right, left, or biventricular support with conventional cannulation techniques and universally available hardware (Table 17-1). Use of the Hemopump has recently been reported in the treatment of cardiogenic shock.[8] This device has been quite successful and has the advantage of peripheral insertion while supporting the circulation to a degree equal to centrally placed pumps.

Table 17-1. BioMedicus support

Reason for assist	IABP	LVAD	RVAD	BiVAD
Postcardiotomy	71	68	6	18
Acute MI	1	3	0	1
Graft failure	7	1	3	13
Bridge to transplant	2	1	5	3
Post-PTCA emergent	2	2	0	0
Other	0	0	0	1
	83	75	14	36

125

Single vs. biventricular support

Both objective parameters and clinical judgment are useful in assessing the need for univentricular or biventricular support. Although theoretical considerations and empirical results have led some centers to use only biventricular support, considerable experience has been accumulated with single ventricle support and this has been shown to be a reasonable option in appropriately selected patients. Patients who have clinically sustained a predominantly single ventricle insult and have hemodynamic data indicating single ventricle dysfunction, will generally do well with single ventricle support. Patients with postcardiotomy shock or left coronary infarctions who show very sluggish left ventricular function with low cardiac output and elevated left atrial pressures may have brisk right ventricular function. These patients generally can be supported with left ventricular support alone. Elevated pulmonary artery pressures caused by elevated wedge with normal pulmonary vascular resistance and a normal PA diastolic wedge gradient will improve with unloading of the left side. "Forward failure" of the right ventricle from left ventricular support is uncommon in our clinical experience. On the other hand, in patients with right coronary infarcts or in cardiac transplant patients with right ventricular dysfunction, the left ventricle may have obvious brisk contractile function with right ventricular distention, elevated CVP, low cardiac output, and low left atrial or pulmonary capillary wedge pressures. These patients will generally do quite well with right ventricular support alone. Patients who have poor contractility of both ventricles, with corroborating hemodynamic data, will usually require biventricular support. In marginal cases the empirical use of biventricular support seems prudent.

OPTIMIZING HEMODYNAMICS

Adequate hemodynamics on mechanical circulatory support has been adequately described in a number of reviews.[1,5,6] Pump flows are adjusted to maintain cardiac index >2.1 L/min/m² with adequate systemic arterial blood pressure (>60 mean) and low

---

BIOMEDICUS SUPPORT

Optimizing hemodynamics

Early application of assist device

Maintain cardiac index over 2.1 L/min/m^2

Minimize pharmacological support

  Inotropic agents

  Vasoactive agents

Optimize fluid and electrolyte balance

  Fluid intake

  Colloid oncotic pressure

  Diuresis and/or continuous arteriovenous hemofiltration (CAVH)

Meet nutritional needs

Support and treat other organ system failure

Anticoagulation

---

atrial filling pressures ($<$20 mm Hg). In addition, the clinical picture of adequate perfusion including warm extremities, adequate urine output, acceptable blood gases, and a normal sensorium are important evidence of optimal hemodynamics. Several seemingly peripheral clinical features bear special emphasis because they frequently determine the likelihood of a successful clinical outcome. (See the box.)

Early institution of support

Early institution of support is important to avoid multiorgan deteriorization, which can result in patient death even with adequate cardiac function. Too often in postcardiotomy patients, cardiopulmonary bypass is prolonged, hoping for ventricular recovery, but leading to further deterioration. If several attempts to wean from cardiopulmonary bypass fail in spite of technically successful surgery, correction of abnormal laboratory values, maximal pharmacological support, and intraaortic balloon pumping, consideration should be given to institution of ventricular assistance. In transplant patients severe organ system failure may exclude the patient as a transplant candidate. In patients who deteriorate despite IABP, early institution of ventricular assistance can reverse renal or hepatic dysfunction, while sustaining the patient until transplantation. With continuous flow-type pumps, the intraaortic balloon pump is used continuously to maintain pulsatile perfusion, helping renal perfusion while decreasing left ventricular work and increasing coronary filling.

Optimizing fluid and electrolyte balance

Optimizing fluid balance is very important in patients who have ventricular assist devices in place. Overzealous use of crystalloids causes increased interstitial and intracellular water, leading to numerous problems that can be obviated with early and vigorous treatment. Hemodilution on pump frequently leads to coagulapathies, necessitating multiple blood transfusions. Coupled with increased intrapulmonary water caused by elevated left atrial pressures or low colloid oncotic pressure, these combine to create respiratory insufficiency in the early postoperative period. Prolonged cardiopulmonary bypass and many hours of open thoracotomy lead to myocardial and mediastinal swelling, which interferes with cardiac function and sternal closure. In patients who have these problems, early attempts should be made to enhance diuresis, removing extra water and electrolytes, using colloid or blood products, as necessary, to maintain adequate filling volumes. Colloid oncotic pressures should be measured and kept in the normal range. Hemoconcentration on cardiopulmonary bypass can help, and this may be continued in the intensive care unit in the face of marginal renal function with continuous arteriovenous hemofiltration. Continuous arteriovenous hemofiltration may be done with arterial and venous cannulation or may be driven directly off the BioMedicus pump tubing.

Pharmacological support

During mechanical circulatory support, efforts are made to minimize the use of catecholamines that increase myocardial oxygen consumption. This may be important in patients with myocardial ischemia to improve favorably the ratio of oxygen delivery to consumption. A notable exception is the common use of low dose dopamine to improve renal perfusion. With adequate cardiac output, vasopressors are used to maintain systemic arterial pressures to exceed 60 mm Hg mean. Peripheral vasodilators are used in the face of increased peripheral vascular resistance to increase marginal cardiac output. Vasodilators such as nitroglycerine or prostaglandin E are more commonly used in an attempt to lower pulmonary vascular resistance to optimize right ventricular function. Heparin may be used 12 to 24 hours following insertion of ventricular assist devices, if surgical bleeding is controlled.

ASSESSING MYOCARDIAL RECOVERY

Although devices for temporary mechanical circulatory support may improve multiple organ system dysfunction by maintaining stable hemodynamics, the possibility of complications caused by the support device dictates removal as soon as practical. Early after insertion, right-sided continuous flow assist devices may generate only nonpulsatile pulmonary artery waveforms. On the left side the intraaortic balloon pump will cause a pulsatile aortic waveform, but no ventricular ejection will be seen. The earliest evidence for hemodynamic recovery is often return of pulsatility with right or left ventricular ejection in patients who have atrial cannulation. With ventricular cannulation for inflow to the pump, this is frequently not present because the ventricle empties into the device, rather than into the aorta or pulmonary artery. Atrial pressures may drop

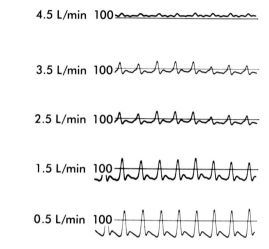

Fig. 17-1. Peripheral arterial waveform with decremental LVAD flows.

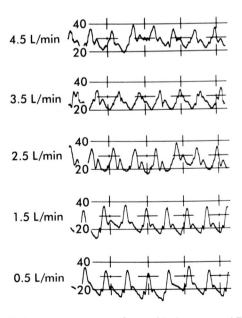

Fig. 17-2. Pulmonary artery waveform with decremental RVAD flows.

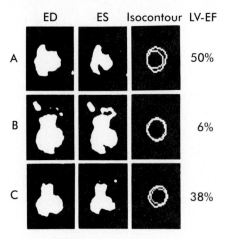

A. Preoperative
B. 1 day postoperative
C. 6 days postoperative

Fig. 17-3. Gated blood pool radionuclide imaging demonstrating left ventricular recovery.

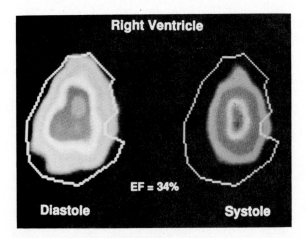

Fig. 17-4. First pass radionuclide right ventricular imaging.

with constant pump flows as ventricular ejection improves, and ejection fraction assessed by radionuclide or echocardiographic study will show improvement in the global and segmental ventricular function. Cardiac muscle shows little tendency to atrophy; so weaning protocols are used only to demonstrate ventricular recovery, rather than recondition the heart to sustain the circulation. With evidence of ventricular recovery, trials of decreasing assist device flow are begun. Pump flows are decreased in 1 liter per minute steps, monitoring hemodynamic parameters, and imaging ventricular

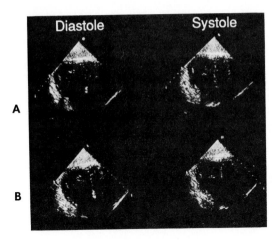

Fig. 17-5. Transesophageal echocardiography. **A**, on RVAD; **B**, off RVAD.

function. Studies in our institution on patients with left ventricular assist devices utilizing left atrial cannulation inserted postcardiotomy for coronary artery bypass demonstrate that increased left ventricular ejection fraction with decreased pump flow indicate a group of patients likely to be weaned from bypass and survive long term.[7] Patients who maintain low ejection fractions or whose ejection fractions decrease with decreasing pump flow are generally not ready to be weaned from the device, regardless of hemodynamic parameters. Full flow is resumed and they are left on the pump another 24 hours before weaning is reattempted. Hemodynamic parameters with decreased pump flows should show a stable blood pressure >60 mm Hg, cardiac index >2 L/min/m^2, $SvO_2 > 60\%$, and little increase in atrial filling pressures (Figs. 17-1 and 17-2). In addition, patients who maintain high pulmonary pressures on full pump flow are unlikely to survive long term after weaning from ventricular assist devices.[7] Intraaortic balloon pumping is continued during the weaning of right and left ventricular assist devices. As a final step, inotropes are used to increase the myocardial contractility to aid in the weaning of ventricular assist devices. With the patient fully anticoagulated, the ventricular assist device is turned off, and cardiac imaging is used to assist global ventricular function. Gated blood pool angiography has been used to image left ventricular fractions (Fig. 17-3), but is less helpful for right-sided imaging because of shielding by the cannulae. First pass radionuclide imaging is very helpful for estimating right ventricular ejection fractions, and may be performed in the ICU. (Fig. 17-4). Echocardiography, either transthoracic or transesophageal, may be used in the intensive care unit to demonstrate myocardial recovery and to aid in weaning ventricular assist devices (Fig. 17-5). Patients who have adequate hemodynamics and noninvasive evidence of improving global ventricular function with decreasing pump flows are returned to the operating room for removal of the support device.

CONCLUSION

Successful use of mechanical circulatory support begins with careful patient selection. Those patients with no chance of myocardial recovery are not appropriate candidates for support unless cardiac transplantation is an option. After institution of support, maintaining adequate, measurable, hemodynamic parameters and a clinical picture of adequate perfusion are important to sustain major organ systems. Hemodynamic and noninvasive evaluation of cardiac function demonstrating myocardial recovery guides device removal.

REFERENCES

1. Adamson RM, Dembitsky WP, Reichman RT et al: Mechanical support: assist or nemesis? *J Thorac Cardiovasc Surg* 98:915, 1989.
2. Ballantyne CM, Verani MS, Short HD et al: Delayed recovery of severely "stunned" myocardium with the support of a left ventricular assist device after coronary artery bypass graft surgery, *J Am Coll Cardiol* 10(3):710, 1987.
3. De Bakey ME: Left ventricular bypass pump for cardiac assistance, *Am J Cardiol* 27:3, 1971.
4. Goldberg RJ, Gore JM, Alpert JS et al: Cardiogenic shock after acute myocardial infarction, *N Engl J Med* 325(16):1117, 1991.
5. Magovern GJ, Golding LAR, Oyer PE et al: Weaning and bridging, *Ann Thorac Surg* 47:102, 1989.
6. Pae WE, Pierce WS, Pennock JL et al: Long-term results of ventricular assist pumping in postcardiotomy cardiogenic shock, *J Thorac Cardiovasc Surg* 93:434, 1987.
7. Sekela ME, Verani MS, Noon GP: Comparison of hemodynamics and ejection fraction during left heart bypass, *Ann Thorac Surg* 51:804, 1991.
8. Wampler RK, Frazier OH, Lansing AM et al: Treatment of cardiogenic shock with the Hemopump left ventricular assist device, *Ann Thorac Surg* 52:506, 1991.

CHAPTER 18

Infection prophylaxis and treatment

Steve H. Dougherty and Richard L. Simmons

INTRODUCTION

Infectious complications persist as a major factor limiting long-term use of the total artificial heart (TAH) and constitute a significant threat even during temporary mechanical cardiac support with the TAH or ventricular assist devices (VAD) (Table 18-1). According to one study, mortality may be as great as 76% for patients who develop infection immediately before or during mechanical cardiac support.[1]

Experience with infection in cardiac support devices, although still limited, parallels clinical experience with infections in other prosthetic devices.[2,3] The presence of the foreign body not only increases the risk of infection, but also promotes the emergence of opportunistic pathogens such as *Staphylococcus epidermidis,* diphtheroids, α-hemolytic streptococci, enterococcus, *Pseudomonas* sp., *Enterobacter aerogenes, Serratia marcescens,* and *Candida albicans. Clostridium difficile* may be recovered from the stool, whether or not there is overt enterocolitis. Such opportunistic organisms often emerge following repeated courses of antibiotics and are likely to be antibiotic resistant, causing superinfection. In addition to prolonged antimicrobial therapy, eradication of infections involving a heart prosthesis usually requires removal of the foreign body and debridement of the surrounding infected tissues—a measure that may be difficult to accomplish with an infected heart prosthesis.

Other factors, such as multiple-organ system failure, hemolysis, aspiration pneumonia, gastrointestinal bleeding, and ultimately global suppression of host-immune defenses, also contribute to the risk of infection in heart prostheses. Devices that are positioned internally, especially in the mediastinum, may impinge on adjacent vital structures such as the lung, causing atelectasis and pneumonia. Even in the absence of postoperative bleeding, clotted blood and serum in the pericardial space inevitably bathe the prosthetic ventricles and vascular conduits, serving as a culture medium for bacteria. Problems such as pneumonia due to prolonged respirator dependency and hematogenous infection from venous access lines, arterial lines, the pump's pneumatic

Table 18-1.   Incidence of infection in heart prosthesis recipients°

Source	No. patients	Device	No. infected patients (%)	Duration of implant (days)
Joyce[1]†	93	TAH	42 (45)	<1-243
Didisheim[29]‡	42	TAH	29 (69)	1-620
	40	VAD	8 (40)	1-74
Muneretto[21]	28	TAH	10 (36)	<1-43
Griffith[6]§	16	TAH	6 (37)	1-35
Copeland[63]	6	TAH	5 (83)	9-244
Starnes[64]	18	VAD	5 (28)	1-90
Farrar[44]	29	VAD	6 (21)	<1-31

TAH, Total artificial heart; *VAD*, Ventricular assist device.
°Not all infections involved the heart prosthesis itself.
†Some infections occurred before TAH implantation.
‡This survey overlaps some of the other reports.
§In four of the six cases, infection followed cardiac transplantation.

drivelines, and urinary catheters may be unrelenting. Aseptic management of access sites and use of preventive antibiotics, although probably effective, tend only to delay the onset of infectious complications unless patients can be weaned from the heart prosthesis by medical management or cardiac transplantation.

RISK FACTORS FOR INFECTION IN THE TAH OR VAD

In general there are many factors that can influence the risk of infection in implanted devices, including contamination of the device during manufacture or implantation (e.g., if the patient is septic at the time of implantation or if the implant bed itself is contaminated), postoperative wound infection, and episodes of remote site infection. Since clinical experience with heart prostheses is limited, however, specific risk factors for TAHs or VADs have yet to be defined. Among 16 patients bridged-to-cardiac-transplantation over an average 9 days (range, 1-35 days) with the Jarvik TAH, Griffith et al.[4] found that age, number of sternotomies, duration of implantation of the TAH, days of mechanical ventilatory support, and duration of preoperative use of inotropic agents and the intraarterial balloon pump did not predict subsequent lethal infection. However, a larger study of longer duration might have revealed such factors to be important. In another report, for example, mortality during mechanical cardiac support was 83% for patients older than 40 years compared with 18% in younger patients.[5] As Griffith observed: In the bridged patient almost every potential factor known to contribute to surgical infection is present.[6]

Percutaneous drivelines

All TAHs or VADs currently in use have percutaneous pneumatic or electrical drivelines that are continuously exposed to contamination from the patient's skin flora.

In spite of considerable study, no completely reliable method of preventing bacterial migration, and subsequent infection, along the transintegumental tracts of such devices has yet been found.[7] Although driveline-associated infection is not a major problem during short-term use of heart prostheses, given enough time such infections are virtually inevitable. Often they cannot be eradicated without removing the bacterial biofilm-laden foreign material.[8-10]

When a percutaneous foreign body is introduced, the epidermis of the cut wound edges and hair follicles proliferates and migrates downward into the space between the wound edge and the implant. If the tract is shallow, epithelial ingrowth may succeed in "marsupializing" the foreign body (i.e., completely surrounding it by an epithelialized surface). If the tract is deep, however, the process of cellular ingrowth appears to arrest at the level of the subcutaneous fat, usually without the establishment of an effective antibacterial barrier between the implant and surrounding subcutaneous tissues.[7] Shear stress between the mobile skin and percutaneous implants apparently discourages the formation of mechanical linkages between the implant and adjacent host tissue. However if the device is fixed to underlying bone so that at least one component of the host/implant interface is immobilized, the epidermis, or connective tissue from the dermis, may anchor at the implant surface, creating an effective antibacterial seal. Several reports provide evidence of clinical success with various bone-anchored prostheses.[11-13]

When skeletal fixation of a percutaneous implant is impractical, however, as is generally the case for drivelines of heart prostheses led out through the chest or abdominal wall, epidermal attachment and a bacterial barrier can still be encouraged by providing a porous or grooved synthetic surface into which dividing skin cells or fibroblasts can migrate. Thus fabrication of catheters with subdermal buttons or collars of porous materials that allow the ingrowth of host tissues leads to a more stable host/implant interface and a longer implant life.[14] Transcutaneous catheter connectors made of ceramics, sintered hydroxyapatite, or porous vitreous carbon, for example, appear to promote tissue attachment, and may discourage infection for as long as 2 years.[15-17] Likewise, the creation of V-shaped microgrooves on metallic surfaces encourages cellular attachment and may have applicability in the design of percutaneous devices.[18]

Dacron velour has been used recently to cover the entire subcutaneous segment (skin edge to peritoneum) of percutaneous drivelines for VADs positioned in the peritoneal cavity. Extending the velour to the skin edge instead of burying it under the skin in traditional fashion apparently encourages direct epithelial invasion of the velour itself, thereby discouraging marsupialization and infection. Whether the excellent antibacterial defenses of the peritoneal cavity also contribute to the success of this approach is unknown. Most VADs are certainly intended for only short-term (days to months) use, a factor that probably also limits the risk of infection.

Because infection can spread along percutaneous drivelines into the mediastinum, however, TAHs that depend on such lines will probably never be truly successful as permanent cardiac replacements. Indeed, virtually all current clinical use of heart prostheses is for bridging to myocardial recovery or cardiac transplantation. It has been possible experimentally, to confine driveline-associated infections to skin access sites, but only for brief periods (months) of time.[19] Some VADs have functioned clinically for nearly a year without significant infectious complications. Eventual success with permanent mechanical cardiac replacement, however, will probably require prostheses that are totally implantable (i.e., do not require percutaneous drivelines). An electric pump powered by an external induction coil, for example, is under development.

Prosthesis design

Some types of cardiac assist devices may be more vulnerable to infection than others. For example, implantable, as opposed to paracorporeal, systems require only one percutaneous driveline and may thus pose less risk of driveline-related infections, particularly during longer periods of implantation. On the other hand, implantable VADs are larger and more difficult to install and require extensive dissection of the anterior abdominal wall and of the diaphragm from the chest wall for apical cannulation of the heart. This increases the potential for bleeding and wound complications, particularly in postcardiotomy patients.[20] The safest designs from the standpoint of infection risk are probably those that eliminate percutaneous drivelines.

Bacteremia associated with invasive monitoring and critical care

Depending on their overall condition, patients being supported with a TAH or VAD are likely to have indwelling venous catheters for fluid management and medications, an arterial cannula for hemodynamic monitoring, a bladder catheter to monitor urine output, and perhaps an endotracheal tube. All such cannulae carry a substantial and often underappreciated potential for producing sepsis—bacteremia or fungemia arising from the cannula that can spread hematogenously to the heart prosthesis.[21] Indeed, **hematogenous** infection of heart prostheses may be even more common than ascending infection via the drivelines.[22] More than 40% of all nosocomial septicemias occurring in the intensive care unit (ICU) are related to intravenous infusion.[23] The incidence of catheter-associated urinary tract infection is about 5% to 10% per day, even with a closed urinary catheter system, and approximately 1% to 4% of such patients develop bacteremia.[24] Patients requiring prolonged intubation and ventilatory support in the ICU often die of pneumonia (the latter accounts for up to 36% of septic deaths during TAH bridging to transplant),[21] and about 6% experience nosocomial bacteremias of pulmonary origin.[25] Thus any remote focus of bacterial infection or colonization, especially from catheters and monitoring devices, has the potential to spread hematogenously to the heart prosthesis. If a VAD is positioned in the peritoneal cavity, even bacterial translocation from the intestinal tract may pose the threat of infection.[26]

Although there is little specific information on the risk of bacteremic infection of heart prostheses from cannula-associated infections, the problem may be somewhat analogous to that of early prosthetic valve endocarditis. Convincing microbiologic evidence suggests that prosthetic valve infections occurring during the first 12 months following valve insertion are apt to have been acquired nosocomially via bacteremic spread from arterial and venous catheters, bladder catheters, endotracheal tubes, tracheostomy sites, or other remote site infections (e.g., wound, lung).[27,28] Compared with a prosthetic valve, a TAH with its much larger surface area may be even more vulnerable to such blood-borne infections.[28] Indeed, thrombi located on the valves and at the vascular anastomoses of TAHs removed at autopsy are often infected, and may even have been caused by bacteria that arrived hematogenously.[22,29,30]

It is possible, although unproven, that risk factors for infection of other percutaneous devices such as intravascular catheters may also influence the risk of infection in heart prostheses. Surveillance studies show a strong correlation between organisms present on the skin surrounding vascular catheter sites and the microorganisms recovered from catheters that produce septicemia; the greater the concentration of microflora on the skin, the greater the likelihood of catheter-related bacteremia. In like manner, accumulation of moisture under the catheter dressing is a powerful predictor of catheter-related infection. Duration of catheterization is of particular importance; the longer a catheter remains in place, the greater the likelihood that it will become infected. In high-risk patients in the ICU, for example, central venous catheters left in place for more than 4 days are associated with a significantly increased risk of septicemia. In debilitated patients especially, intravenous cannulae are a common portal of entry for fungi such as *Candida* organisms, and even transient cannula-associated candidemia is a potentially serious clinical event.[31] Still the risk of catheter-associated bacteremia is low in patients whose health is generally good, suggesting that the likelihood of hematogenous infection probably varies with the seriousness of the underlying illness and the state of the host's immune defenses. The relevance of such factors to infections of the drivelines of TAHs or VADs unfortunately remains unknown.

Multiple organ system failure and host immunodepression

Mortality during bridging to transplantation with the TAH ranges from 30% to 50%.[1,5] Sepsis and multiple organ system failure (MOF), especially liver and kidney failure, are among the leading causes.[1,21] In older patients especially, MOF is often precipitated by chronic heart failure, with immunodepression and infection occurring later as secondary complications.[32−35] Use of mechanical cardiac support may lead to improved nutritional status and vital organ function, which in turn presumably reduces the risk of infection. Indeed, preoperative pneumonia has sometimes been seen to resolve after institution of mechanical cardiac assistance.[36,37]

However, the longer the duration of mechanical support, and the more blood transfusions the patient receives, the more likely it becomes that ensuing MOF and sepsis are related to the pump itself.[38,39] The need for hemodialysis (associated with a high perioperative mortality in TAH patients[1]) or for total parenteral nutrition arising from renal or intestinal failure are probably also risk factors for infection.

Studying two TAH heart recipients for periods of 8 and 10 months respectively, Stelzer et al.[40] found a progressive decline in the number of peripheral blood helper/ inducer T cells. A large number of activated suppressor/cytotoxic T cells were also noted, together with a progressive decrease in B cells. Total IgG and IgM levels, however, were not decreased, and there were no changes in neutrophil phagocytic or respiratory burst capacity. Similarly, Kaplan et al.[41] found that peripheral blood neutrophils from patients with implanted left ventricular assist devices exhibited normal superoxide release and chemotaxis. Although plasma concentrations of C3a may be slightly elevated, significant activation of the complement system has not generally been observed.[42]

In another report, autopsy examination of two TAH heart patients who survived long term revealed reduced numbers of lymphoid germinal centers and atrophy of the T lymphocyte-dependent areas.[42] The patients' reticuloendothelial systems were found to be engorged with degenerated erythrocytes, suggesting that the multiple blood transfusions necessitated by device-associated hemolysis and coagulopathy may have caused reticuloendothelial blockade. Such changes could potentially lead to a progressive loss of content of the antigen-specific lymphoidal elements and, perhaps, to a reduced ability to ingest microbe-antibody complexes and clear microorganisms from the circulation.[22] Indeed, blood transfusion per se is known to be a risk factor for infection.[43]

Thus the clinician must often contend simultaneously with two circumstances in which the prevention and treatment of infection are especially difficult: the presence of the prosthetic device itself and the presence of host immunodepression.

Note that cardiac support devices may themselves be a risk factor for infection following heart transplantation. According to some authors, if mechanically supported patients are not transplanted during episodes of active infection, their incidence and type of infection following transplantation is similar to that of recipients who do not require pretransplant mechanical support.[44,45] In contrast, however, Hsu et al.[46] compared patients receiving pretransplant mechanical support (VAD or TAH) to patients undergoing elective heart transplant and found, in the bridged patients, a significant increase in perioperative infectious complications, such as mediastinitis, urinary tract infection, and thoracic cavity infection (but not pneumonia). Bridged patients also experienced an increase in perioperative infection-related mortality.[46]

PREVENTION OF INFECTION IN THE TAH OR VAD

Prevention of infection in heart prosthesis recipients is often a challenge. Careful timing of the procedure and selection of the patients may help to reduce the risk. For example, some workers regard the presence of infections associated with bacteremia, including pneumonia, as a contraindication to use of TAHs as a bridge to transplantation—not only because of the risk of hematogenous spread to the device itself, but also because of potential infectious complications following the transplant procedure.[4] In some centers, immunosuppression (e.g., in a heart transplant patient) is considered a contraindication to mechanical cardiac support. Indeed mortality resulting from sepsis is very high in transplant patients with acute, accelerated rejection who receive mechanical cardiac support.[47,48] Still, success with mechanical support in such patients, especially when instituted for only brief periods of time, is occasionally reported.[49]

Superficial infection of the skin or wounds, urinary tract infections, or mild pneumonia with low-grade fever, however, are not necessarily contraindications to the use of mechanical cardiac support.[50]

Early institution of mechanical support before circulatory deterioration may reduce the overall risk of complications, including infection. Likewise, short-term use of mechanical support is associated with less risk of infection than long-term use. Ideally, bridging to transplant with the TAH should proceed for no more than 28 to 30 days, although for VADs, longer periods of support may be feasible.[9,51] In one report only 5% of TAH patients who were bridged for an average of 16 days experienced a driveline infection.[51]

Although infections of driveline and cannulation sites are often considered late complications of TAHs or VADs, administration of perioperative antibiotics, plus meticulous care of the driveline access sites, are still probably worthwhile.[3] In one center a regimen of perioperative cefamandole (1 g intravenously every 6 hours) plus vancomycin, continued until all invasive catheters have been removed, has been used.[46] Cefuroxime might be substituted for cefamandole. Some clinicians use only perioperative vancomycin. Care of driveline access sites may vary among institutions. One successful regimen incorporates wound cleansing with peroxide, followed by application of silver sulfadiazine cream and dry gauze two to three times per day. After several days, a healthy-looking access site should require only once-daily dressing changes.

Early extubation and mobilization of the patient are important goals of management.[20] Some authors place patients with implanted heart prostheses in reverse isolation. However, the value of this practice is questionable because most infections probably arise from the patient's endogenous flora. Detailed discussions of infection prevention in prosthetic device surgery are available.[52,53]

TREATMENT OF INFECTION IN THE TAH OR VAD

Patients with a heart prosthesis are often immunodepressed and vulnerable to infection. Multiple episodes of sepsis and antibiotic therapy may eventually lead to the emergence of antibiotic-resistant, opportunistic bacteria, both Gram-negative and Gram-positive, and also to colonization and infection by fungi.[54] Because a complete discussion of all such potential pathogens and their treatment is beyond the scope of this chapter, only a few of the most common and virulent organisms will be mentioned. Discussions of the microbiology and therapy of implant infections are available elsewhere.[55,56]

Staphylococcus aureus and *Staphylococcus epidermidis*

S. aureus, which colonizes the skin, frequently infects prosthetic devices, including heart prostheses and their drivelines. The organisms probably spread to the device either directly by contamination during operative placement or postoperatively by extension from superficial wound infections. *S. epidermidis* and other coagulase-negative staphylococci, on the other hand, more often contaminate intravascular devices by bacteremic spread from catheters, lines, and monitoring devices. They are also more likely than *S. aureus* to be resistant to methicillin and other antibiotics.

Antibiotic therapy for intravascular infections due to staphylococci is controversial. Infections caused by methicillin-susceptible *S. aureus* should probably be treated with oxacillin or nafcillin (1.5 to 2.0 g intravenously every 4 hours), perhaps with the addition of gentamicin (1 mg/kg intravenously every 8 hours) for the first 5 days of therapy. Methicillin-susceptible *S. epidermidis* infections require oxacillin or nafcillin (as above), plus rifampin (300 mg orally every 8 hours), plus gentamicin (as above, except for the initial 2 weeks of therapy). Infections due to methicillin-resistant *S. aureus* typically require treatment with vancomycin (7.5 mg/kg intravenously every 6 hours). Methicillin-resistant *S. epidermidis* infections are treated the same as those due to sensitive *S. epidermidis,* but with the substitution of vancomycin for semisynthetic penicillins.[57] Other agents, such as teicoplanin or minocycline, may also be useful for staphylococcal infections, particularly those due to resistant organisms.[58,59]

Pseudomonas aeruginosa

Infections due to *P. aeruginosa* may be acquired from environmental sources, from the patient's endogenous flora, or by nosocomial spread from other patients. Like all Gram-negative infections associated with prosthetic devices, those due to *P. aeruginosa* are extremely difficult—perhaps even the *most* difficult—to treat and can seldom be controlled without removal of the infected device. Indeed, the frequent recovery of *P. aeruginosa* and other Gram-negative organisms from the flora of TAH-associated infections may help to account for the extreme lethality of this problem.

Antibiotic therapy for established intravascular infections due to *P. aeruginosa* should be initiated with high-dose aminoglycoside (e.g., tobramycin 8 mg/kg intravenously per day) plus an extended spectrum penicillin (e.g., ticarcillin 18 g intravenously per day). Serum aminoglycoside levels and bactericidal activity should be monitored to maintain peak gentamicin or tobramycin levels in the range of 12 to 20 μg/ml, and at least 10 times the minimum bactericidal concentration of an infecting blood isolate, respectively. These higher dose and peak serum concentrations of gentamicin or tobramycin, compared with the doses and levels usually recommended, have demonstrated efficacy in *P. aeruginosa* endocarditis.[60]

Candida albicans

Like infections due to *Pseudomonas* sp., candidal infections associated with TAHs are difficult to treat and lethal. An established infection of a TAH due to *C. albicans* requires therapy with high doses of amphotericin B (as much as 1 mg/kg per day) given in combination with oral flucytosine (dose adjusted for renal function). Even then the chances of cure without removal of the infected prosthesis are poor.[61]

Unfortunately, infections of cardiac prostheses are often polymicrobial with a complex "consortium" of organisms incorporated in the bacterial biofilm. Thus they may defy treatment with predetermined drug regimes. Furthermore, antibiotic concentrations that appear effective under standard laboratory testing conditions may be ineffective against organisms ensconced in surface biofilm. In vitro studies suggest that early treatment of such infections, while the biofilm is still "young," would produce the best results.[62]

In addition to prolonged antimicrobial therapy, eradication of infections associated with heart prostheses often requires removal of the foreign body and debridement of the surrounding infected tissues. It is paradoxical that surgical removal of the infected device, for obvious reasons of physiology, may be just as incompatible with survival as in situ preservation of the device.

REFERENCES

1. Joyce LD, Johnson KE, Toninato CJ et al: Results of the first 100 patients who received Symbion Total Artificial Hearts as a bridge to cardiac transplantation, *Circulation* 80:(III)192, 1989.
2. Dougherty SH, Simmons RL: Infections in bionic man: the pathobiology of infections in prosthetic devices—Part I. *Curr Probl Surg* 19:217, 1982.
3. Dougherty SH, Simmons RL: Infections in bionic man: the pathobiology of infections in prosthetic devices—Part II. *Curr Probl Surg* 19:265, 1982.
4. Griffith BP, Kormos RL, Hardesty RL et al: The artificial heart: infection-related morbidity and its effect on transplantation, *Ann Thorac Surg* 45:409, 1988.
5. Muneretto C, Solis E, Pavie A et al: Total artificial heart: survival and complications, *Ann Thorac Surg* 47:151, 1989.
6. Griffith BP: Interim use of the Jarvik-7 artificial heart: lessons learned at Presbyterian-University Hospital of Pittsburgh, *Ann Thorac Surg* 47:158, 1989.
7. von Recum AF, Park JB: Permanent percutaneous devices, *Crit Rev Bioengineer* 5:37, 1981.
8. Kunin CM, Dobbins JJ, Melo JC et al: Infectious complications in four long-term recipients of the Jarvik-7 artificial heart, *JAMA* 259:860, 1988.
9. Dobbins JJ, Johnson GS, Kunin CM et al: Postmortem microbiological findings of two total artificial heart recipients, *JAMA* 259:865, 1988.
10. Gristina AG, Dobbins JJ, Giammara B et al: Biomaterial-centered sepsis and the total artificial heart. Microbial adhesion vs tissue integration, *JAMA* 259:870, 1988.
11. Albrektsson T, Dahl E, Enbom L et al: Osseointegrated oral implants. A Swedish multicenter study of 8139 consecutively inserted Nobelpharma implants, *J Periodontol* 59:287, 1988.
12. Gregory M, Murphy WM, Scott J et al: A clinical study of the Branemark dental implant system, *Br Dent J* 168:18, 1990.
13. Holgers KM, Tjellstrom A, Bjursten LM et al: Soft tissue reactions around percutaneous implants: a clinical study of soft tissue conditions around skin-penetrating titanium implants for bone-anchored hearing aids, *Am J Otol* 9:56, 1988.
14. Allan A, Graham TR, Withington PS et al: Development of a polyurethane percutaneous access device for long-term vascular access, *ASAIO Trans* 36:M349, 1990.
15. Amano I, Katoh T, Inagaki Y: Clinical experience with alumina ceramic transcutaneous connector to prevent skin-exit infection around CAPD catheter, *Adv Perit Dial* 6:150, 1990.
16. Aoki H, Akao M, Shin Y et al: Sintered hydroxyapatite for a percutaneous device and its clinical application, *Med Prog Technol* 12:213, 1987.

17. Krouskop TA, Brown HD, Gray K et al: Bacterial challenge study of a porous carbon percutaneous implant, *Biomaterials* 9:398, 1988.
18. Chehroudi B, Gould TR, Brunette DM: Titanium-coated micromachined grooves of different dimensions affect epithelial and connective-tissue cells differently in vivo, *J Biomed Mater Res* 24:1203, 1990.
19. Murray KD, Abbott TM, Olsen DB et al: Correlation of gross and microscopic appearance of skin buttons in total artificial heart animals, *ASAIO Trans* 36:825, 1990.
20. Ott, RA, Mills TC, Eugene J et al: Clinical choices for circulatory assist devices, *ASAIO Trans* 36:792, 1990.
21. Muneretto C, Pavie A, Solis E et al: Special problems in use of the total artificial heart as a bridge to transplantation, *Transplant Proc* 21:2551-2, 1989.
22. Ward RA, Wellhausen SR, Dobbins JJ et al: Thromboembolic and infectious complications of total artificial heart implantation, *Ann N Y Acad Sci* 516:638, 1987.
23. Maki DG: *Pathogenesis, prevention, and management of infections due to intravascular devices used for infusion therapy.* In Bisno AL, Waldvogel FA, eds: *Infections associated with indwelling medical devices,* Washington, DC, 1989, American Society for Microbiology.
24. Hessen MT, Kaye D: *Infections associated with foreign bodies in the urinary tract.* In Bisno AL, Waldvogel FA, eds: *Infections associated with indwelling medical devices,* Washington, DC, 1989, American Society for Microbiology.
25. Scheld WM: Developments in the pathogenesis, diagnosis and treatment of nosocomial pneumonia, *Surg Gynecol Obstet* 172 (suppl):42, 1991.
26. Mora EM, Cardona MA, Simmons RL: Enteric bacteria and ingested inert particles translocate to intraperitoneal prosthetic materials, *Arch Surg* 126:157, 1991.
27. Archer GL: *Staphylococcus epidermidis and other coagulase-negative staphylococci.* In Mandell GL, Douglas RG Jr., Bennett JE, eds: *Principles and practice of infectious diseases,* New York, 1985, Wiley & Sons.
28. Dougherty SH: Pathobiology of infection in prosthetic devices, *Rev Infect Dis* 10:1102, 1988.
29. Didisheim P, Olsen DB, Farrar DJ et al: Infections and thromboembolism with implantable cardiovascular devices, *ASAIO Trans* 35:54, 1989.
30. Weidemann H, Muller KM, Hennig E et al: Experience with vascular grafts in total artificial heart replacement, *Int J Artif Organs* 13:288, 1990.
31. Komshian SV, Uwaydah AK, Sobel JD et al: Fungemia caused by Candida species and Torulopsis glabrata in the hospitalized patient: frequency, characteristics, and evaluation of factors influencing outcome, *Rev Infect Dis* 11:379, 1989.
32. Kawaguchi AT, Gandjbahch I, Pavie A et al: Liver and kidney function in patients undergoing mechanical circulatory support with Jarvik-7 artificial heart as a bridge to transplantation, *J Heart Transplant* 9:631, 1990.
33. Solis E, Leger P, Muneretto C et al: Clinical application and patient selection in the use of a total artificial heart as a bridge for transplantation, *Eur J Cardiothorac Surg* 2:65, 1988.
34. Muneretto C, Rabago G Jr, Pavie A et al: Mechanical circulatory support as a bridge to transplantation: current status of total artificial heart in 1989 and determinants of survival, *J Cardiovasc Surg (Torino)* 31:486, 1990.
35. Termuhlen DF, Pennington DG, Roodman ST et al: T-cells in ventricular assist device patients, *Circulation* 80:(III)174, 1989.
36. Vega JD, Poindexter SM, Radovancevic B et al: Nutritional assessment of patients with extended left ventricular assist device support, *ASAIO Trans* 36:M555, 1990.
37. Friedel N, Viazis P, Schiessler A et al: Patient selection for mechanical circulatory support as a bridge to cardiac transplantation, *Int J Artif Organs* 14:276, 1991.
38. Pierce WS, Gray LA Jr, McBride LR et al: Circulatory support 1988. Other postoperative complications, *Ann Thorac Surg* 47:96, 1989.
39. Moritz A, Rokitansky A, Trubel W et al: Timing for implantation and transplantation in mechanical bridge to transplantation, *Int J Artif Organs* 14:270, 1991.
40. Stelzer GT, Ward RA, Wellhausen SR et al: Alterations in select immunologic parameters following total artificial heart implantation, *Artif Organs* 11:52,1987.
41. Kaplan SS, Basford RE, Kormos RL et al: Biomaterial associated impairment of local neutrophil function, *ASAIO Trans* 36:M172, 1990.

42. Wellhausen SR, Ward RA, Johnson GS et al: Immunologic complications of long-term implantation of a total artificial heart, *J Clin Immunol* 8:307, 1988.

43. Tartter PI: Immune consequences of blood transfusion in the surgical patient, *Surg Immun* 2:13, 1989.

44. Farrar DJ, Hill JD, Gray LA Jr et al: Heterotopic prosthetic ventricles as a bridge to cardiac transplantation. A multicenter study in 29 patients, *N Engl J Med* 318:333, 1988.

45. Pifarre R, Sullivan H, Montoya A et al: Use of the total artificial heart and ventricular assist device as a bridge to transplantation, *J Heart Transplant* 9:638, 1990.

46. Hsu J, Griffith BP, Dowling RD et al: Infections in mortally ill cardiac transplant recipients, *J Thorac Cardiovasc Surg* 98:506, 1989.

47. Cabrol C, Gandjbakhch I, Pavie A et al: Is the use of artificial hearts the future solution for interim treatment of patients awaiting retransplantation? *Transplant Proc* 21:3658, 1989.

48. Cabrol C, Solis E, Muneretto C et al: Orthotopic transplantation after implantation of a Jarvik 7 total artificial heart, *J Thorac Cardiovasc Surg* 97:342, 1989.

49. Ott RA, Mills T, Allen B et al: Successful treatment of acute allograft failure using pneumatic biventricular assistance, *J Heart Lung Transplant* 10:264, 1991.

50. Reedy JE, Swartz MT, Termuhlen DF et al: Bridge to heart transplantation: importance of patient selection, *J Heart Transplant* 9:473, 1990.

51. Gaykowski R, Taylor KD, Yates WG: Cumulative clinical experience with the Symbion J7 TAH, *ASAIO Trans* 34:455, 1988.

52. Dougherty SH, Simmons RL: *Prosthetic devices.* In Wilmore DW, Brennan MF, Harken AH, Holcroft JW, Meakins JL, eds: *Care of the surgical patient, vol 2, Elective care,* New York, 1989, Scientific American.

53. Kaiser AB: *Antimicrobial prophylaxis of infections associated with foreign bodies.* In Bisno AL, Waldvogel FA, eds: *Infections associated with indwelling medical devices,* Washington, DC, 1989, American Society for Microbiology.

54. Burns GL, Olsen DB: Patterns of bacterial infection in calves implanted with artificial hearts, *ASAIO Trans* 36:M138, 1990.

55. Dougherty SH: *Microbiology of infection in prosthetic devices.* In Wadstrom T, Eliasson I, Holder I, Ljungh, A, eds: *Pathogenesis of wound and biomaterial-associated infections,* London, 1990, Springer-Verlag.

56. Bisno AL, Waldvogel FA, eds: *Infections associated with indwelling medical devices,* Washington, DC, 1989, American Society for Microbiology.

57. Karchmer AW: Staphylococcal endocarditis. Laboratory and clinical basis for antibiotic therapy, *Am J Med* 78:116, 1985.

58. Lawlor MT, Sullivan MC, Levitz RE et al: Treatment of prosthetic valve endocarditis due to methicillin-resistant Staphylococcus aureus with minocycline *J Infect Dis* 161:812, 1990 (letter).

59. Venditti M, Micozzi A, Serra P et al: Intraventricular administration of teicoplanin in shunt associated ventriculitis caused by methicillin resistant Staphylococcus aureus *J Antimicrob Chemother* 21:513, 1988 (letter).

60. Pollack M: *Pseudomonas aeruginosa.* In Mandell GL, Douglas RG, Jr., Bennett JE, eds: *Principles and practice of infectious diseases,* ed 3, New York, 1990, Churchill Livingstone.

61. Threlkeld MG, Cobbs CG: *Infectious disorders of prosthetic valves and intravascular devices.* In Mandell GL, Douglas RG, Jr., Bennett JE, eds: *Principles and practice of infectious diseases,* ed 3, New York, 1990, Churchill Livingstone.

62. Anwar H, Costerton JW: Enhanced activity of combination of tobramycin and piperacillin for eradication of sessile biofilm cells of Pseudomonas aeruginosa, *Antimicrob Agents Chemother* 34:1666, 1990.

63. Copeland JG, Smith R, Icenogle T et al: Orthotopic total artificial heart bridge to transplantation: preliminary results, *J Heart Transplant* 8:124, 1989.

64. Starnes VA, Oyer PE, Portner PM et al: Isolated left ventricular assist as bridge to cardiac transplantation, *J Thorac Cardiovasc Surg* 96:62, 1988.

CHAPTER 19

Role of FDA in a ventricular assist device program

Abhijit Acharya and Bette Lemperle

INTRODUCTION

The 1976 Medical Device Amendments to the Food, Drug, and Cosmetics Act authorize Food and Drug Administration (FDA) to (1) approve and oversee ventricular assist device (VAD) and total artificial heart (TAH) clinical trials, and (2) evaluate these heart-assist and replacement devices for safety and effectiveness before they may be marketed.[1] Up to 35,000 patients in the United States may benefit from temporary or long-term VAD or TAH assist[2] for uses such as weaning from cardiopulmonary bypass, staged transplantation, long-term heterotopic assist, or orthotopic replacement. Formal clinical trials of these devices started in 1981. Since then a significant evolution has occurred in device design and the sophistication of clinical trial protocols.

FDA's role in the development and clinical characterization of VADs and TAHs has involved issues of law, regulation, engineering, clinical trial design, risk/benefit analysis, patient rights, and quality of life, as well as public and media expectations of these technologies. This chapter primarily addresses clinical trial design and data analysis. However, an examination of the FDAs overall involvement in the VAD/TAH program provides a paradigm that illustrates a science-based regulatory agency in the development and assessment of high technology, life-sustaining medical devices.

The level of FDA's involvement in developing sound engineering and animal testing protocols for TAHs and VADs was not unusual for intracorporeal life-sustaining devices, and parallels the requirements for prosthetic heart valves. Clinical, ethical, societal, and quality-of-life aspects of the artificial heart trials posed the most difficult and unprecedented challenges to FDA's regulatory role. Issues confronted included (1) the ability of a patient, on the verge of death, to give truly informed consent; (2) whether quality of life, in addition to its continuation, should be an important factor in a decision to continue or expand clinical trials; (3) fear that distribution of scarce donor hearts may be skewed in favor of VAD/TAH recipients; and, (4) whether FDA should even be regulating clinical trials of last-ditch devices such as VADs and TAHs.

Although there is general agreement with the basic principles underlying FDA's oversight of clinical research, not everyone agrees on how these principles should be translated into the specifics of an investigation, such as patient selection criteria, definition of success, and follow-up protocol. This has been true of the VAD/TAH studies as well. In the early days many investigators, enthusiastic about these new technologies, viewed them first as potentially life-saving therapy for their dying patients, with data collection and protocol compliance being distinctly secondary concerns. Potential investigators did not appreciate FDA's role in limiting the availability of these yet unproven investigational devices. There was resistance to FDA insisting on a degree of uniformity in study protocols and data collection to decrease the potential for bias in these multicenter trials. FDA, on the other hand, contended that by not conforming to these requirements, investigators were adding to the delay in getting potentially useful devices to the market and restricting their availability for wider use.

The "paperwork burden" has been another issue. There is no question that writing an investigational device exemption (IDE) application, an annual report, or a premarket approval application (PMA) is time consuming and an exacting task. Collecting and analyzing scientific data, followed by a written presentation in a scientific format, is akin to developing a research proposal or writing a scientific paper for a peer review journal. Eventually the PMA application for a VAD or TAH will be reviewed by a peer group of scientists and physicians on FDA's Circulatory System Devices Panel for objective evidence of safety and effectiveness, and for scientific validity of the proposed labeling claims.

Emergency use of the investigational TAHs as a bridge-to-transplant proved to be a difficult regulatory and public relations problem for FDA in 1985 and 1986. A typical scenario was as follows:

FDA would get a call from a surgeon saying that he or she had a patient in heart failure about to expire while waiting for a donor heart. It would also be revealed that the institution had previously applied to participate in the TAH study while the surgeon had completed the manufacturer's required training and was ready to implant the TAH device as a bridge, to keep the patient alive until a donor heart became available. Under these circumstances, with a patient about to expire, FDA had no choice but to allow the implantation.

As these emergency requests became more frequent, it was evident that FDA needed to take action to prevent this activity from compromising the TAH program, by inhibiting an orderly collection of data for appropriately selected patients under a uniform protocol. This was an issue fraught with multiple problems. On one hand, the agency could be accused of denying a last resort, potentially life-saving device to a dying patient and of meddling in the practice of medicine. On the other hand, approval of these numerous requests could quickly undermine investigational protocol and weaken the IDE structure because all TAH bridge to transplants were emergency implants by definition.

FDA has attempted, with considerable success, to address these difficult issues through a continuing dialog with the clinical investigator community, professional societies, and consumer groups, while pointing out that some of the societal and health economic issues are beyond the scope of FDA's legislated mandate. As a result of this cooperative dialogue, scientific documentation of the device's clinical safety and effectiveness has evolved to the point that market release of one or more short-term use VADs appears to be near.

MEDICAL DEVICE AMENDMENTS OF 1976 (PUBLIC LAW 94-295) AND SAFE MEDICAL DEVICES ACT OF 1990

The Medical Device Amendments of 1976 and the Safe Medical Devices Act of 1990 defined a medical device, clearly distinguishing it from a drug, and established a three-tiered system for regulating devices. In this three-tiered system, each tier or class is based on the extent of control necessary to reasonably ensure device safety and effectiveness. Class I devices (e.g., surgical scissor, manual stethoscope) are subject to general controls only, such as good manufacturing practices, quality assurance in manufacturing, and labeling. Class II devices (e.g., x-ray, ultrasound) can be marketed subject to general controls and special controls, such as compliance with performance standards, postmarket surveillance, and additional preclinical and clinical performance data requirements that FDA may consider necessary. Class III devices (e.g., heart valve, implantable defibrillator) are life-sustaining or life-supporting devices for which general controls and special controls are insufficient to ensure safety and effectiveness; therefore these must undergo the premarket approval process. Total artificial hearts and ventricular assist devices fall within the Class III regulatory category.[1]

Regulations promulgated to enforce the Amendments of 1976 and 1990 provide for three types of medical device application: (1) to legally ship a device, (2) to conduct a clinical investigation of a device, or (3) to seek approval to market a device. These applications include (1) investigational device exemptions (IDEs), (2) premarket approval (PMA), and (3) the 510(k) or premarket notification. IDEs are intended to study medical device safety and effectiveness in humans after sufficient preclinical data demonstrates the device's relative safety. For certain Class III devices, the manufacturer then submits device preclinical and IDE clinical data in a PMA application. The PMA application is reviewed by FDA scientists and may be submitted to an advisory panel at FDA discretion. Advisory panels (composed of physicians, scientists, consumers, and industry representatives) regularly assist the agency by making recommendations on the safety and effectiveness of new devices. Their participation in this approval process adds a critical perspective from the academic community and the everyday world of medical practice, as a complement to FDA's scientific and technical review. The PMA application process allows the agency to determine if a Class III medical device has been shown to be reasonably safe and effective for its intended use, and is therefore suitable for marketing.[1]

The act and subsequent regulations mandated that clinical trials of medical devices meet certain requirements for the protection and welfare of human subjects, and for an orderly collection of clinical data. Three basic requirements are (1) a risk/benefit analysis, based on objective criteria, must be conducted (i.e., benefit to the individual patient in terms of likely therapeutic value, and to the society in terms of knowledge to be gained, outweighing the foreseeable patient risks, must be demonstrated); (2) informed consent must be obtained; and (3) an institutional review board (IRB) and FDA must provide peer review of the proposed clinical trial. These legal requirements are not very different from those imposed by the National Institutes of Health (NIH) for funding clinical research, and are derived from landmarks such as the Nuremberg Code, the Declaration of Helsinki, and the Ethical Guideline Statement of the American Medical Association. Indeed, these are the requirements of good science and good clinical research.

INITIAL EXPERIENCES

FDA approved the first VAD studies in 1980 and 1982 when William Pierce, Glenn Pennington, and William Bernhard initiated their clinical trials with VADs. The first approval of an investigational TAH as a permanent implant occurred in 1982 and was followed by four patient implants in the United States between 1982 and 1985. In 1985 with transplantations becoming increasingly successful, demand increased, causing a longer wait for transplant hearts. FDA approved the Jarvik-7 and Penn-State TAHs for clinical trials as bridge devices. At that time VADs were already being used as bridges-to-transplant, with far less publicity than the TAHs generated.

During these early years of clinical trials, FDA did not play a very active role trying to define clinical protocols or data analysis strategies. Rationale for device design, assessment of blood and tissue-contacting materials compatibility, evaluation of such design/material factors as resistance to thrombus formation, evaluation of potential causes for damage to blood components, characterization of the device, assessment of device durability, reliability, and in vivo performance were the focus of FDA's review. The box on p. 248 summarizes preclinical characterization data and testing requirements for the VADs and TAHs. This was a learning period for sponsors, investigators, and FDA. New and unique questions and concerns were addressed and procedures and policies were progressively developed. Sponsors were relied on to do what was necessary to optimize the scientific yield from these clinical trials.

Patient enrollment was slow 5 years ago when VADs were being used by only a few investigators at a few centers, with rarely more than three or four patients per center entering a study in a year. To gather more information regarding VAD utility in appropriate patient populations, it was necessary to include many more centers in each study than is generally considered desirable with a new device. Although these devices were in the early stage of clinical use, 10 or as many as 20 centers, were approved for participation in an attempt to increase VAD experience.

SUMMARY OF PRECLINICAL DATA REQUIREMENTS

A detailed description of the total system (pump, controller, software, and connectors) (e.g., design, design validation test results, dimensions, materials, engineering drawings and photographs, operation, safety features, and rationale for each feature)

The pump

Characterization of the materials and demonstration of acceptable biocompatibility for all implanted components (emphasis on blood contacting surfaces)

Description of the placement of the pump (internal and external), location in the body, and connection to the body. Are thermal effects a concern? Is there a limitation on patient size? How is fit determined?

Description of the mechanism of action. Will it operate synchronously or asynchronously to the natural heart?

Description of anticipated transvalvular pressures, loads, and the designed safety factors, including real time or accelerated valve test data

Description of the worst cases and normal physiological conditions under which the pump can operate

Description of the conditions that will cause the pump or the pump valves to fail

Description of the design features fashioned to address known clinical complications (e.g., thromboembolism, hemolysis, bleeding infection, calcification, device failure), including flow visualization test results

Description of specific application parameters (e.g., drive pressure limit vs. expected arterial pressure, back pressure on valves, peak pulsatile flow at outflow, peak pressure drop across valves, regurgitation, maximum pressure the diaphragm can withstand compared with its burst pressure, and pump housing pressure limit)

The console

The tests used to qualify the design (e.g., mechanical, electrical, component, pressure, dynamic, environmental, software)

Description of the labeling and engineering specifications (i.e., electrical, mechanical, pneumatic), including the tolerance of error for each specification

Description of the backup system and the potential causes of console failure

Description of the accuracy of the console in estimating blood flow, pressures, and durations

The methods used to validate accuracy of the console and assurance that test equipment has been adequately tested, calibrated, and/or standardized

The software/firmware program validation, including the inputs used to evaluate boundary conditions

The software requirements, specifications, and methods used to verify software performance

Description of the software safety features and an analysis of possible errors and failures (i.e., hazard analysis, failure mode and effects analysis)

The system

Characterization

A description of the experimental protocol, test conditions (e.g., mock loop, test fluid, operating temperature range, measurement instrumentation, calibration equipment) and test results for the evaluation of a final clinical model for which no changes were made during the period of testing. This includes the following:

SUMMARY OF PRECLINICAL DATA REQUIREMENTS—cont'd

Data on use of the device in all modes of synchronous and asynchronous operation

Data showing value ranges (e.g., air pressure, beats per minute, RA pressure, LA pressure, percent systole, suction) required to attain the cardiac outputs anticipated in the clinical setting

Data showing the peak pressure gradients across the valves and the peak pressures at the exit ports for each cycle, for the parameter ranges noted above

Data showing the parameters of operation at the worst case physiological conditions (extreme flows and extreme pressures) under which the pump can operate, and the threshold conditions which will cause the pump to fail

Description of Starling's curves for the operation of the device

Durability and reliability testing

The experimental protocol, a description of the test apparatus (diagrams, methods of operation), test conditions, test equipment calibration, and test results for the evaluation of a final clinical model for which no changes were made during the period of testing

Test results for a minimum of eight systems, remove and examine four after 6 months, and allow four to run to failure. Conditions for running the systems (worst case and normal) should be based on results of the characterization study

Description of the model used to predict reliability (currently 80% reliability, with 95% confidence or better, is acceptable)

Test results of a detailed examination of all components for wear, cracks (with special emphasis on the diaphragm and the valves using SEM, thermal imaging, and/or other high magnification examinations), fatigue, predicted system life, predicted component life, and maintenance schedule

Description of all failures, including when they occurred, why they occurred, whether they could be resimulated, whether the component could be changed, potential effect on a clinical situation, whether the reliability test was continued after the failure, and action taken to prevent recurrence of the failure

In vivo studies

Animal studies

The protocol used to study the physiologic aspects of the use of the final clinical model of the device in eight animals. The device must be in its final configuration with no changes made to it during the period of testing. Testing must be performed on a minimum of eight animals for no less than 4 months, which, based on the information provided to us by those researchers conducting animal studies, is the appropriate period for obtaining meaningful information on how the design performs in a physiological environment and how the animal responds to the device. After 4 to 5 months, the animal usually outgrows the capacity of the device. Also:

Description of the type of animal used in the study and any aspect of animal care that could affect the results of the study

Discussion of the implant procedure and any effects it could have on the study outcome

Summarization of the course of events for each animal

Discussion of hematology and blood chemistry study results for each animal, including the normal ranges for the type animal in the laboratory where the studies were performed, the baseline findings for each animal, and the level at which a parameter is considered clinically significant for hemolysis, kidney failure, etc.

Continued

SUMMARY OF PRECLINICAL DATA REQUIREMENTS—cont'd

Summary of hematology and blood chemistry data for all animals, including the mean preimplant parameters and the mean on-device parameters at regular intervals, including the number of animals represented by interval values

Discussion of all complications using graphs/tables to demonstrate the rate of occurrence

Submission of the explanted device reports for each animal including a gross description of each device, using diagrams and photographs, as necessary, to illustrate the appearance, results of microscopic and SEM/EDAX examinations of component wear and deterioration, a description of the location and size of thrombus formation, and results of histopathological studies

Submission of autopsy reports for each animal, with pictures of the device in situ, gross necropsy examination with conventional histological studies of major organs, and histological evaluation of all areas of grossly evident pathology

Descriptions of changes made as a result of experiences during the animal implants

Cadaver studies

Discussion of the protocol for and the results of human fit studies, including recommendations on patient size, placement location, placement parameters, and measurements required to determine adequacy of fit

---

In 1985 the Society of Thoracic Surgeons testified at an FDA advisory panel review of a TAH as a permanent implant. The Society urged continuation of the investigation under "rigid" controls and a broadening of scientific information collected (e.g., operative techniques, coagulation, neurological and immunological responses, renal function, infection) to facilitate development of improved devices for wider use. FDA was in full agreement with these recommendations and held that the same scientific considerations applied to VAD/TAH clinical trials design for short-term use as in bridge-to-transplant patients.

In 1988 as VAD patient enrollment started to rise and FDA began to see clinical data on a regular basis, FDA asked the Cardiac Assist Advisory Committee of the Society of Thoracic Surgeons to respond to multiple issues consuming FDA's attention. After appropriate interaction and consideration, this committee responded to our numerous questions in writing, providing us with a clearer understanding of the investigators' views on issues such as (1) questions they believed should be answered in clinical trials; (2) the importance of standard testing procedures; (3) minimum acceptable survival rates for weaning and bridging studies; (4) preimplant data to be collected; (5) length of patient follow-up; (6) the importance of implantation technique to patient outcome; and (7) how different VAD pump operative modes should be evaluated. We believed that the increased participation of investigators regarding protocol issues fostered mutual understanding and established a dialog that will be expanded in the future.

CURRENT STATUS OF IDE STUDIES

In 1986 and 1987 FDA concluded that VAD study sponsors were not defining, directing, or monitoring their studies with the kind of control and goal orientation necessary to develop scientific data for eventual determination of safety and effectiveness. As a result, in the past 3 to 4 years, FDA encouraged study sponsors to write comprehensive annual progress reports, with up-to-date aggregate data and preliminary analyses. Scientists and clinicians in the Center for Devices and Radiological Health, members of the Circulatory System Devices Panel, and consultants from other medical device panels, were consulted for data analyses. These reviews indicated that as much clinical and physiological information as possible should be gathered on VAD patients during these early studies of emerging technology. These reviews also supported FDA opinion that the structure originally proposed for these studies was not adequate, given the complex, multicentered trials that evolved. It appeared that the data submitted to FDA was preliminary and could be best utilized as a baseline for formulating questions to be answered about device clinical effectiveness and utility in appropriately designed second-phase clinical trials.

FDA maintains that a pilot study is valuable, and that a second-phase trial, with experienced investigators implanting devices in appropriate patients, can be conducted expeditiously. The anticipated result is data of a quality suitable for a final analysis to determine VAD safety and effectiveness as a bridge-to-transplant or for weaning from bypass. Some sponsors have completed this process, and a satisfactory overall result and conclusion to the evaluation is anticipated, despite initial frustrations.

Today VADs have been used experimentally at about 60 centers in this country, and knowledge and experience concerning their clinical utility is rapidly expanding. With so many centers involved in clinical trials, it has been prudent for study sponsors to bring investigators together regularly, usually on an annual basis, to share experiences in their studies. As a result, investigators are participating in a broader range of investigational issues and activities and are more aware of the clinical trial issues that challenge study sponsors and FDA.

From the IDE inception, new study sponsors are encouraged to design studies using sound scientific principles appropriate to multicentered trials. Although this is a reasonable expectation for a study in support of marketing a device, in practice, protocols are regularly encountered that do not systematically consider targeted study populations. Unaddressed are (1) questions that need to be answered about a device and the effect on the intended population; (2) general and specific study objectives based on these questions; (3) how success or failure of study objectives will be demonstrated; and (4) how specific data parameters will be collected to demonstrate success or failure.

Some new study sponsors simply state that the trial is expected to demonstrate device safety and effectiveness in a general patient population such as one with "low cardiac output." A data collection form may be included in the submission, or data collection may be presented as optional. The FDA encourages sponsors to establish continuity among questions to be answered, data to be collected, size of the study, and the steps leading to the proposed analysis. Otherwise, conclusions drawn from the study may be unacceptable.

Collection of control and reference group data is essential and should be collected from the outset of clinical implantation. If patients are their own controls, as is common with the VAD weaning indication, time frames for attempted weaning with drug therapy and intraaortic balloons (IABs) before VAD therapy must be established and adhered to. The assumption is that before entrance into the study, no apparent, irreversible, end-organ function has occurred and the device may be evaluated by its ability to maintain appropriate pressures, flows, and patient hemodynamics; to protect endorgan function; to promote myocardial recovery; and thereby to promote survival. With the bridge indication, we expect clinical centers to track patient transplant populations who meet the same study criteria as bridge patients but who do not receive the bridge device.

Uniform study criteria, entrance criteria, procedures, and interpretation of adverse events are essential for both intracenter and intercenter pooling of data. Justification must always be given for pooling among study centers. With the large number of study centers and investigators in VAD studies, uniformity becomes a critical issue when justifying pooling of data for analysis (e.g., data has been reviewed by the FDA in which as many as half of enrolled patients did not meet entrance criteria). This can be attributed in part to the tendency of some investigators to reason that if the device has worked well for long periods to bridge patients who meet standard heart transplant criteria, it may work well in patients who do not meet transplant criteria, reversing severe endorgan dysfunction and allowing sufficient recovery to permit a transplant weeks or months later. This may be true and may identify a subsequent group of patients to be studied. However, by adding a new group of patients, a separate study has been initiated before the original study questions have been answered; it is likely that both study and premarket approval will be delayed.

Both bridge-to-transplant and recovery protocols require patients who enter studies to have adequate end-organ function or dysfunction considered reversible. Every attempt should be made to document end-organ function accurately before device implant. Consequently, when a patient is on a device beyond the time it normally takes to recover from the effects of cardiopulmonary bypass and other hematologic assaults, hematology and blood chemistry parameters that reflect end-organ function status are expected to be maintained at reasonable levels or improved compared with preimplant levels. Therefore patients with irreversible end-organ function are not eligible for these studies, and if they are implanted as emergency use protocol deviations, their data should be analyzed separately from the core patient group.

Another uniformity issue concerning study entrance criteria is defining heart transplant candidates. When bridging was initiated in 1985, each heart transplant center's criteria for transplant were based on the Stanford criteria and varied little from center to center. At that time it was sufficient to state that patients who met their center's heart transplant criteria could be entered into a bridge-to-transplant study. Today, however, transplant criteria vary from center to center and it is no longer sufficient, in a multi-centered study, to state that a patient may enter the study after meeting the heart transplant criteria at his or her center. Study entrance criteria must incorporate those heart transplant criteria that define a specific study population. This does not mean that all centers must use the same heart transplant criteria as those specified for the study. Rather, patients who enter the study must meet study transplant criteria.

Evaluation of adverse effects also has limited use when each event is not specifically defined. Although accepted uniform definitions are lacking within the medical community at this early stage of emerging technology, each investigator must have a basis for making a declaration about an event that ensures conformity or at least comparability with such decisions at other study centers. Definitions developed for these early studies may be the basis for generally accepted definitions across all VAD studies in the future.

The issue of uniformity extends to implant procedures, patient management, autopsy protocols, and explanted device analyses. When uniform procedure is not followed, the reason must be documented. This information is extremely important to the overall analysis.

In addition to appropriate study design and procedures to ensure collection of reliable data, FDA has also focused attention on actual data collection used to evaluate study endpoints and to answer the important questions about device function in the indicated patient population. For valid conclusions to be drawn, this data must be collected for all patients, at specified times, in the same manner. Otherwise, use of the most appropriate statistical methodology to support a conclusion is worthless. If the study is supposed to demonstrate that the device can increase cardiac output to levels consistent with survival in hemodynamically compromised patients, data must be collected to demonstrate patients' hemodynamic parameters before implant and at regular intervals after implant. Likewise, if demonstrating that the device does not cause hemolysis, kidney failure, or untoward neurological effects, data must be collected for baseline information before device implant, during device use, and after device removal. When data are aggregated to demonstrate device effects on patients, only data for those patients for whom all of the data were collected can be used in the analysis. Sometimes data from autopsy reports or device analysis studies are used to demonstrate that a particular anticipated effect or patient injury was not observed in the study. Such data must be qualified with information on the number of autopsies and device analyses that were actually performed.

These are a few examples of VAD protocol issues with which FDA has been grappling in its regulatory role. There has been progress amidst these many complexities; it is anticipated that the Circulatory Systems Panel will soon be evaluating data in preparation for making recommendations on several systems under study. Based on our experience with these issues, FDA can offer advice to sponsors and investigators who are embarking on VAD/TAH projects.

PMA FACILITATORS

To move a study smoothly through the FDA approval process, from IDE state to PMA filing and subsequent review by the Circulatory System Device Panel, there must be high-caliber study leadership. The study manager, in addition to understanding all of the preclinical technology aspects (e.g., design, materials, device qualification, manufacturing, quality control, animal studies) must be proficient in the field of clinical trial design and have practical experience in orchestrating an appropriate device study. This person will have to convene committees to address different study aspects, recruit technical persons to carry out tasks, work with FDA, and enroll and train reliable investigators. These tasks do not get easier with time because once the centers are enrolled in the study, constant monitoring is required to assist teams as they get started, and to ensure collection and submission of the necessary data without institutional censoring regarding validity. Aggregating data begins with the first subjects and controls. Preliminary analyses are required for progress reports. The study manager must be a scientist, a communicator, an organizer, and more. Once a competent manager is appointed, it behooves the sponsor to support this person. This support must have at least two prongs: (1) encouragement in using sound scientific principles in the conduct of the study, and (2) the provision of adequate staff to accomplish the job. The most capable study manager cannot remedy problems encountered during the trial course without complete cooperation of an administrator who takes time to follow the trial progress and who will make required decisions to ensure its success.

Investigators must be committed to the PMA process, thus ensuring steady progress. For multicentered studies, investigator steering committees offer an effective technique for gaining clinical input into study designs; it also fosters uniformity and cooperation among the centers. Investigators should agree on study objectives, endpoints, and definition of success. Based on their experiences and data collected in the pilot study, investigators can help determine the most appropriate indication for use, and for the patient population in whom it should be utilized. Investigators should also develop and define study inclusion and exclusion criteria, write the implantation procedure, and define adverse events. Patient management, autopsy, and device analysis protocols also benefit from their input.

The best study plan can go astray for any number of reasons. The way to prevent this from happening and to ensure overall study integrity is to design and carry out an effective monitoring plan. Data managers must have knowledge and commitment to do the job properly. Loss of such a person at one study center, particularly if it is an active center, can create considerable confusion. A common problem is the tendency for a committed clinical investigator, with genuine enthusiasm for the device, to broaden indications for use. If the approved study protocol is modified by each investigator to adapt to specific center-related therapy regimens, then as many separate and distinct studies as there are investigators will develop. There is a strong possibility that data collected at each center will be invalid for pooling. As a consequence, device marketing approval will be delayed.

Assertive monitors must visit study centers regularly to review data collected for accuracy and completeness, and to interview the study team. During these visits, protocol violations are discussed. This is also the time to assess new investigators and arrange for training of new team members in device use. Many issues that can affect trial length and outcome are detectable through these regular monitoring reviews.

As a final step, to facilitate the PMA process, sponsors must stay in touch with the data base. Some groups wait until it is time to submit a PMA application before taking stock of data quantity and quality collected to demonstrate safety and effectiveness in the intended patient population. After finally aggregating the information they have been collecting, everything suddenly starts to shift—the study design, the patient population, and more. When this happens, the information submitted to FDA to support device safety and effectiveness for one indication may be more suitable as justification for a new study. Several experiences such as this have persuaded us to acknowledge that frequent data aggregation and preliminary analyses are absolutely necessary and time saving. A pilot study may be one way to prevent this from occurring. Another measure that is particularly useful is the progress report. When all of the data are aggregated and preliminary analyses are performed at regular intervals, a sponsor acquires a "feel" for the data and can sense whether study objectives are being met. Such an evaluation, and subsequent feedback from FDA, may be instrumental in the early correction of an erroneous course.

CONCLUSION

Use of permanently implantable LVAD systems is on the horizon. Manufacturers who have worked for years developing their systems with private and NIH funding are advancing rapidly toward implantation of their first clinical models. FDA looks forward to working with the medical community and industry to ensure the safety and effectiveness of these new circulatory assist systems as they enter the clinical phase of development and move into the market place.

REFERENCES

1. US Department of Health and Human Services: *Regulatory requirements for medical devices: a workshop manual,* FDA 89-4165, Center for Devices and Radiological Health, Rockville, Md.
2. US Department of Health and Human Services: *Artificial heart and assist devices: direction, needs, costs, societal and ethical issues,* NIH 85-2723, National Heart, Lung and Blood Institute, Bethesda, Md.

PART THREE

DEVELOPMENT AND SUPPORT OF A VENTRICULAR ASSIST DEVICE PROGRAM

CHAPTER 20

The process of experimental cardiovascular device development for clinical use

George M. Pantalos

The past several years have provided me with an opportunity to participate in artificial heart and ventricular assist device development and to observe similar efforts by colleagues affiliated with other organizations. I am by no means an expert in the process of cardiovascular device development. However, certain recurrent patterns have emerged with many of the device development programs I have examined. The steps delineated below will seem second nature to the experienced developer. An entrepreneur or beginner requires reckoning of each step in the process if a cardiovascular device has any hope of moving from the drawing board into clinical application. Although the steps identified in this process are not intended as a plan for success, it is hoped they will serve as a useful guide for cardiovascular device development.

Step 1. Design conception and design definition

The "light bulb" and "napkin-to-notebook" stages. No one knows when a lightning bolt will strike. It is invariably during a moment of need in the operating room, laboratory, or during lively discussions at the lunch table, or during happy hour. The classic comment, "I wish I had a gadget that would do thus and so" immediately results in a sketch, frequently on a napkin or the back of an envelope. Further contemplation of device design requirements simultaneously refines conception and definition of the new cardiovascular device. Sooner or later the design concept congeals and needs to be appropriately recorded in a notebook or other appropriate place of documentation. One of the most difficult parts of this stage is clarifying exactly what the device will do. A few examples of the design goals that need to be clarified include how many liters of blood per minute should it pump and at what range of pressures? At what range of beats per minute does it need to function? What current and voltage stimuli does it need to provide? What are its power requirements? How long should it be expected to function?

Step 2. Prototype development and concept validation

"Fabrication-to-feasibility" stage. Mental images or napkin sketches eventually need to be translated into a tangible object to evaluate if (1) the device looks like what was anticipated, (2) it works, and (3) the idea is worth pursuing. In time-honored tradition, building a prototype is usually a bootlegged affair that one is obliged to tackle in the attic, garage, basement, or in the laboratory after hours. Surplus material is pilfered from here, and interchangeable parts are borrowed from there. Sooner or later (and often much to one's amazement), a device takes form and adds new dimensions beyond the initial conceptualization.

This prototype will invariably need to be reworked many times before it finally reaches the point where it can be turned on to do whatever was intended. Although a prototype may exhibit sufficient promise of functioning, anxiety is heightened at the moment of in vitro preliminary device performance, durability, and reliability assessment. If one is lucky, the device may even work the first time it is turned on. If not, do not be dismayed. There is always a detail that has been overlooked, but can hopefully be rectified. During preliminary device performance evaluation, one will begin to get an idea of whether the device has any hope of functioning and approaching design goals originally proposed. At this stage, it may be necessary to reevaluate erstwhile design goals, which may have been too ambitious. Many deficiencies may be recognized. Assuming this initial device is not completely hopeless, a multitude of design and fabrication iterations are undertaken, followed by retesting to determine if design goals can be met. Sometimes monumental changes are needed; other times a little improvement here and there will do the job. It is hoped this prototype will resemble its original design and have some chance of functioning as originally intended.

Step 3. Sponsorship acquisition

"Fun to finance" stage. Thus far device development has been subsidized in stages by bootlegging here and there, tapping into a development fund, and often dipping into personal finances. Although frustrating, the work has also been fun because an idea has reached a certain level of reality. However, challenges on the road ahead bring into focus the hefty requirements for device development support needed to move from the prototype stage through preclinical testing and into initial clinical trials. Depending on the complexity and design goals, one should expect that further cardiovascular device development and testing will cost from hundreds of thousands to several million dollars, just to advance into clinical trials.

Many potential sources of funding exist. Proposals may be submitted to federal granting agencies, particularly the National Heart, Lung and Blood Institute (NHLBI). Although the NHLBI's philosophy is to fund only a limited amount of pure device development, funds can often be obtained if an application is congruent with investigation of well-developed scientific hypotheses. Another avenue available from several federal agencies is the Small Business Innovation Research Program (SBIR). Many governmental agencies have SBIR programs established for the purpose of assisting small businesses to obtain start-up funds (Phase I as much as $50,000) to develop devices with the potential for ultimate commercialization. Private foundations can often be approached, particularly when a foundation has an expressed interest in the advancement of cardiovascular medicine. If handled properly, one might also consider approaching a corporate entity, which could provide both dollars and Research and Design (R&D) resources, useful for advancing the device to clinical readiness. However, one must approach these arrangements with caution. Who possesses the technology rights and how the royalties may be awarded must be clearly delineated.

Clinicians sometimes have development funds, program R&D funds, or other sources of financial support from practice groups that may be used to finance cardiovascular device development. This approach may be more successful if a clinician conceives the original idea or provides substantial early phase development input. Clinicians may be more apt to support device development if they perceive its chances of reaching clinical application are promising and are offered an opportunity to conduct initial clinical trials. Of course, when all else fails, there is always that phone call to a rich uncle. When things become really desperate, one can organize bake sales, car washes, and other innovative approaches to raising funds such as garage sales, yard work, begging, and assigning the kids a paper route.

Step 4. Preclinical in vitro device evaluation

"How much for how long" stage. By this time, device development has shown a fair amount of functional promise. It is now important to verify how well the device will perform and for how long. This will ultimately be done through in vivo testing, but extensive in vitro testing can provide a valuable evaluation of the device. A bench setup, when possible, should attempt to duplicate the physical environment in which the device is expected to perform (e.g., when testing an artificial heart or ventricular assist device, it is desirable to test the device submerged in a saline bath, heated to body temperature). The device should pump a blood analog solution in typical hemodynamic conditions. Performance range should be clearly defined. Multiple test setups will also need to be devised so that several duplicate devices can pump continuously to establish test device durability and reliability. It is essential to implement a monitoring scheme for recording key performance parameters. Glitches in function can be documented so that their solution can be sought. A large enough test sample size will be needed so that durability and reliability statistical techniques can be used to establish a certain percentage confidence level for your device.

Step 5. Preclinical in vivo device evaluation

"Proof-of-the-pudding" stage. Early successful preclinical in vitro device evaluation can then lead to initial in vivo device evaluation. In general, Steps 4 and 5 will occur with a certain degree of overlap because device modifications from early animal

implantation testing may warrant repeating performance and durability-reliability tests with the most recent device configuration. The goal of animal implantation testing is to demonstrate safe and effective device performance with desired device function. Early implantation results will probably indicate where iteration on device design, material selection, fabrication, implantation technique, and postoperative management will be needed; device retrieval analysis is a very important tool in this process. The final preclinical device version will emerge for a well-defined series of in vitro and in vivo evaluations.

Step 6. Device modification for clinical trial

"Patient has two legs, not four" stage. Cardiovascular devices whose design is essentially species independent will generally be appropriate for human clinical trials without a change in the animal test version. However, devices that are species dependent, such as an artificial heart or ventricular assist device system, may require the development of a human version to accommodate human anatomy, which may substantially depart from the anatomy of the in vivo test animal. There must, however, be substantial testing that indicates that a human model will demonstrate equal or superior performance characteristics compared with the animal version.

One example from our experience in developing total artificial hearts has been the design of inflow and outflow port orientation and location for both animal and human versions. The human heart lies primarily anterolaterally; as heart size increases with progression of end-stage heart disease, enlargement progresses laterally, toward the chest wall. The calf and sheep hearts lie more longitudinally in their orientation, with limited lateral space due to a narrow chest cavity. The consequence of these differences is that the calf version may fit poorly, or not at all, within the cardiac cavity of the human mediastinum and vice versa. Because it may be difficult to demonstrate human model function in an animal because of poor fit, additional in vitro testing that demonstrates equivalent or superior device performance will be necessary before entering clinical trials (e.g., additional human artificial heart model testing entails generating ventricular function curves, durability-reliability data, and intraventricular flow visualization tests to verify that no adverse flow patterns have been introduced by relocating human configuration inflow and outflow ports).

Step 7. FDA clinical trial application formulation

"Renegade to regulated" stage, or the "you want to know what?" stage. By the time Stage 7 is reached, a lot of time, money, and effort have already been expended in perfecting the device. Therefore researchers become confident that the device is ready for clinical trials. It is at this time that too many people start to think about meeting requirements for U.S. Food and Drug Administration (FDA) device approval. If the prototype is substantially equivalent to a device already in existence before the 1976 Medical Devices Act, researchers may apply for a 510K device approval. This approach gener-

ally requires less animal, bench, and clinical evaluation before market approval. Many new devices, however, are not substantially equivalent to preamendment devices, and must proceed through the Investigational Device Exemption (IDE) FDA evaluation route. An IDE is sought to demonstrate device safety and efficacy for a specific indication to initiate clinical trials. Data must be submitted to document in vitro and in vivo device performance, along with the anticipated protocol for the clinical investigation. There are several drafted or completed guidance documents that already exist for different classes of cardiovascular devices. This literature is readily available upon request from the FDA Office of Device Evaluation.

On receipt of the guidance documents, an inexperienced cardiovascular device developer may experience "regulatory cardiogenic shock." A plethora of data is recommended for submission with the IDE application, including extensive documentation of (1) in vitro performance, test protocols, and test results, (2) in vivo experiments, including in vivo performance and parameters evaluating animal health, and (3) substantial data from device explant retrieval analysis. This work needs to be conducted with adherence to Good Laboratory Practice Regulations (GLP). At this time device developers realize they have failed to collect data that the FDA will expect them to include with the IDE submission. Exhuming buried data is an arduous task, but will sometimes be sufficient to fill in the gaps. However, too often the data plainly and simply do not exist, necessitating more in vitro and in vivo experiments, which translate into a major expense of time, effort, and money. To avoid regulatory cardiogenic shock, it is prudent, very early on, to become familiar with guidance documents closely associated with the investigational device. It is also helpful, at that early stage, to schedule a meeting with the FDA Division of Cardiovascular Devices, to educate them about the theory and current state of device development, for the purpose of soliciting their input on specific kinds of data they will expect to be submitted with a 510K or IDE application. A second FDA visit may prove beneficial as one anticipates formulating a 510K or IDE application. In addition, Division of Cardiovascular Devices members frequently attend major cardiovascular and artificial organs meetings. Researchers will benefit by attending the sessions on regulatory affairs, which often involve participation of one or more FDA members, as well as having the opportunity to chat with them informally out of session.

An important perspective to have while developing a cardiovascular device is the anticipation of the next level of regulatory requirements. To receive FDA IDE approval, adherence to GLPs is required. To receive FDA Premarket Approval (PMA), adherence to Good Manufacturing Practices (GMP) is required. Establishing compliance with GMPs is a long and involved process. If their organization does not already meet the GMP requirements, many developers have found that it is helpful to begin the implementation of GMP requirements while also preparing for the initiation of their clinical trial, rather than putting it off until the time of PMA application formulation.

Step 8. Initiation of clinical trials

"Heifer" to "human" stage or the "responsible leap of faith" stage. The goal of the clinical trial is to demonstrate device safety and effectiveness when used in humans. Committing to initiating a clinical trial represents a "responsible leap of faith" that is well-grounded in successful test results of animal and bench experiments that document device safety and efficacy to this point of development. This is no small undertaking, especially when the clinical trial will involve multiple centers. From the device developer's perspective, a clinical trial actually commences with center preparation. Protocols must be drafted that include (1) patient selection criteria, (2) surgical implantation technique, (3) data to be collected during the postoperative period, (4) patient follow-up, and (5) explant device analysis obtained during surgical removal or post-recipient death. Complex cardiovascular devices may require special training sessions for a clinical trial team. Goals to be accomplished include briefing on detailed device function and monitoring, surgical implantation technique, and postoperative patient care.

Refresher courses may be necessary along with periodic visits to each clinical trial center to help attain and maintain proficiency in clinical trial conduct. It is imperative before clinical trial initiation that the center have an understanding of precisely what data are needed to demonstrate device safety and efficacy. Failure to do so may result in essential data not being collected. This anecdotal patient data, although helpful in understanding device operation, may not be deemed sufficient by the FDA to support an IDE application. The clinical trial sponsor must therefore have sufficient personnel resources to provide periodic on-site clinical monitoring to ensure that essential data are being collected. This point cannot be overemphasized because denial of premarket approval or clinical trial cessation can occur, not only because of grave device deficiencies, but because of deficient clinical trial conduct.

A clinical trial requirement is the periodic FDA data reporting. An anticipated schedule and format for reporting data should be established with the FDA, who may also request additional clinical trial data. Enactment of the Safe Medical Devices Act of 1990 has enabled the FDA to request data directly from the clinical trial centers. Presentation of this data is essential to document device safety, efficacy, and proper clinical trial conduct. Previous FDA experience concerning clinical trials conduct can actually be very helpful in providing valuable guidance to enhance the value of the clinical trial.

The initial clinical stage is very helpful in validating device design and function, or indicating where minor or major changes are required. Device iteration may then take place. Minor device modifications, backed up with sufficient in vitro testing, may be permissible within a clinical trial context. However, major device changes may require temporary clinical trial cessation until further in vitro and in vivo evaluation qualify the device for clinical investigation.

Major device changes should immediately raise the question of whether clinical trials should be continued or suspended. This decision-making process needs to seriously consider input from the clinical trial center's participating investigators, FDA, and from a critical biomedical engineering performance assessment.

Step 9. Premarket device modification

"What they really wanted was this" stage. Following extensive clinical trials, necessary refinements of a device and its associated systems will become apparent. Often these modifications will make the device easier for clinicians to use, but may also require alterations to improve its performance. Radical modifications may necessitate additional in vitro and in vivo testing, followed by clinical trial testing. Less substantial changes such as fine tuning of software programming, clarification of labeling, or improvements on a device's control console may require less evaluation. Here again, a visit to the FDA would be helpful in understanding regulatory implications of these modifications, and may help one delineate between modifications that are essential and those that are desirable but not essential.

Step 10. Licensing the technology

"Prospect to product" stage. This stage may come at any number of steps throughout this process. When working solo or within a small organization, technology licensing rights may come early on so that one may gain the benefit of acquiring substantial resources that will promote device development. However, if one is part of a large corporation venture group, chances are the technology will remain within the company. It is important to understand that by licensing the technology, one may lose control over further device development and testing, depending upon the licensing arrangement. Generally, the earlier in this process that technology is licensed, the less one will have to gain because the licensor will have to bear the majority of program development and testing. The later in the developmental pathway a device is licensed, the more confidence one has in the device's future; by absorbing more developmental costs, one stands to gain more if the licensing is handled skillfully. It is generally safer to license the technology on a device-by-device basis, rather than on a family of devices.

Step 11. FDA premarket approval

"Was it really safe and effective" stage. Step 11 is similar to Step 7 in concept, but requires an order of magnitude more work because now one must substantiate that the device was safe and effective in clinical trials. Compliance with GMP requirements must also be demonstrated, following a PMA panel review that recommends approval. Periodic reports on clinical trial conduct will have helped to establish the format for reporting data to the FDA. At this time, a presubmission FDA meeting will prove helpful in receiving guidance on PMA application preparation.

A review of all device performance data, patient data, and device related and non-related adverse events that need to be submitted in a PMA application is beyond the scope of this chapter. This information is described in available FDA documents (FDA 87-4214, FDA 89-4158, and FDA 87-4179 listed in the resource materials at the end of this chapter). There is, however, a recurrent issue that merits discussion. A plethora of patient data needs to be presented to document that, first and foremost, study patients meet entry criteria. Although this may sound obvious, a discrepancy in this criteria is one of the major reasons for a clinical trial to be extended beyond the point where the sponsor believed they would have enough patients to receive PMA. It is important to keep in mind that the device needs to have demonstrated its safety and efficacy for a specific indication. In the effort to gain device clinical trial experience rapidly, it will be tempting for clinical investigators to include borderline entry criteria patients. This approach will be useful in clarifying entry criteria limits, but may not add to the number of appropriate patients needed to obtain PMA. A responsible assessment of this data has the potential to redefine entry criteria that will expand or possibly reduce the patient population. As the IDE sponsor, it is in one's highest interest to promote only *appropriate* device use for the identified indication or indications.

Step 12. Approved clinical use

"Will it really continue to be safe and effective" stage. Obtaining FDA Premarket Approval successfully is perceived as reaching the summit. Indeed, this is a monumental achievement to be celebrated, but not for long. Once the pinnacle is reached, one realizes that one is not at the top, but at the entry to a gradually upward sloping path marked "continuous improvement." It is on this path that device refinement, in its many dimensions, occurs. Obtaining PMA does not mean that your device is perfect, only that it is safe and effective as proven to date, and that it must continue to be safe and effective if marketing is to be maintained. This is the stage at which information desired about your device, but not necessarily submitted for PMA, can be acquired. It is also the time to refine all aspects of device documentation, production, quality assurance, training new users and updating current users, and accumulation of clinical experience for presentation at professional meetings and in professional journals. Rigorous clinical follow-up is imperative to continuously verify results that demonstrate safety, efficacy, and appropriate device use. This effort is particularly useful because the long-term device use may reveal deficiencies not found during the preclinical and clinical evaluation. A rapid, credible response to address any deficiencies may well make the difference between the device maintaining its market approval or being removed from the market temporarily or permanently.

CONCLUSION

The 12 steps identified in this scheme represent a long and demanding path requiring an immense commitment of resources. For many devices, the scheme will span 5 to 10 years or more and will cost from several hundred thousand to several million dollars. With the United States trend toward more rigorous medical device regulation, the process of device development is going to become even more difficult, more expensive, and more time-consuming. This will regrettably make it even harder for the developer with a great device, but limited resources, to get beyond Steps 1 and 2.

The good news is that with good financial, material, and personnel resources and with a well thought-out, disciplined developmental plan, these steps can be successfully accomplished. With a deficiency of any of these components, the path will be constantly uphill and possibly too steep to reach the goal. Good Luck!

RESOURCE MATERIALS

Questions on general policies, procedures and administration of the PHS SBIR Program should be directed to:

Office of Research Training and Special Programs
National Institutes of Health
Room 5B-44-Building 31
Bethesda, MD 20205
(301) 496-1968

The U.S. Food and Drug Administration has a number of useful resource materials that can be requested.

U.S. Food and Drug Administration
Center for Devices and Radiological Health
Division of Small Manufacturers Assistance
5600 Fishers Lane, HFZ-220
Rockville, MD 20857
(301) 443-6597
(800) 638-2041

Questions specific to cardiovascular devices can go to:

U.S. Food and Drug Administration
Office of Device Evaluation
Division of Cardiovascular Devices
1390 Piccard Drive, HFZ-450
Rockville, Maryland 20850
Telephone: (301) 427-1205
FAX: (301) 427-1957

The following resource material is available from the FDA.

Regulatory Requirements for Medical Devices (FDA 85-4165)
Good Laboratory Practice Regulations (Federal Register December 22, 1978, pp 59986-60025)
Device Good Manufacturing Practices Manual (FDA 87-4179)
Premarket Approval (PMA) Manual (FDA 87-4214)
Premarket Notification: 510(k)—Regulatory Requirements for Medical Devices (FDA 89-4158)

Investigational Device Exemptions—Regulatory Requirements for Medical Devices (FDA 89-4159)

Replacement Heart Valves—Guidance for Data to be Submitted to the Food and Drug Administration in Support of Applications for Premarket Approval

Draft Guidance for the Preparation and Content of Applications to the Food and Drug Administration for Ventricular Assist Devices and Total Artificial Hearts

Draft Guidance for the Preparation and Content of Applications to the Food and Drug Administration for Vascular Grafts

Additional FDA guidance is available from the following resources:

- Tripartite Biocompatibility Guidance (obtained through the Division of Small Manufacturers Assistance (301) 443-6597 or (800) 638-2041
- Guideline for Monitoring Clinical Studies
- 43rd Annual Quality Congress Transactions-Regulatory Submission for New, Improved Devices; by Drs. Chiacchierini and Busher
- Statistical Aspects of Submissions to FDA: A Medical Device Perspective; by Dr. Chiacchierini and Henry Lee, Jr.
- Reviewer Guidance for Computer Controlled Medical Devices

FDA instructional videos are available from the following:

Investigational Device Exemptions (IDE)

Statistical Aspects of Submissions to FDA: A Medical Device Perspective

The Association for the Advancement of Medical Instrumentation (AAMI) has a number of useful resource materials that can be requested.

AAMI

3330 Washington Blvd.

Suite 400

Arlington, Virginia 22201-4598

Telephone: (703) 525-4890

FAX: (703) 276-0793

- Blood Pressure Transducers—General ... AAMI/American National Standard (BP22-058)
- Blood Pressure Transducers—Interchangeability and Performance of Resistive Bridge Type:
  AAMI/American National Standard (BP23-058)
- Cardiac Monitors, Heart Rate Meters and Alarms: AAMI/American National Standard (EC13-058)
- Diagnostic Electrocardiographic Devices: AAMI/American National Standard (EC11a-058)
- ECG Electrodes, Disposable Pregelled: AAMI/American National Standard (EC12-058)

- Testing and Reporting Performance Results of Ventricular Arrhythmia Detection Algorithms:
  AAMI Recommended Practice (ECAR-058)
- ECG Connectors: AAMI Standard (ECGC-058)
- NonAutomated Sphygmomanometers: AAMI/American National Standard (SP9-058)
- Electronic or Automated Sphygmomanometers: AAMI/American National Standard (SP10-058)
- Cardiac Valve Prostheses: AAMI/American National Standard (CVP3-058)
- Vascular Graft Prostheses: AAMI/American National Standard (VP20-058)
- Design, Testing, and Reporting Performance Results of Automatic External Defibrillators: AAMI Technical Information Report (TIR2-058)
- Cardiac Defibrillator Devices, Second Edition: AAMI/American National Standard (DF2-058)

REFERENCES

Kessler DA, Pape SM, Sundwall DN: The Federal Regulation of Medical Devices, *N Engl J Med* 317(6):357, 1987.

Kahan JS, Holstein H, Munsey R: The Implications of the Safe Medical Devices Act of 1990, *Medical Device and Diagnostic Industry,* February 1991.

Holstein HM: The Safe Medical Devices Act of 1990, *Regulatory Affairs* 3:91, 1991.

CHAPTER 21

Design and management of ventricular assist device clinical trials

The corporate sponsor's view

Bruce J. Shook and Janice T. Piasecki

INTRODUCTION

Ventricular assist device (VAD) clinical trials are much like modern art; their beauty depends largely on the viewer's perspective, and there is no shortage of perspectives.

An astute observer at one of the "regulatory sessions," which are occasionally appended to relevant scientific meetings, will quickly discover that a spectrum of opinions exists regarding the current system for evaluating ventricular assist devices. Physicians will frequently voice their frustration with regulatory restraints on their use of these devices because their patients are critically ill; ventricular assist device technology may be their only hope. Government should not stand between the physician and his or her best efforts to save a human life.

The Food and Drug Administration (FDA) will emphasize their charter; they must protect the public health. They cannot carry out their mission without valid scientific evidence establishing a device's safety and efficacy. The only way to get such evidence is through a thoughtfully designed, well-controlled clinical trial.

Corporate sponsors of these VAD trials also have distinctive viewpoints. Their viewpoints are shaped by an eclectic assortment of responsibilities, unique to the corporate sponsor, who must satisfy needs of both clinical investigators and the FDA. Thus the clinical trials process becomes more than device evaluation for the corporate sponsor. It is a juggling act requiring the sponsor to be part scientist, part engineer, part clinician, and part regulator. The sponsor also has a unique stake in clinical trial outcome. Success can mean financial prosperity; failure can mean loss of the product, or worse.

What follows is an attempt to bring elements of this juggling act together, and to review what is required to navigate the clinical and regulatory maze associated with VADs.

CLINICAL TRIAL DESIGN

So, what does the FDA really want? This is a question that many people, inside and outside of the FDA, have spent much time pondering. For devices such as PTCA catheters or pacemakers, the answer is straightforward. But for ventricular assist devices, this query is left at least partially unanswered.

Ventricular assist devices have been used clinically since the 1960s. However, none has successfully made its way through the regulatory process. This leaves the FDA with no precedent and many open questions. A multitude of questions are easily identified, but answering them is frequently difficult. FDA prefers to concentrate more on broad scientific issues and less on details. To be sure, some details are available in the "Draft Guidance on Ventricular Assist Devices and Total Artificial Hearts," but this document is a work in progress (as its title implies). It does not touch on some of the more critical questions for sponsors such as how many patients are required before premarket approval (PMA) submission.

The FDA's focus on the general need for sound science is apparent in the area of clinical trial design. It is essential that the clinical trial design be carefully thought out; this thinking process must include the FDA. They will emphasize the importance of certain trial design elements, such as the definition of hypotheses, methods used to test these hypotheses, control methods, and the importance of indications and contraindications. The FDA cannot define the details associated with each issue for each trial. The sponsor must take the initiative and craft a clinical study that deals directly with these important questions. If the study design is built on firm scientific ground, the FDA will most likely accept it with limited comment.

One of the key clinical study design issues is the formulation of coherent hypotheses. It is impossible to answer a question that has yet to be asked. The sponsor must have a clear vision of what questions are being investigated, and that vision must be articulated as the study design's cornerstone. Most of the remaining study design issues revolve around getting the answers. A clear statement of the hypotheses being tested is essential. Assuming the hypotheses have been thoroughly thought out, such a clear statement will be the sponsor's ally as time goes on. A well-defined target is always easier to hit. Conversely, a target that is poorly defined at the outset can become a major impediment to progress because the questions are likely to change just as they are being answered.

How one goes about testing a hypothesis is, of course, hypothesis dependent. Most VAD trials will focus on a few general themes:

1. Does the VAD provide sufficient circulatory support?
2. Is the VAD associated with an unacceptable level of adverse effects?
3. Is survival increased by VAD support?

The first question can be directly answered by comparing the key hemodynamic parameters (mean arterial pressure [MAP], cardiac index [CI], and pulmonary capillary wedge pressure [PCWP]) during VAD support with the same parameters immediately before VAD support. The "permanence" of any circulatory improvement noticed during VAD support should also be assessed by comparing these hemodynamic values following VAD support with those recorded before VAD support.

The second hypothesis can be addressed only through a careful assessment of adverse effects occurring before, during, and after VAD support. Suggested methods for accomplishing this important task are reviewed later in this chapter. The relationship of these adverse effects to the VAD or the patient's underlying conditions can be established by the clinical investigators, but the judgment of what is an acceptable level of complications (and what is not) is ultimately a subjective one.

The third hypothesis seems simple enough on the surface, but it can actually lead to some difficult questions to which there are only subjective answers. First, a reasonable survival definition must be set forth. Survival for 30 days is typically not very meaningful for VAD trials. Patients are frequently hospitalized for extended periods and those that survive for 30 postoperative days may not live to go home. A much more meaningful endpoint is hospital discharge. Second, there must be some identification of what constitutes an acceptable survival rate, which is inextricably tied to the patients being treated. Indications for use play an essential role in establishing the expected survival rate.

Assessment of a VAD's performance can easily be clouded by the variability of cardiac disease and the patients' response to treatment. However, control methods can frequently help lift this fog and turn gray areas to white or black. Development of a control population that has not been subjected to treatment with the VAD being tested can be accomplished in several ways: (1) patients can be prospectively randomized to the VAD or some accepted therapy; (2) a nonrandomized group of concurrent controls can be developed; (3) the patient can be used as his or her own control; or (4) a historical control group can be developed from the literature.

The gold standard against which all clinical studies are judged is the prospective randomized trial. Prospective randomization removes any bias from assignment of patients to control or VAD groups. It also produces groups that are comparable because patients are equally likely to be assigned to one group or another. This is an attractive approach for the corporate sponsor because (if the study is executed properly) the results will be unequivocal. The sponsor will know whether his or her VAD is better, worse, or no different from the existing treatment, and the results will stand on firm scientific ground. If the news is positive and the study has been properly executed, the FDA will have little cause for doubt. If the news is negative, at least the trial produced the information necessary to make a difficult business decision.

A primary drawback associated with randomized trials is time. Only half of the patients enrolled will actually be treated with the VAD, and this increases time required to accrue sufficient VAD experience. Nonetheless, if the nature of the device being studied lends itself to a prospective randomized trial, then this should be the control method of choice.

For VADs that are not readily studied in a prospectively randomized fashion, other approaches must be considered (e.g., if the VAD is applied as a last resort, randomization obviously cannot occur). The development of a nonrandomized concurrent control group in this setting raises ethical questions because the control group is allowed to die. Such a study may also produce groups that are not sufficiently comparable. Historical controls can be dredged up from the literature, but this is scientifically weak, and is unlikely to hold up under FDA scrutiny. This leaves use of each patient as his or her own control.

This method of controlling the study is attractive because it permits a relatively objective assessment of VAD impact, and does not raise the ethical issues previously described. Such a study design has been employed by sponsors who wish to evaluate a new VAD technology, but are limited to treating patients who have failed all conventional therapies. The basis for such a study is a complete and accurate collection of data before enrollment of each patient, and during and after the period of VAD support. Pre-VAD data are taken as a baseline against which the on-VAD and post-VAD data may be compared. This strategy very clearly depends on collection of complete pre-VAD data, a sometimes elusive commodity (more on this later).

Indications and contraindications are another cornerstone of clinical study design. A precise definition of who is to be treated and who is not is essential for success. This definition affects the study in many ways. It strongly influences time required to complete the study by limiting patients who are suitable. It affects survival rate expectations. It influences the way in which adverse effects are viewed. If critically ill patients with no therapeutic alternatives are being studied, a higher frequency of some adverse effects is expected. And most important for the sponsor, indications and contraindications will eventually constitute the permissible labeling and marketing claims. The sponsor must be sure at the outset that the patients being studied are the patients who will ultimately be targeted as customers once clinical trials are done.

CLINICAL TRIAL START UP AND MANAGEMENT

After clinical trial design has properly evolved and FDA has had their say, it is time to put the plan into action. The first and most vital step is locating and recruiting the best possible group of clinical investigators. Leads can come from many different sources, including physicians with whom the sponsor has prior experience, literature searches for investigators who have published their previous experience with VADs, exhibition of a VAD at scientific meetings producing interest among potential investigators, and physicians contacting the sponsor on their own once they become aware of a trial.

Regardless of how candidates materialize, they must be carefully screened and selected. If this is done well, the trial is far more likely to proceed according to plan. Some guidelines for selection follow.

1. Do not become enamored with fame. Although it is certainly important to have

investigators who are respected, the fact that they are widely known does not mean that they will be productive investigators.

2. Take a close look at support staff. VAD trials are very data- and paperwork-intensive. They usually require at least one person other than the principal investigator who will be responsible for administrative issues.
3. Pay close attention to numbers. Patient enrollment is frequently a limiting factor in VAD trials, and estimates from individual investigators may vary widely. It is unwise, generally speaking, to assume that the total potential population at a given center is likely to be enrolled. Actual enrollment numbers are almost always a subset of the total number of patients fitting the protocol's description.

Training the team

Once selected, key members of each clinical team must be trained. It is generally best to conduct training sessions away from the hospital to obtain team members' undivided attention. Personnel attending these session(s) should represent a cross-section of the hospital services that will be participating in the VAD trial. Principal and co-investigators, perfusionist(s), operating room staff, intensive care unit staff, and the study coordinator should be represented at the training session.

Extent of training required will vary from device to device, but there are several important elements that should be reviewed in any training program. First, device design must be clearly explained. It is easier for the clinical team to understand how to operate a given system if they understand why it works like it does. The sponsor's challenge is to impart the basic design philosophy without clouding the issue with technical complexities.

Second, the clinical application of the system must be taught by doing. The team should implant the VAD in an appropriate animal model and take the system through all of its operational paces, including alarm and failure scenarios. This experience is invaluable, particularly for teams that do not have significant prior experience with other VAD technologies.

Third, the lessons learned by other investigators must be passed on. As the trial progresses, many details will emerge that make VAD implant and explant, and patient management, easier and more effective. These nuances are important and should be communicated at every opportunity.

Fourth, clinical study requirements must be reviewed in detail. The participants must walk away with a clear understanding of what is expected from them. Participants must understand study design, indications and contraindications, data collection requirements, and record keeping requirements.

Getting the data

One of the most important elements of a VAD trial is also the most elusive, data collection. No study, no matter how large or well designed, will get anywhere with the

FDA if the necessary data are not collected. Only objective clinical data will serve to answer the questions posed by the study's designers.

It is up to the sponsor to ensure that data collection happens. This is a seemingly straightforward task for many clinical trials, but VAD trial sponsors cannot afford laxity when it comes to data collection. The nature of VAD application is typically emergent. A patient is in dire hemodynamic straits and circulatory support must be instituted immediately. This is not a scenario conducive to orderly data collection, so the sponsor must make it as easy as possible.

Repeated training plays an important role in data collection. The principal and co-investigators must be aware of both the parameters to be followed and the schedule for their collection. In addition, there must be a "data champion." This important role is usually played by the study coordinator who takes data collection as a personal responsibility. This data champion is thoroughly familiar with data requirements and goes to great lengths to obtain necessary numbers.

The sponsor can also facilitate data acquisition through a couple of simple but important actions. First, data forms should be logically designed, with simplicity as a key design criterion. Second, any data form(s) used at the time of VAD implant should be packaged with the device. Packaging should be arranged so that anyone who opens the box sees the data form staring back at them. This one single act eliminates a commonly encountered excuse: "We didn't have the form."

Assessing adverse effects

One of the most difficult aspects of a VAD study is assessing device safety. The clinical study must demonstrate that the device is not associated with an unacceptable level of device-related adverse effects. There is, however, no precedent to suggest what is acceptable or unacceptable.

To successfully assess VAD safety, a sponsor must confront this problem in the early phases of study design. It is vital that several issues be sorted out when drafting the protocol. First and foremost, adverse effects that are expected (e.g., bleeding) must be clearly defined, and all investigators should be instructed to judge presence or absence of individual effects according to established definitions. These definitions should be developed with the aid of the investigators and an awareness of expanding VAD literature. Investigator input during formulation of definitions is vital, but once the definitions are set, all investigators should put aside their own personal opinions and adhere to the definitions.

It may also be helpful to classify each adverse effect by cause (e.g., the patient's underlying condition, or the device). Such judgments should be the investigator's domain, but the sponsor must ensure uniformity between centers. Thus definitions of what is patient related and what is device related should also be established early.

Once the study is up and running and data are rolling in, close sponsor surveillance is extremely important. Despite development of lucid definitions, it is human nature to make judgments based on one's own opinions. The sponsor must critically review the entire patient record to verify that reported adverse effects match other available facts in the context of the definitions.

These activities will ensure uniform and accurate reporting of adverse effects from center to center, but the problem of defining what is acceptable still remains. Any discussion of the acceptability of adverse effects must first return to the patients being treated.

Patient selection criteria for VAD studies typically require that VAD-supported patients be in the most desperate circumstances. Chronic congestive heart failure, cardiogenic shock, long cardiopulmonary bypass times, and perioperative complications can result in an impressive array of adverse effects. Selection criteria also typically require that patients fail "accepted" therapies, thus ensuring that mortality without some extraordinary intervention is very high, if not 100%. This lack of alternatives tends to put adverse effects statistics in perspective.

It would be ideal if the sponsor could look to some gold standard to define what is "normal." For example, sponsors of percutaneous transluminal coronary angioplasty catheters can look to the National Heart Lung and Blood Institute Registry and to numerous previously approved PMAs for such a reference point. For VADs there is no real gold standard. The Combined Registry of Mechanical Ventricular Assist Devices and Artificial Hearts, compiled by Penn State University, is the largest VAD registry. It is strictly voluntary, however, and does not employ a system of adverse effects definitions. It is therefore almost impossible to interpret any differences or similarities between registry data and one's own.

In the end, assessment of adverse effects is a subjective one that must consider all of the aforementioned factors. The sponsor must strive to chronicle experiences of trial participants objectively and uniformly, and report them in the light of patients being treated.

Dealing with federal regulation

The first rule of dealing with FDA regulation is to remember that FDA staff members are people too. As such, they are most likely to respond in a positive manner if they are well informed and comfortable with the sponsor's plans. This is attainable only through frequent interaction between sponsor and FDA reviewer(s). Presubmission meetings are a key part of this important communication.

These meetings allow the sponsors to review their thoughts on the spectrum of topics affecting ultimate VAD approval, including device design, in vitro and in vivo testing, clinical study design, and clinical results. If the FDA is informed of the sponsor's plans at the outset, they then have an opportunity to comment and solicit input from other groups, such as the Food and Drug Administration's Office of Science and Technology or the Devices and Technology Branch of the National Heart, Lung and Blood Institute. This builds familiarity among those who will ultimately play a role in VAD evaluation. This familiarity is invaluable when dealing with technologies that have little to no regulatory track record.

Once requirements for a given submission have been worked out to everyone's satisfaction, the next task is compiling and presenting all of that information in an easily assimilated form. Particular attention should be paid to delivering what was promised, and to overall submission organization.

An FDA reviewer should be able to find items promised easily in the presubmission meeting. If 10 devices were to be tested for reliability, then data from 10 devices should be clearly presented. If the VAD was intended to increase mean arterial pressure significantly, then an appropriate analysis showing that it does so should be presented. In short, submissions should be structured around delivering what was expected.

Submissions must also be well organized (e.g., use tabs, page numbers, and diagrams), well written (use consistent terminology), and reviewed carefully before submission. Review by persons not involved with the submission can provide valuable insights into how understandable the material is. The importance of this step should not be underestimated. A submission could contain a wealth of important and relevant data, but still get bogged down in the review process if the information is not presented properly.

Interaction with the FDA is, of course, not limited to presubmission meetings. It is also important to communicate with the FDA as the trial progresses. Sponsors must be candid with clinical trial results, sharing the good news, as well as the bad. Real-time communication between the sponsor and the FDA greatly facilitates the regulatory process.

CONCLUSION

Ventricular assist device trials are a unique entity. In some cases devices have been in clinical use for years. However, regulatory experience with VADs has been limited, and there is little precedent for the FDA and corporate sponsors to rely on for guidance. In the absence of precedents, sponsors must rely on sound science and a great deal of common sense to successfully travel the path to approval.

Sponsors must work closely with the FDA to define questions to be answered, and methods required to obtain the answers. Once defined, the plan must be executed with close cooperation of the clinical investigators. Last, sponsors must take great care in delivering to the FDA what was promised, in a form that can be readily understood. The sponsor must combine all of these ingredients, in careful balance, to ultimately achieve success.

CHAPTER 22

Clinical engineer's role in ventricular assist device support

Marilyn Cleavinger, Richard G. Smith, David H. Loffing, and **George J. Olding**

INTRODUCTION

Ventricular assist device (VAD) clinical trials have presented us with many challenges. As with any complex system, a management approach that fosters multidisciplinary collaboration enhances the successful application of these devices. Cooperation among cardiovascular surgeons, clinical engineers, nurses, and many other specialists and ancillary care personnel is required to give optimal care to this patient group.

Centers active in VAD trials usually designate a core group of personnel familiar with VAD problem solving to facilitate patient care during the implant and participate in ongoing data collection required by the clinical trial format.[1] Composition of the core group varies between centers, but most teams include at least one clinical engineer with significant responsibilities for device and patient management. This chapter will present the background and skills that clinical engineers bring to the team and discuss the experience at University Medical Center's Artificial Heart Program.

WHAT IS A CLINICAL ENGINEER?

Clinical engineering is a relatively new profession, having come into existence in the past 20 years. Healthcare professionals are rarely familiar with clinical engineering since medical training programs do not routinely expose them to this specialty. The basic role of clinical engineers is to be a "technical problem solver" within the hospital, a position that is likely to expand as new technologies continue to develop.[2]

Estimates are that at least 100,000 different machines are currently being offered to hospitals by more than 3000 manufacturers.[3] Medical professionals find it difficult to keep up with the volume of new technologies and instrumentation being introduced. Clinical engineering developed to meet a need to safely use, maintain, and manage complex instrumentation found within today's healthcare facilities.

Clinical engineering is a subspecialty of biomedical engineering, a field defined as that branch of science concerned with understanding and solving problems in biology and medicine using principles and methods drawn from engineering, science, and technology. Clinical engineering involves the application of engineering methods and technology to healthcare delivery. Most major medical centers today have clinical engineering departments whose function is to help effectively utilize existing technology and efficiently incorporate new technological innovations.[4]

EDUCATION AND TRAINING FOR CLINICAL ENGINEERS

The interdisciplinary nature of biomedical engineering requires a solid background in engineering skills and specialized knowledge in the life sciences. Clinical engineers are further specialized in clinical medicine, healthcare systems, and administrative skills. Minimum training requirements for clinical engineers are a bachelor's degree in engineering (typically biomedical, chemical, electrical, or mechanical engineering), with additional coursework in life sciences plus direct experience in design, modification, and testing of medical instrumentation. Most educational programs that provide specialized training in clinical engineering are at the master's level and include intensive hospital exposure via clinical internship experience.[5]

TYPICAL COURSEWORK FOR CLINICAL ENGINEERS

Advanced chemistry
Advanced physics
Advanced mathematics
Biological or life sciences
Engineering core courses:
    Statics
    Dynamics
    Electrical networks
    Fluids
    Thermodynamics
Advanced engineering specialty courses
    (i.e., electrical, mechanical,
    biomedical, or chemical)
Computer languages and applications
Physiological systems modeling
Biomaterials
Biomechanics
Signal processing
Medical imaging
Device design
Medical instrumentation
Clinical engineering fundamentals
Clinical internship

The box on p. 279 provides a brief list of coursework required to obtain a biomedical engineering degree with specialization in clinical engineering. This list was compiled from the requirements in place at a number of the biomedical engineering programs in existence today[6] and represents a typical curriculum. Some terminology found in the box may be unfamiliar to the reader who is not an engineer. It is perhaps appropriate here to expand on two subjects that are more relevant to practicing clinical engineers—medical instrumentation and clinical engineering fundamentals.

Today's medical instrumentation expands the five senses with a wide variety of transducers and signal processing devices that convert information about living systems into a form that can be used for diagnostic or monitoring purposes. Instrumentation design includes: (1) studying biopotentials such as electrocardiograms and electroencephalograms, (2) techniques to acquire these signals safely, (3) understanding how to convert one type of energy into another using transducers, and (4) techniques to amplify and process these signals into meaningful information. Understanding the components and principles used to design medical equipment is required to assess device functionality or to apply devices to patient care.

Courses in clinical engineering fundamentals and clinical internships expose students to the practical side of operating a clinical engineering department. Standard topics for these classes are listed in the box below.[7] These courses provide an understanding of healthcare delivery systems, and methods for technology introduction and management in that environment.

THE CLINICAL ENGINEER'S ROLE IN TECHNOLOGY MANAGEMENT

Clinical engineers have a number of roles in technology management. To direct patient care providers, their most visible contributions are (1) performance and safety testing medical devices, (2) training operators to use medical devices safely and effectively, and (3) maintaining functional equipment. Clinical engineers also provide (1) design, custom modification, or repair of sophisticated medical instruments; (2) pre-

---

CLINICAL ENGINEERING FUNDAMENTALS

Healthcare delivery systems
Hospital organizational structure
The economics of healthcare
Codes, standards, and regulations in the healthcare environment
Management of equipment, preventive maintenance, and repair
Training for medical equipment users
Planning for facilities development and equipment acquisition
Legal and ethical issues in clinical engineering

purchase evaluation and planning for new medical technology; (3) facilities modifications; (4) cost-effective management of equipment repair; and (5) incident investigation, risk management, and liability control.

Most clinical engineers manage technology on a hospital-wide basis. There are certain medical departments such as anesthesiology and radiology that are so technology-intensive that engineers are frequently dedicated solely to those departments.

Clinical engineering practice has always been shaped and developed by the changing needs of healthcare professionals. Its interdisciplinary foundation allows it to be dynamic. Thus this profession can and has easily adapted to managing problems posed by the introduction of ventricular assist device technology.[8]

THE EMERGING TECHNOLOGY OF VENTRICULAR ASSIST DEVICES

Outside the medical field, businesses developing technological innovations can be rapidly rewarded by commercialization of their products. Newly emerging technologies may undergo numerous refinements as they mature. This process provides an opportunity for basic scientific and engineering research to play an important role in expanding new technologies.[9]

Within the medical device field, this process still takes place, but at a much slower rate. Because risks are inherent in technologies such as VADs, use of these devices is carefully regulated in the United States by the Food and Drug Administration (FDA). Pulsatile ventricular assist devices are available only in limited numbers at clinical sites chosen for participation in carefully controlled trials allowed for by the Investigational Device Exemption (IDE) process.

Conducting successful IDE studies has proven to be a monumental task. Proper patient selection, appropriate data collection, and distinguishing among device, procedure, and patient-related complications present special challenges. Comparison of study parameters across all patients at all sites has been difficult. VAD manufacturers have found it difficult to maintain financial solvency for the length of time required to complete these studies.

During clinical trials, device changes cannot be made solely for the purpose of innovation. All device modifications require prior FDA approval. However, it is still possible for users to make limited innovations to this technology. These may come in the form of improvements to surgical techniques, patient management, or engineering changes external to the device, which enhance its monitoring or diagnostic capabilities. Clinical engineers have developed systems to provide remote patient monitoring and adaptations that allow long-term patients to reside outside the hospital during VAD support.[10] These projects may help direct the future of VAD development by controlling costs and providing a better quality of life for VAD implanted patients.

Despite many restrictions limiting VAD use at this stage of development, many proponents support their continued use. National Institutes of Health (NIH) funds have recently been designated to support initial clinical trials of implantable ventricular assist systems in human subjects with chronic refractory heart failure.[11] Permanently implantable VAD systems should provide new opportunities for technological innovations in this area.

It has been suggested that clinical engineers can play an active role in addressing several issues that might improve clinical testing required to reasonably ensure the safety, effectiveness, and potential benefits of these new technologies. Engineers can help physicians design valid clinical studies and define state-of-the-art in vitro procedures for evaluating device performance. This may decrease time required to make devices commercially available.[12]

CLINICAL ENGINEERING IN VAD SUPPORT

Application of a new technology such as ventricular assist devices carries with it requirements for support that do not correlate well with volume of patients supported. Active ventricular assist device programs generally devote substantial resources to support a specialized team composed of physicians, nurses, clinical engineers, and various other medical support staff.[13] University Medical Center's VAD support team relies heavily on clinical engineers to perform many of the functions necessary to the program. Specific responsibilities delegated to engineering staff include (1) maintaining device readiness; (2) operating, monitoring, and troubleshooting device equipment; (3) providing education to patients, family members, and hospital staff; (4) managing patient transport logistics; (5) preparing the facility for device patients; (6) acting as a liaison between device manufacturers and users, and (7) collecting and disseminating IDE required data.

Engineering resources are organized within a group known as the Artificial Heart Program. Two full-time and two part-time clinical engineers are available to support this program. During implants, these engineers are on round-the-clock call to provide device monitoring and troubleshooting. Our program has supported 38 patients for a total of 1278 days using three types of pulsatile assist devices: (1) Symbion J-7 Total Artificial Heart (TAH), (2) Symbion Acute Ventricular Assist Device (AVAD), and (3) Novacor Left Ventricular Assist System (LVAS).

Remote monitoring and data collection

Our engineering team has developed an extensive information network for our assist device patients. This network, shown in Fig. 22-1, uses the Artificial Heart Laboratory as a centralized location for patient monitoring and data collection. The system duplicates information displayed at the patient's bedside monitor for the Artificial Heart Laboratory. Device controller information is also reproduced via either hard wiring, a network link to the patient monitoring system, or by modem transmission.

This remote monitoring system allows clinical engineers to check on device per-

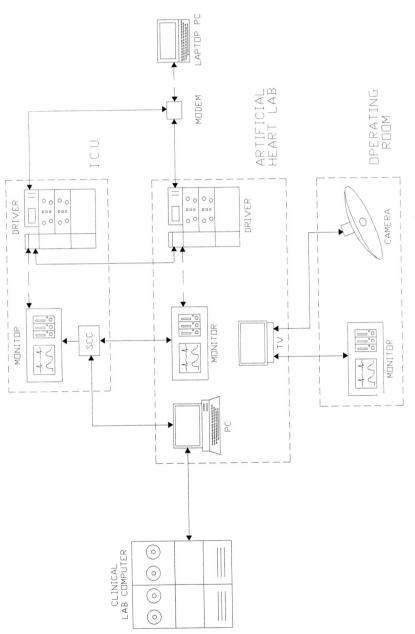

Fig. 22-1. Artificial heart information network.

formance at any time either from the Artificial Heart Laboratory or from home. Engineers can therefore be on call for medical staff consultation regarding assist device patients without physically remaining at the bedside. In this manner, the program can maintain an increased level of technical support without requiring all device patient care providers to be intensively trained to reach that same level. We believe that this provides a desirable continuity of care to our patients at the level of device management. It also greatly reduces the level of resources devoted to constant retraining of staff because of infrequent contact with assist device patients, staff turnover, or moving patients from ICU to a less intensive monitoring environment such as a general care unit.

In addition to remote monitoring, the Artificial Heart Laboratory also has a data link to the clinical laboratory computer, which provides access to patient laboratory results. Thus complete data gathering for assist device patients can be done in the Artificial Heart Laboratory.

Training activities

The Artificial Heart Laboratory also serves as a training and resource center for potential assist device patients, their families, and patient care providers. Laboratory equipment includes a Donovan mock circulation with each type of assist device attached, as shown in Fig. 22-2. Mock circulation and drivers are used to demonstrate device operation for training purposes.

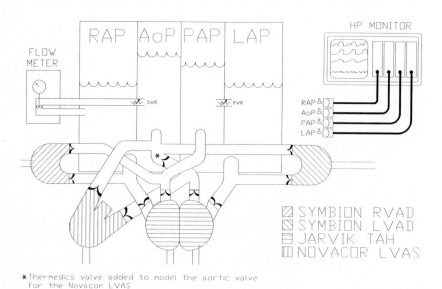

Fig. 22-2. Configuration of Donovan mock circulation with training circulatory assist devices attached.

ARTIFICIAL HEART
NURSING CHECKLIST

DO NOT MAKE DRIVER ADJUSTMENTS.
CONTACT ARTIFICIAL HEART ENGINEERING
FOR ASSISTANCE AT 6-6455 OR 6-7735
    OR PAGE_____ ON BEEPER_____

DATE _____
NAME _____
PATIENT # _____

	06:00	08:00	10:00	12:00	14:00	16:00	18:00	20:00	22:00	24:00	02:00	04:00
ARE WAVEFORMS OK ?												
HEART RATE (bpm)												
SYSTOLIC DURATION (%)												
LEFT DRIVE PRESSURE (mm Hg)												
RIGHT DRIVE PRESSURE (mm Hg)												
IS EXTERNAL SYNC LAMP OFF ?												
VACUUM (INCHES WATER)												
ARE AC POWER LAMPS ON (X 3) ?												
DO BATTERIES CHECK OK (X 3) ?	▨			▨			▨		▨		▨	▨
ANY VISIBLE OR AUDIBLE ALARMS ?												
IS BACKUP DRIVER READY ?												
IS HOURLY AVG C.O. PRINTING OUT ?												
DISK % FULL												
PRIMARY AIR TANK PRESSURE (psi)	▨			▨			▨		▨		▨	▨
RESERVE AIR TANK PRESSURE (psi)	▨			▨			▨		▨		▨	▨
DO YOU SENSE ANY AIR LEAKS ?												
DRIVELINE CONNECTORS AVAILABLE ?												
ARE DRIVELINES OK ?												
ARE WHEELS LOCKED ?												
RN SIGNATURE												

TAHCKLST   Rev. 4/28/87

Fig. 22-3. Nursing checklist for total artificial heart implant.

This equipment is utilized during a 1-day workshop given in conjunction with our Nursing Staff Development Department. Participants are afforded an opportunity to acquire hands-on experience as they perform exercises designed to gain familiarity with the device system. They practice emergency response procedures such as how to switch controllers in the event of a malfunction. Additional topics include a review of the theory and practice of device use, patient selection criteria, nursing care plans, and selected case studies.

Mock circulation simulations include the effects of (1) AVAD position on filling (patient transfer from supine to upright position); (2) driveline kinking on pneumatic devices; (3) inflow obstruction on device output; (4) hypertension on device output; (5) unloading the left ventricle by selecting the fill and eject endpoints for the LVAS.

During each implant, additional training is provided by engineering personnel. Nursing staff are instructed in device operation and basic troubleshooting throughout each assist device implant. The process of checking equipment function has been simplified by implementing nursing checklists (Fig. 22-3). This close collaboration between clinical engineers and medical staff has resulted in a high level of proficiency with respect to assist device management.

Device management

Artificial Heart Program engineers provide device start-up in the operating room and driver management throughout the implant period. Engineers are also responsible for the logistics involving patient transports. Mobilizing these patients involves providing adequate power during transit, moving bulky equipment along with the patient, ensuring that both patient and equipment can fit along the designated path, and making any driver adjustments required. We routinely accompany patients to diagnostic testing sites, or provide exercise or a change of scenery for mental health purposes. Because transport requires interruption of device primary power sources, we believe that it is prudent for an engineer to accompany patients during this time, in case troubleshooting becomes necessary.

Study of thrombus formation and flow patterns

Thrombus development within an assist device is influenced by many factors, including material surfaces, patient variables, infection, anticoagulation regimens, and flow properties within the device.[14] Assist device design should minimize areas of stasis.

Frequent observations of thrombus formation on the Symbion AVAD diaphragm-housing junction adjacent to the outflow orifice (Fig. 22-4) prompted us to search for an explanation of this phenomenon. Based on flow studies and diaphragm visualization during device operation, we concluded that thrombus formation is enhanced because of a localized area of low flow. Several factors contribute to this phenomenon. These are depicted in Fig. 22-5. During diastole, diaphragm movement on the outflow side does not occur to the same degree as on the inflow side. As ejection begins during sys-

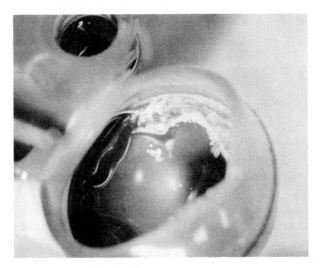

Fig. 22-4. Thrombus (white crescent-shaped area) at the Acute Ventricular Assist Device (AVAD) diaphragm-housing junction, outflow side.

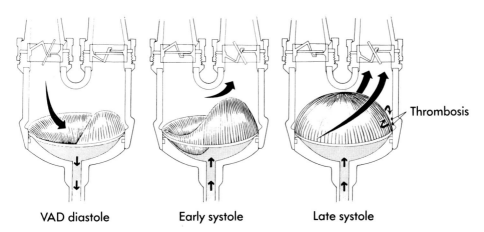

VAD diastole   Early systole   Late systole

Fig. 22-5. Diaphragm positions during AVAD cycle.

tole, blood flows around the housing circumference from the inflow to the outflow side. As these flows meet near the outflow side, they are significantly slowed down and change from laminar to turbulent. Both diaphragm position and the turbulence created in the area of the outflow contribute to the likelihood that thrombus will form in this area.

This information has led us to modify our driver management to maximize motion in the area labeled in Fig. 22-5 as "thrombosis." We formerly allowed the AVAD to fill to an average of 70% to 80% of its total stroke volume. We can now adjust the driver parameters to allow it to fill beyond that point. This leads to a greater downward diaphragm displacement during diastole, and also opens up the area around the diaphragm-housing junction outflow orifice, which enhances the surface washing effect in this area.

Diaphragm movement is also increased when the patient is in an upright position. This AVAD orientation produces greater hydrostatic pressures within the AVAD and causes the diaphragm to move downward more uniformly. For this reason we try to get our patients out of bed and mobilized as rapidly as possible.

Study of hemolysis and housing-diaphragm clearance

Several of our early AVAD implants produced significant hemolysis. We observed that the amount of hemolysis correlated with variables such as cardiac output, left AVAD pneumatic drive pressure, and amount of vacuum applied during diastole. We also noted that the use of two AVADs did not increase the levels of hemolysis seen, which would be expected if the hemolysis were related to damage caused by the artificial valves or the exposure of blood to an artificial surface.

After studying the AVAD diaphragm position at the end of systole, we found that at increased drive pressures (200 mm Hg), the AVAD diaphragm and housing actually made contact. Shear forces generated in areas of decreased clearance between the diaphragm and housing were excessive. We were able to demonstrate that hemolysis levels correlated with parameters that affected the amount of clearance between the AVAD diaphragm and housing.

Again, conditions leading to decreased diaphragm-housing clearance can be minimized by manipulation of driver parameters. We have established guidelines for driver management to control hemolysis as (1) left drive pressures less than 180 mm Hg, (2) VAD heart rate below 80, and (3) vacuum less than 15 mm Hg. We have been successful in controlling AVAD patient hemolysis using this management scheme; however, it does limit the maximum AVAD output flow to no greater than 5 L/min.

CONCLUSION

Use of temporary assist devices has allowed us to rapidly expand the knowledge base regarding patient selection criteria, device complications, and device management. Refinements in these areas such as those examples discussed above have been proposed by experienced users. As the study of these devices continues, additional innovations should make further progress possible.

With permanent cardiac assist devices now on the horizon, a commitment to ongoing technological innovations in this field seems obvious. Although today's patients are in the hospital and closely monitored by medical staff, it is our hope that tomorrow's patients will be out leading normal, active lives. These patients are sure to challenge us in many ways. As patients move devices further from the realm of research work, new methods for assessing the performance of many different device system components will be required. Noninvasive device monitoring, long-distance monitoring, and new power systems will be required for permanently implanted devices. Effects of environmental factors will also require study. Collaboration between engineers and other medical staff will continue to be important. The experience gained during the temporary use of assist devices should provide a good foundation for this work to proceed.

REFERENCES

1. Swartz MT, Ruzevich SA, Reedy JR et al: Team approach to circulatory support," *Critical Care Nursing Clinics of North America* 1(3):479, 1989.
2. Newhouse VL, Bell DS: The future of clinical engineering in the 1990s, *J Clinical Engineering* 14(5):417, 1989.
3. Goodman G: The profession of clinical engineering, *J Clinical Engineering* 14(1):27, 1989.
4. Bronzino JD: Education of clinical engineers in the 1990s, *J Clinical Engineering* 15(3):185, 1990.
5. Newhouse VL, Mylrea KC, Topham WS et al: Clinical engineering, an academic discipline, *J Clinical Engineering* 10(3):203, 1985.
6. Browneller PA: Bioengineering education, 1986—Part I, *J Clinical Engineering* 11(1):39, 1986.
7. Webster JG, Cook AM: *Principles and practices of clinical engineering,* Englewood Cliffs, N.J., 1979, Prentice-Hall.
8. Bernstein MS: A changing role for the clinical engineer: the artificial heart, *J Clinical Engineering* 14(5):423, 1989.
9. Roberts EB: Technological innovation and medical devices. In Ekelman K, ed: *New medical devices: factors influencing invention, development and use,* Washington, DC, 1988, National Academy Press.
10. Kormos RL, Borovetz HS, Pristas JM et al: Out-of-hospital facility for the Novacor bridge to transplant patient: the Pittsburgh family house (FH) experience, *ASAIO* 20:13, 1991 (abstract).
11. Smith RG, Cleavinger M: Current perspectives on the use of circulatory assist devices, *AACN Clinical Issues in Critical Care Nursing* 2(3):488, 1991.
12. Rahmoeller GA: Ethical issues in the regulation and development of engineering achievements in medical technology—a regulatory perspective, *IEEE Engineering in Medicine and Biology Magazine* 7(2):94, 1988.
13. Cleavinger M, Smith RG, Loffing DH et al: The circulatory assist device program at University Medical Center: clinical training and technical support, *Critical Care Nursing Clinics of North America* 1(3):515, 1989.
14. Icenogle TB, Smith RG, Cleavinger M et al: Thromboembolic complications of the Symbion AVAD system, *Artif Organs,* 13(6):532, 1989.

CHAPTER 23

Perfusionist's role in a centrifugal ventricular assist program

Dennis Mills, Tom Golden, Roxi Wolfe, Keith Johansen, John Shafer, and **Marv Gohman**

INTRODUCTION

In early 1985 our perfusion practice elected to replace the primary arterial roller pump with a centrifugal pump (Sarns/3M, Ann Arbor, Michigan). Prompted by encouraging reports from other centers, we also evaluated the centrifugal pump as a ventricular assist device (VAD).[1] The theoretical basis for ventricular assist after insult is to "rest" the myocardium for a time so ventricular function can recover. Centrifugal pumps, by providing all or part of the energy required to move blood through the circulatory system, can rest the myocardium.

CENTRIFUGAL BLOOD PUMP

In many cardiac centers the centrifugal pump has replaced the conventional roller pump as the main arterial pump. Centrifugal pumps have proved to be safe, reliable, inexpensive, and offer advantages over roller pumps. A positive displacement roller pump will continue to pump fluid or air until it is turned off. By design it is capable of generating tremendous positive and negative pressures. With centrifugal pumps, on the other hand, air entering the pump head displaces its prime, creating an airlock. It cannot pump air after it loses its prime, nor can it exceed a positive pressure greater than 600 mm Hg, and its maximum output is 7 L/min.

Deleuze et al.,[2] who compared pneumatic ventricle and centrifugal pumps, found comparable left ventricle unloading. Gentle blood handling, elimination of tubing spallation, compact size, and portability are a few more reasons why the centrifugal pump lends itself so well to ventricular assist. Other authors agree "the simplest, most accessible inexpensive support system at present seems to be the commercially available centrifugal force pump."[1]

A series reported by Emery et al. demonstrated excellent late function in nine patients who have returned to the mainstream of life following the use of mechanical circulatory support after cardiac transplantation.[3] "We believe that aggressive measures of myocardial support are warranted in patients in the posttransplantation period should univentricular or biventricular dysfunction occur. A variety of devices are available and the simplest device that will support the patient's circulation should be used," they declared.

In 1985 we began using Centrimed/Sarns/3M centrifugal pump systems for assisted circulation in patients unable to be weaned from cardiopulmonary bypass (CPB). Between May 1985 and August 1991, 32 patients were supported with the VAD system assembled by our perfusion staff. All patients were postsurgical and represented an incidence of 0.55%, or 32 of 5859 patients perfused during this 6¼ year period. Of these 32 patients, 20 were successfully weaned, 14 survived to hospital discharge, and 13 remain alive and well.

Considerations for centrifugal pump

Many factors were considered before the centrifugal pump was selected as our choice for ventricular assist applications.

1. The more sophisticated ventricle pumps are very expensive, ranging in price from $5000 to $25,000 per application.
2. Perfusionists are more familiar with centrifugal pumps because they are used daily for CPB. Although the VAD application differs from routine CPB, the clinician is not required to retrain on basic operations of the equipment but must only review the VAD protocol.
3. Centrifugal pumps in VAD applications do not produce a pulsatile flow. However, intraaortic balloon pumps (IABP) are most often a component of ventricular assist therapy and can provide pulsatility, if desired.
4. Some degree of anticoagulation is necessary to reduce risk of thrombogenesis when centrifugal pumps are used.
5. Centrifugal pumps can be safely replaced during patient assist without surgical intervention.
6. Centrifugal pumps restrict patient mobility. If long-term assist (e.g., weeks) is needed, patient ambulation would be possible though difficult.
7. Centrifugal pumps are simple to operate and are "user friendly."
8. Pneumatic VADs are not available to all clinicians and remain investigational devices.
9. Centrifugal pumps are able to generate a pulsatile flow pressure curve but do not synchronize with the electrocardiogram (ECG).

VAD CIRCUIT

The VAD circuit for right, left, or biventricular assist is simple to assemble and identical for all applications (Fig. 23-1). One coil of polyvinyl chloride (PVC) tubing (⅜ inch inside diameter x ³⁄₃₂ inch wall thickness) is aseptically presented to the operative field with one sterile centrifugal pump. The surgical nurse attaches one end of the PVC tubing to the pump head inlet connector and the other end to the outlet connector of the pump head. This "loop" is now cut in the center, leaving the inlet tubing and outlet each 4 to 5 feet long. The circuit, tubing, and pump head are filled with sterile saline or electrolyte solution. Care is taken to remove all air from the circuit before placing clamps on inlet and outlet tubing ends. The surgical nurse labels the pump head (left or right) and also labels the tubing to indicate flow direction to and from the pump. Labelling will reduce the risk of an incorrect connection at the operative site and the risk of confusing a right ventricular assist device (RVAD) with a left (LVAD).

The perfusionist attaches one or two tethered drive motors to an IV pole and positions it/them close to the operative field. The surgical nurse passes to the perfusionist the primed pump head and just enough tubing to accommodate interfacing the pump head with the drive motor. When tubing connections to the inflow and outflow cannulae are complete, the pre-pump checklist should be complete. Only one tubing clamp is needed for each VAD circuit; removing unnecessary clamps will reduce confusion in this nonroutine procedure.

To begin assist, the centrifugal pump is started and its revolutions per minute (RPM) are increased to a level adequate to generate forward flow, usually 1800 RPM, before the clamps are removed and flow to the patient is initiated.

Considerations for VAD circuit

Note that the PVC tubing used in the VAD circuit should use ³⁄₃₂ inch wall thickness and not ¹⁄₁₆ inch, which becomes too soft and flexible when it reaches body temperature. This limpness increases the risk of kinking or collapsing.

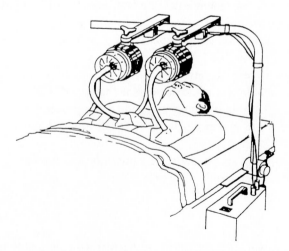

Fig. 23-1. The biventricular assist device in use.

Limiting the number of connections in the VAD circuit reduces the sites at which turbulence and/or flow stasis may form. However, connectors are necessary to attach the pump head to the inflow and outflow patient cannulae. Connectors with integral Luer port and stopcocks provide a convenient access for dialysis and/or hemoconcentration. There is the added risk of air embolism from these access sites, so one should consider restricting these connectors to the right heart assist circuit.

CANNULAE AND CANNULATION

Oxygenated blood is withdrawn from the left atrium by a cannula especially designed for this application (Research Medical, Salt Lake City, Utah). The wire-wound cannulae are 50 to 60 cm long, providing adequate length for the cannulae to exit the chest cavity via a subcutaneous tunnel, passing through the skin below the sternotomy. Pulling the distal tip of the cannula into the chest before cannulating the heart chamber reduces risk of inadvertent decannulation later in the procedure.

Cannulae should exit the chest via separate incisions, allowing more complete closure of the chest and reducing the potential for infection.[4] Magovern observed that closing the chest could also minimize bleeding.[5] If the sternal closure seemed to compromise pump inflow, only the skin was closed.

The left atrial drainage cannula is available in several French sizes and distal tip-angle configurations from 10 degrees to a full 180 degree arc. Usually, a 30 French cannula with a 45 degree angle is passed through the superior pulmonary vein into the left atrium. A pursestring suture snared with a disposable Rummel tourniquet (DLP, Grand Rapids, Michigan) secures the cannula in place. To maintain tension on the pursestring, the suture tails are securely wrapped on the locking spool of the Rummel tourniquet. Large hemoclips are placed on the Rummel to reduce the possibility that the pursestring will loosen during assist.

Adamson et al. generally accomplished left atrial cannulation through Saunderguard's groove, with care taken not to occlude the right superior pulmonary vein.[6] As an alternative, cannulation via either the roof of the left atrium between the superior vena cava and the aorta or the left atrial appendage was acceptable. If the patient is being supported by total CPB during VAD cannulation, the perfusionist is directed to partially occlude the venous line—this will distend the atria. Combining atrial distension with the Valsalva maneuver will limit the risk of air embolism during cannulation.

Aortic cannulation

If the aorta is not already cannulated, a wire-wound, 40 cm long cannula with a rigid tip, size 22 French (Research Medical, Salt Lake City, Utah), is introduced into the ascending aorta in the usual manner. The cannula's configuration allows it to lie under the closed sternum without compressing the heart. Its added length permits it to exit the chest via a separate incision inferior to the sternotomy.

Cannulating the pulmonary artery

A 55 cm long cannula with a 14 degree angled tip (Research Medical, Salt Lake City, Utah) is pulled through a skin incision inferior to the sternotomy and into the thoracic cavity. A Teflon felt doughnut may be placed on the cannula before its insertion into the heart chambers to facilitate suture placement at cannulation site, useful if bleeding cannot be controlled via the pursestring.

Right heart cannulation

If the decision to support the right heart is made while standard venous drainage cannulae are in place in the right atrium, only the pulmonary artery needs to be cannulated. When right arterial venous drainage cannulae must be inserted, longer (50 to 60 cm) wire-wound cannulae (Research Medical, Salt Lake City, Utah) with a smaller French size (30 French) may be considered because the VAD does not rely on gravity drainage for flow but instead relies on the negative pressure generated by the centrifugal pump.

VENTRICULAR ASSIST PROTOCOLS FOR THE PERFUSIONIST
Safety

Patient safety undergoes many challenges during a prolonged period of around-the-clock pumping. We have developed a checklist of *do's* and *dont's* to minimize the patient's exposure to danger.

Setup

1. Minimize the use of connectors in the circuit to limit the areas of turbulence at the connector-tubing interface.
2. Employ Luer-Lok connectors in the RVAD circuit to accommodate such services as hemoconcentration or hemodialysis.
3. Ensure that all stopcock ports are "dead-ended" with nonporous Luer-Lok port protectors to prevent inadvertent air aspiration into the system.
4. Assemble the entire circuit in a sterile field using sterile technique.
5. Have two perfusionists involved in changing pump heads; this is most efficiently accomplished at the changing of shifts.
6. Label VAD drive motors, pump drive consoles, and inflow and outflow tubing clearly regarding function (right or left) and blood flow direction to minimize confusion.
7. Check console alarms to ensure that minimum flow value is entered on the console and audible alarm volume is set at the maximum.

Equipment available at bedside

1. Cart containing supplies, spare disposables, and everything necessary to change a pump head

2. "Mini-lab," including equipment to measure (a) blood gases, (b) electrolytes, (c) activated clotting time, and (d) hematocrit
3. Battery pack, which is plugged in and charging when not in use
4. Hand crank(s) for manual pump operation
5. Name and paging number of the perfusionist on call
6. All forms for adequate charting; a complete record is maintained from the initiation of assistance; data is to be recorded every 2 hours or when there is a change in the patient's status

Monitoring the VAD patient

1. Anticoagulation: the goal is to prevent thrombogenesis while retarding bleeding from the many potential bleeding sites. We have adopted the following protocol:
   a. Heparinization to an activated clotting time (ACT) of 480 sec before initial insertion of assist device.
   b. Heparin is reversed with protamine after VAD support is begun and ACT is allowed to return to normal limits (about 120 sec). When hemostasis is achieved or when chest drainage is less than 100 ml/hr, heparin therapy is resumed.
   c. During ventricular assistance, the degree of anticoagulation is geared to the flow rate:

   4.0 L/min = ACT of 180 to 200 sec
   1.5 L/min = ACT of 480 sec

   Note that all pump heads are examined carefully for evidence of thrombus after use. In 83 pump heads examined, only one 3-4 mm thrombus was discovered.
2. Pressures: to achieve adequate flows, we maintain mean filling pressures of at least 10 mm Hg by patient volume loading. Lower filling pressures may result in insufficient flows, as well as "chattering" outflow line(s). Other desired pressure ranges include:
   a. Arterial pressure: 100 to 150 mm Hg
   b. Left atrial pressure: 5 to 15 mm Hg
   c. Central venous pressure: 5 to 15 mm Hg
   d. Pulmonary artery pressure: 10 to 20 mm Hg
3. Urine output: if urine output is less than 25 to 30 ml/hr, the physician is notified.
4. Patient temperature: the physician is notified if the temperature reaches 100°F or above.
5. ECG: routinely monitored in the intensive care unit (ICU).
6. Blood gases: blood gases are recorded every 2 hours, unless abnormal values require more frequent monitoring.
7. Drugs: drugs and dosages are recorded every 2 hours.
8. Blood loss: recorded and replaced according to physician's orders.
9. Patient's skin: observed closely for mottling or any change in color.
10. Pump head(s): inspected for seal leaks every 8 hours or when one suspects potential pump failure.

HEMOCONCENTRATION

Hemoconcentration is the method we use to remove excess water from the vascular compartment during ventricular assistance. Most likely the VAD patient has been on and off CPB several times, has experienced several incidences of low blood pressure, and has compartmentalized significant amounts of fluid. Edema may often be visually observed in the skin, as well as noticed in the lungs on chest films. Excess fluid is also sequestered in the myocardium and other organs/tissues to some degree. Renal function may be depressed and other means of ultrafiltration are needed to resolve tissue edema. For this reason, hemoconcentrators play a major role in managing our VAD patients.

Materials needed to perform hemoconcentration

1. Hemoconcentrator
2. ¼ inch tubing set with lines for inlet, outlet, and effluent ports (inlet and outlet lines should have male Luer-Lok ends) to reduce risk of connection separation
3. 1 L bags of 0.9% sodium chloride (NaCl) solution, used to prime the circuit
4. 10 ml of heparin, 1000 units/ml
5. Two 2-way (ideally) or 3-way Luer-Lok stopcocks (if a 3-way stopcock is turned incorrectly air can be entrained into patient)
6. Two ⅜ inch x ⅜ inch straight tubing connectors with Luer Lok side ports
7. One Hoffman-style screw clamp used to control effluent water from hemoconcentrator
8. Slow-flow infusion pump and tubing set (i.e., IMED pump) to be used in place of Hoffman clamp for more accurate control of effluent water over time
9. Graduated canister, used to collect shed saline during prime procedure

The VAD circuit provides access to the patient's circulatory system. If an RVAD is being installed, we insert two ⅜ inch x ⅜ inch connectors (with 2-way stopcocks connected to each Luer side port) into the circuit. One connector is placed on either side of the pump, creating a high and low pressure differential that drives the circuit. An RVAD is the preferred site because any air inadvertently introduced will be halted at the lungs. If only an LVAD is in use, these connectors should be inserted into corresponding positions on the LVAD circuit. Although having these ports on LVADs carries an increased risk, we believe the need to remove body water outweighs the risk. Inserting these connectors under sterile conditions in the operating room precludes the perfusionist from inserting the connectors in the ICU under less optimum conditions.

Primary indications for hemoconcentration are a poor urine output or presence of significant edema—patient weight gain of 10 or more kilograms. When connecting the primed hemoconcentrator circuit to the VAD, note that the hemoconcentrator's inlet line connects to the outlet or high pressure side of the centrifugal pump. The hemoconcentrator's outlet line connects to the inlet or low pressure side of the centrifugal pump. Be sure air-free connections are made and all connections are tight. Stopcocks should remain closed until all connections are secure. If the stopcock on the low pressure side is opened before the connection is secure, the unit will deprime and/or pass air to the patient.

ACT should be maintained at 1½ times normal when using the hemoconcentrator. If VAD flow decreases because of lack of intravascular volume, volume is usually replaced with a colloid osmotic agent such as 5% albumin or fresh frozen plasma. Serum albumin, total protein, hematocrit, hemoglobin, and other blood component levels determine which components need replenishment. With proper osmotic pressure restored in the vascular space, water will continue to move from intracellular spaces into the vascular space and out the hemoconcentrator. We have employed hemoconcentration for as long as 7 days.

If renal failure persists, the patient may require hemodialysis while on the VAD. This can be accomplished using the same access connections. In some cases, costly dialysis can be avoided by making use of the hemoconcentrator. If weight loss is the primary goal, hemoconcentration is more effective because it can be run 24 hours a day with

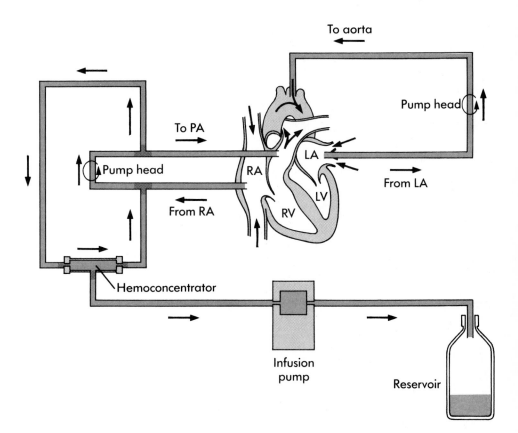

Fig. 23-2. Schematic representation of basic ventricular assist circuitry. Note the hemoconcentrator positioned in the RVAD circuit.

continuous, less dramatic shifts in weight loss. Even in the face of high metabolite levels, the hemoconcentrator can obviate dialysis using the continuous arteriovenous hemofiltration (CAVH)-method. With this technique, clear fluids are infused into the patient and act as a transport mechanism, passing such molecules as BUN and creatinine through the hemoconcentrator's membrane (Fig. 23-2).

STAFFING

Staffing for nonroutine procedures taxes the imagination of the schedule maker and wears down the staff if it has not been done properly. VAD monitoring is included as a regular case on day-to-day scheduling. In our practice, only perfusionists monitor VADs. Although some institutions have used nurses and other ancillary personnel, we believe this procedure requires the expertise of trained perfusionists. As long as the VAD is in use, the perfusionist must be immediately available, either in the patient's room or in the hospital.

CHANGING PUMP HEADS DURING VAD
Indications

Pump heads should be changed (1) when moisture is observed in the magnet compartment, located on the back side of the pump head, (2) when the pump has run for more than 48 hours, or (3) if there is any unusual pump head noise; a chirping or squealing noise may indicate imminent bearing failure.

Necessary supplies

1. 500 ml normal saline 0.9%
2. Sterile Asepto syringe
3. Sterile towels
4. Sterile gloves
5. Four tubing clamps
6. Betadine prep solution
7. Surgical cap and mask

Procedure

Requires the assistance of a nurse or perfusionist. Note that profound hypotension may occur during the interruption of VAD. This period may be kept as short as possible by practicing the technique for proficiency and carefully reviewing each step with the team before making the pump change.

1. Put on surgical cap and mask and wash hands well.
2. Carefully swab the two tubing connection sites with Betadine solution. Allow adequate time for solution to dry (about 2 minutes) before separating tubing from pump head.

3. a. Open gloves, sterile towels, and new pump head.
   b. Don sterile gloves.
   c. Use sterile towels as drapes to delineate immediate work area around drive motor.
   d. Using sterile technique, fill Asepto with saline.
4. Review the steps with assistant before proceeding.
5. a. Clamp outlet and inlet tubes with clamps; note time.
   b. Direct assistant to stop the pump and separate the "old" pump head from drive motor.
   c. Remove tubing from old pump head. Some perfusionists cut the tubing with sterile scissors or a surgical blade, others carefully pry off the tubing to remove the old pump head.
6. a. Connect tubing to inlet of new pump head.
   b. To prime a new pump head by back-filling (1) hold pump head below patient's right heart level, (2) instruct assistant to slowly open tubing clamp proximal to this connection, and (3) back-fill the new pump head from the patient. Instruct assistant to reapply clamp when pump head is full (60 ml).
   c. If the atrial pressure is insufficient to back-fill the pump head, reclamp and slowly fill the pump with saline from the Asepto syringe.
   d. Tap newly primed pump head gently to release any trapped air.
7. a. When making the second connection, have the assistant pour saline over the site to ensure an air-free connection.
   b. If saline is unavailable, lower pump below patient's right heart level and have the assistant slowly declamp the tubing distal to this connection. Blood will flow, exiting the connection site, until tubing is forced over the barbed connector. This alternative also ensures an air-free connection.
   c. Inspect the newly primed and connected pump head for trapped air, and remove the air as necessary.
8. Reconnect new pump head to drive motor.
   a. At the console, start the pump at a speed of at least 1800 RPM and remove all clamps from circuit.
   b. Confirm positive directional blood flow in pump by checking the flowmeter and patient's pressure.
9. Note time required to replace pump head and record procedure on permanent record. A well-practiced team should complete a pump head change in 30 to 90 seconds.

WEANING FROM VAD

Most sources agree that weaning should not begin before a support period of at least 24 hours.[7] It is hoped that patients will be stabilized during that time. Most survivors of VAD support share these characteristics[7]: (1) they have undergone fewer than 75 hours of pump support, (2) right ventricular failure is mild or absent, (3) signs of recovery of left ventricular function are evident within 24 hours, and (4) there is no ECG evidence of postoperative myocardial infarction. Sometimes conversely, after 24 to 48 hours of support, the ventricles look hopelessly damaged, but after 72 to 96 hours, function returns.[6]

The decision to wean from VAD is based on hemodynamic parameters. A left atrial catheter and a Swan-Ganz catheter are normally in place. Monitoring left atrial (LA) pressure is much more accurate than the pulmonary capillary wedge pressure (PCWP) obtained from a Swan-Ganz catheter, which must also be used to determine cardiac output in these patients. Periodically the VAD and IABP are halted briefly to assess ventricular recovery as indicated by the magnitude of ejection on the arterial wave form. When the unassisted ventricle can maintain (1) a cardiac index of 2.0 L/min/m^2, (2) a mean arterial pressure greater than 60 mm Hg, and (3) an atrial pressure below 20 mm Hg, weaning from VAD can begin.[6] Transesophageal echocardiography is also useful in determining ventricular function in VAD patients. Intraoperative echocardiograms were used for LVAD patients to exclude the presence of a patent foramen ovale and a subsequent right-to-left shunt.

1. a. The weaning process is begun by gradually decreasing the output of the VAD by 500 ml/min every hour over a 6 to 8 hour period until a flow of just 1500 ml/min is reached.
   b. When both ventricles have been assisted, the patient is simultaneously weaned from both systems.
2. At a flow of 1500 ml/min and below, the level of anticoagulation must be augmented with heparin to an ACT of 480 seconds to avoid stasis thrombosis.
3. a. When the patient has tolerated a flow of 1500 ml/min for a period of 1 to 2 hours, ventricular assist may be terminated and the pump turned off.
   b. IABP should remain operating at 1:1, and inotropic agents are generally required.
4. a. An observation period of 1 to 2 hours, with the ACT remaining at 480+ seconds, is required to ensure maintenance of adequate hemodynamics.[8]
   b. The patient is then returned to the operating room for removal of the VAD cannulae.
   c. VAD cannulae are removed with the patient in the head-down position during temporary occlusion of the carotid arteries to protect from cerebral emboli.
   d. The IABP should be left in place for at least 24 hours after removal of the VAD.

ANTICOAGULATION

The anticoagulation protocol in our practice is at the discretion of the surgeon. It is the perfusionist's responsibility to see that this protocol is followed. By monitoring the patient's ACT and observing any bleeding, the perfusionist should be able to recommend the appropriate heparin infusion rate.

Patients that prove to be unweanable from the heart-lung bypass machine following surgery represent the vast majority of those who receive a centrifugal type ventricular assist device. Our protocol for anticoagulation in these cases is as follows:

1. *Full anticoagulation* is achieved before CPB with the administration of 3 mg of heparin per kilogram of patient body weight, which extends the ACT to about 480 seconds; this level is maintained during the initiation of ventricular assist.
2. When CPB is discontinued, heparin is neutralized with protamine sulfate at a ratio of 1:1, or 1 milligram of protamine for every milligram of circulating heparin.
   a. When hemostasis is evident at surgical sites, usually 3 to 6 hours after protamine infusion, heparinization is reinstated.
   b. The ACT should now be maintained at 180 to 200 seconds via a continuous heparin infusion; usual infusion rate is between 500 and 1200 units per hour.
3. When attempting to wean the patient from the VAD, or if the blood flow rate is less than 1.5 L/min, heparinization should be increased to attain an ACT of 480 seconds. Note that a bolus injection, as well as an increase in the heparin infusion rate, may be needed to achieve the desired ACT quickly.
4. If the patient is actively bleeding, a variation in protocol is prescribed by the attending physician. The heparin infusion may be discontinued until bleeding stops.
5. ACTs are the primary means of monitoring anticoagulation and may be measured more frequently when VAD flow is reduced.

Although this protocol has successfully controlled thrombogenesis in our VAD circuits, a time of especially high risk is the period of interrupted flow during the changing of pump heads. The level of anticoagulation is minimal and the perfusionist must work quickly to mitigate the potential for clot formation.

Stagnant blood in the heart chambers is a more likely source for clot formation than the centrifugal VAD circuit. The resting LV chamber should be carefully watched when the native LV displays only minimal movement. In one series of 22 LVAD patients,[9] 7 yielded evidence of LV thrombus and systemic embolism to the brain or kidney as revealed at necropsy. Positioning the left atrial drainage cannula across the mitral valve into the left ventricle may eliminate areas of stagnant blood that could be possible sources of emboli.

For VAD patients with mechanical heart valves, it is recommended that only partial assist, if feasible, be employed. This may help to "wash out" both the valve and also the ventricle. Otherwise, the valve would remain closed, allowing the blood in the ventricle to stagnate. Therefore some ventricular ejection would be beneficial.[10]

NURSE/FAMILY RELATIONSHIPS

It is extremely important that explicit communications are maintained between the perfusionist monitoring the VAD and the nurses and other personnel who are caring for the patient. It must be a team approach with each care group—perfusionists, nurses, respiratory care, renal, infectious disease, cardiology, and surgery personnel—involved in the patient's care. In our practice, a "primary care-giver" is designated to coordinate all orders and procedures. This reduces the number of conflicts and mitigates their dimensions. The primary care-giver is usually the attending surgeon or cardiologist. We also have a set of standing orders for ventricular assist that defines most of the parameters we strive to maintain.

Although perfusionists are usually quite comfortable working with other caregivers within the hospital setting, we are, as a rule, less at ease when relating to patients' families. During assists, which can last from 2 to 7 days or longer, we often become well acquainted with family members, which may present a problem if the patient is unable to be weaned from the VAD. It is important to maintain an attitude of compassion without losing our professionalism, an attitude that assures family members we cared and did all we could, even if the outcome did not include patient survival.

TRANSPORTING THE VAD PATIENT

Extreme care must be taken when moving the patient from bed to bed. Be sure that all lines and tubing will reach or be able to move along with the patient. Instant exsanguination can occur if the VAD tubing is inadvertently disconnected. Also, any infusion or monitoring lines that become dislodged may be very difficult to replace with a VAD in operation.

The ultimate transport is moving a VAD patient to a distant hospital. This may be necessary if the patient requires a transplant or bridge-to-transplant that the present hospital cannot offer. If the distance dictates air transport, there are several considerations that apply.

1. The lack of available space requires that only three medical personnel travel with the patient.
   a. One nurse meets the direct nursing needs of the patient.
   b. A second nurse runs the infusion pumps and ventilator.
   c. The third person is the perfusionist who manages the VAD and IABP. A transportable model balloon pump is a definite advantage because of space and weight requirements.
2. All infusions must be changed to syringe-type and completely debubbled. At high altitudes, low atmospheric pressure allows air to expand; therefore all infusion and monitoring lines should be scrutinized for air, which must be eliminated.
3. FAA rules dictate that the patient and all equipment must be properly secured in the aircraft.

It is a challenge to move these patients, but it is also a rewarding experience when it leads to a better outcome for the patient.

CONCLUSION

Our perfusion practice incorporates the centrifugal pump for both routine CPB and nonroutine VAD support. This pumping modality is always readily available, reliable, simple to use, relatively low in cost, and is proven to perform well in both total and partial circulatory support.

REFERENCES

1. Lammer D, Frazier O, Igo S et al: Total artificial hearts and ventricular assist devices as bridges to heart transplantation, *Texas Medicine,* Vol 84, December 1988.
2. Deleuze P, Liu D, Tixler J et al: Centrifugal or pneumatic pump experimental comparative study. *Proceedings of the International Workshop on Rotary Blood Pumps,* Vienna, 1988.
3. Emery RW, Eales F, Joyce L et al: Mechanical circulatory assistance after heart transplantation, *Ann Thorac Surg* 51:43, 1991.
4. Rose D et al: Conference on circulatory support, St. Louis, Feb 6-7, 1988.
5. Magovern G et al: Conference on circulatory support, St. Louis, Feb 6-7, 1988.
6. Adamson R, Dembitsky W, Reichman R et al: Mechanical support: assist or nemesis? *J Thorac Cardiovasc Surg* 98:915, 1989.
7. Magovern GJ, Golding LAR, Oyer PB et al: Weaning and bridging, *Ann Thoracic Surg* 47:102, 1988.
8. Mills D et al: Techniques involved in a ventricular assist program using a centrifugal pump in a community-based practice, *J Extra-Corp Technol* 20:72, 1988.
9. Nakatani T, Noda H et al: Thrombus in a natural left ventricle during left ventricular assist; another thromboembolic risk factor, *ASAIO Trans,* 36:M711, 1990.
10. Mesana T, Monties T Jr, Blim D et al: Thromboembolytic complications during circulatory assistance with a centrifugal pump in patients with valvular prostheses, *ASAIO Trans* 36:M525, 1990.

CHAPTER 24

Nurse training and preparation to implement a ventricular assist device program

Marilyn Hravnak and Elisabeth George

INTRODUCTION

Ventricular assist devices (VADs) are currently used to support some patients with myocardial failure. Current indications range from acute right or left ventricular failure that is not responsive to conventional therapy to chronic bridge to transplantation. Preparation of the intensive care unit (ICU) environment, and even more important, the staff caring for the patient with a VAD, is essential to VAD program success. When in place, the VAD becomes an extension of the patient's anatomy; thus it is essential that personnel caring for the patient understand the purpose and function of the devices and care considerations, and train to institute emergency measures in the event of device malfunction.

BACKGROUND

The cardiac transplantation program at the University of Pittsburgh Medical Center began in 1980. Since that time 596 heart transplants have been performed; 40 have occurred within the past year. Patients awaiting transplantation are suffering end-stage cardiac dysfunction without other significant organ disease, and may deteriorate before a donor heart can be obtained. In some cases mechanical assistance may be indicated until a donor heart can be located.

In 1985 use of the Symbion Total Artificial Heart (TAH), Symbion, Inc., was instituted as a bridge-to-transplant option at the University of Pittsburgh Medical Center. To date 20 individuals have been implanted with this device. Length of implant has ranged from 2 to 48 days. Indications in the early stages of use were for patients requiring longer term mechanical assistance; but as of late, the TAH has been limited to patients with biventricular failure. In 1987 use of the Novacor Left Ventricular Assist System (LVAS) (Novacor Division of Baxter Healthcare Corp., Oakland Calif.) was instituted. This device, also intended as a bridge to transplantation, has currently been implanted in 24 patients at UPMC. Length of implant has ranged from 2 to 303 days. The intended application is for those patients requiring cardiac transplantation with exacerbation of left ventricular failure. Use of a third device at UPMC, the Thoratec Ventricular Assist Device (Thoratec Laboratories Corp., Berkeley, Calif.), was begun in 1990. In addition to use as a bridge to transplantation, it may also be implemented in patients with acute right or left ventricular failure. To date one patient has been implanted with the device at the University of Pittsburgh Medical Center, with a length of implant of 226 days.

PREPARATION TO BEGIN THE PROGRAM

The decision to implement a VAD program affects multidisciplinary members of the healthcare team. Included are the obvious choices of surgeons, intensivists, anesthesiologists, nurses, biomedical engineers, and respiratory therapists. Also involved are social workers, dietitians, radiology technicians, and physical therapists. In addition, members of housekeeping, central distribution, and plant services, as well as security and public relations, must be included. Support is required of the hospital's infectious disease department and pharmacy. Depending on the type of monitoring or research studies to be conducted, the clinical and pathology laboratories may also be involved. It is apparent that the effect of such a program is wide and requires the commitment of many. Initial inclusion of as many of these personnel and departments as possible is important for the development of a functional, creditable multidisciplinary program.

Once the VAD program need is identified, the surgical team pursues the feasibility of using available devices. As principal investigators for these as yet experimental devices, they must apply to the manufacturer and the Food and Drug Administration (FDA) for permission to use the device. They must submit a variety of information concerning use of the device and implementation and on-going support of the program, as well as outline the experience of all levels of team members, and previous statistics. Approval by the university's Investigational Review Board must also be gained.

When determining the postimplantation course of care for these patients, it is important to understand that the commonalities between the care needs of these patients and other cardiothoracic surgical patients are far greater than the differences. Although importance must certainly be placed on the unique requirements or limitations imposed by the devices, the basic care tenets to be provided remain the same. Indeed, if too much emphasis is placed on the equipment compared with the basic overall patient care needs, the outcome may be impaired for the implanted patient and other intensive care patients deserving of the healthcare team's time and attention. In addition, overemphasis on the uniqueness of this particular patient jeopardizes the emotional well-being of both patient and his/her family and impairs their ability to cope with the situation. Likenesses rather than differences should be emphasized, with the goal of returning to a normal lifestyle.

Nursing should be involved in the project at its inception. Nurses may be included in the advance team sent to the manufacturers to learn about the devices. They should supplement this knowledge through analysis of information provided by the manufacturer and review of the literature. It is also helpful to contact other centers using the devices, to draw on their experience and expertise. Networking can help through sharing ideas and information that one may not have originally thought of addressing, as well as validating decisions already made. In the early evolution of VAD therapy the ability to share information was limited by the small number of centers approved to use the devices. As more centers use devices, this is now less of a problem, and most are willing to share information and welcome site visits to advance knowledge dissemination.

It is important to note that a program begins with one patient. Plans that are made at the beginning may not meet the needs a few years in the future because of changing practices, administrative and physical environments, numbers of implants done, morbidity and mortality, and information gained by personal and institutional experience. Sometimes your best guess will be right, and sometimes it will be wrong. It is important to continuously evaluate what you have implemented and alter practices or policies to achieve your desired outcome. In the following sections we will relate our experiences in establishing environmental preparation and nursing practices and training, and illustrate how they required change over time as the program grew and we learned.

PREPARATION OF THE ENVIRONMENT

When determining what, if any, changes or additions must be made to the Cardiothoracic ICU environment when beginning a VAD program, the following questions should be asked:

1. How is the device driven and powered, and is an uninterrupted supply available?
2. In the opinion of the team is protective isolation required?
3. Will patient privacy be adequate?
4. Is there sufficient space available to store emergency supplies and backup equipment?

At the University of Pittsburgh Medical Center, the first device implemented was the Symbion TAH. This device required a continuous supply of dry compressed air at a delivery pressure of 100 psi for its function. Since medical gases available at the bedside in most ICUs have been downregulated to 50 psi, it was necessary to install a compressed air line that was fed from the compressed air generator, but bypassed the downregulator. Piping and valves were installed to accommodate two devices at a time, and an air dryer was installed to remove moisture before air entry into the device. Small openings were created in the walls of the two rooms selected to house the patients so that air hoses and electrical cords could be passed without interference to door closure or doorway traffic. Although in some institutions separate air compression generators were installed to isolate the TAH from the common compressed air supply, it was thought that backup mechanisms for loss of air pressure were sufficiently secure to ensure function for prolonged periods of time in the event of failure of the main generator. In retrospect, this decision has proved sound. Although the main generator has never failed, there have been times of unusually high patient occupancy when increased usage of the compressed air has caused the available air pressure to dip below 100 psi, with subsequent intermittent activation of the backup tanks. Activation of the backup has never failed. Four backup tanks are available in the ICU, with an additional 14 tanks in a nearby storage closet, thus providing approximately 20 hours of function. In addition, compressed air provided by H-cylinders may also be used, with each one providing approximately 2 hours of pressure. These sources provide a wide margin of comfort in the event of main air compressor malfunction, and seem to make questionable the cost of a separate air delivery system. (Although later modification of the Symbion TAH permitted a gas source at 50 psi to be utilized, I included the above information as an example of the process one should go through when making decisions best fitted to each institution and one's own sense of comfort.)

The Thoratec pump is also air driven, although an internal compressor provides the air supply, and the Novacor LVAS is electrically driven. However, all three rely on electricity to power the consoles. At the institution of the program, an isolated power line to the two selected rooms was provided. In time however, it was not always possible for the VAD patients to be housed exclusively in these rooms. Devices are now therefore plugged into circuits common to other ICU equipment. All circuits in the ICU are backed up by the emergency power generator, with a 30 second delay. Each device has battery backup that is activated immediately on loss of AC power (Symbion TAH with 48 hours of support for each module when fully charged, Novacor with 2 hours, and the Thoratec with 2 hours for each module and 45 minutes for the air compressor). In the University of Pittsburgh Medical Center experience, failure of normal or emergency power that exceeds the availability of battery power has never occured. Electrical cords should be positioned so that they are protected from traffic to facilitate staff safety and equipment longevity.

In the beginning, at the University of Pittsburgh Medical Center, patients with assist devices were placed in a protective isolation environment. There is some evidence that presence of the devices themselves may somewhat impair the immune system, although not to the degree that drug-induced immunosuppression posttransplant would. In addition, presence of infection would prevent or delay transplantation. However, evidence gathered at the University of Pittsburgh Medical Center shows that protective isolation does not significantly affect or curtail infection rates in the heart transplant population.[1] In our observation healthcare workers have less likelihood of changing gloves when going from task to task than they do of washing hands. Although this same study has not been conducted in the VAD patient population, VAD patients are no longer kept in protective isolation. It is important to use clean technique as one would with any other ICU patient. Emphasis is to be placed on thorough handwashing of all healthcare personnel in contact with the patient. The main mechanisms of preventing infection should be through minimizing the risk factors of immobility, prolonged mechanical ventilation, and inadequate nutrition. Early mobilization, extubation, and nutritional support are of utmost importance.

Patient privacy should be ensured. Once the program is underway and the uniqueness of the situation diminishes, the inevitable appearance of the curiosity seeker lessens. However, at the beginning of the program, it may be important to place the patient in an area of the unit that is more private and out of the mainstream. Only those healthcare workers whose function is essential to patient care or monitoring should enter the room, and there may be a need to monitor this activity.

As a final step, space should be available for storage of backup equipment. In all cases a backup console is located within the Cardiothoracic ICU. Other supplies that are not needed in the emergent situation may be stored in a more remote area.

EVOLUTION OF THE NURSE'S ROLE

At the University of Pittsburgh Medical Center, nursing has historically taken an active role in pursuing accountability and responsibility for patient care in the Cardiothoracic ICU. Use of the intraaortic balloon pump is longstanding, with nurses responsible for timing, assessing waveforms, assessing equipment function, identifying malfunction, and troubleshooting alarms. It is our particular philosophy that the symbiotic relationship between the patient and the machine necessitates that the scope of nursing practice includes both, and it is logical to extend this thinking to the VAD program.

To determine the nursing care needs of VAD patients, an in-depth understanding of the physics and mechanics of the device is necessary to synthesize information concerning function or malfunction, driver console function and malfunction, waveform analysis, and institution of emergency procedures. Mastery of this information is essential for clinical nurse managers to make decisions regarding the role that nursing will play in the VAD program of their particular institution.

A question that must be addressed at the outset of the program is who does what? It is of importance for the primary investigator (usually the attending surgeon) and the clinical nurse manager to discuss what the responsibilities of the nurse will be and what other types of support will be available. If around-the-clock, on-site support is intended by a group such as clinical engineering, biomedical engineers, or perfusionists, the accountability of nursing for the equipment may not be as intense. If, however, other means of in-house support are not available, it is important for nursing to prepare to assume more responsibility for equipment, function assessment, emergency procedure institution, and setting adjustment. There should be no difference between nursing function on "daylight" and on off shifts or weekends. The patient should be offered, and indeed deserves, the same level of skill and expertise 24 hours a day, 7 days a week. If nurses are to assume this responsibility, then they must prepare for it through education and staffing availability. Only by working with the equipment continuously and becoming intensely familiar with its normal function will nurses (or anyone) become expert and comfortable in dealing with the abnormal or emergent situation.

At the inception of the program, limited usage of the device did not justify full-time engineering support. In discussion between attending surgeons and the clinical nurse manager it was determined that nursing would assume a large amount of responsibility for the equipment, with in-house support by the cardiac surgical resident. Nursing responsibilities included direct patient care, dressing changes at device insertion sites, and documentation. Documentation consisted of recording current settings, waveform analysis, and patient outcome. Nurses performed and recorded safety checks of the equipment in use, as well as of the backup equipment. They performed setting changes in consultation with physicians and documented need for changes, changes made, and patient outcome. They were responsible for recognizing and troubleshooting alarms, and implementing emergency procedures when necessary. It was with this definition of the role of the nurse that the initial training program could then be developed, and nursing care guidelines and protocols put into place.

At present, however, the current size of the program justifies the existence of an engineering staff for the Artificial Heart Program. The engineers are available on site around the clock. Their responsibilities include equipment setup and monitoring, assessment of function, timing adjustments, and documentation with respect to current therapy, FDA required information, and data collection for various ongoing studies. They are responsible for equipment availability and maintenance.[2] When the patient is mobilized or transported, they are responsible for movement of the equipment and setting adjustments. They are available at the bedside for the first 24 hours of implant or until patient stability no longer requires frequent setting adjustments or excessive consumption of nursing time. Thereafter they are available in-house around the clock and are accessible by pager. They assess the patient and equipment routinely or on the nurse's request and are available for consultation with the nurses or surgeons. Most setting or mode changes thereafter are made collaboratively.

Adding a clinical engineer has changed the role of the nurse with respect to equipment. The nurses may focus on the patient in more depth. They are still responsible for (1) assessing function of the equipment, (2) monitoring patient tolerance, (3) making setting adjustments, although there is usually consultation with the engineers if the situation permits, and (4) knowing and instituting emergency procedures in the event of equipment malfunction. It is not believed that the implementation of the engineer's role in any way diminishes the scope of nursing practice. Indeed, the collaborative and collegial effort between the two departments serves only to enhance patient care.

Recently a nurse coordinator has also been added to the Artificial Heart Program staff, and off-site support of some VAD patients is now available.

When implementing a VAD program, it is important that these roles and responsibilities be defined ahead of time. The areas and degree of responsibility defined for each category of healthcare worker will then determine the type of individualized training that must take place.

PREPARATION FOR TRAINING

At the program onset, target dates should be set for the animal implants and the first clinical implant. Once these dates have been projected, a timeline for training may be developed. Milestones along the timeline should include (1) review of manufacturer's information and published literature, (2) networking, (3) definition of roles, (4) trainer training, (5) development of policies and procedures, (6) development of course materials, (7) training, (8) implantation.

The trainer for each category of personnel should be identified. At the University of Pittsburgh Medical Center, the clinical educator (instructor) for the Cardiothoracic ICU served as nurse trainer. Operating manuals were obtained from the manufacturer, and a literature search and review were conducted. Nurses were included in the animal implant trials and performed functions dealing with adjustment and timing similar to projected postimplant duties. Additional practice time in the artificial heart laboratory's mock circulation loop also occurred. The trainer must have a full understanding of teaching concepts to be effective; adequate educator training should also be included on the timeline.

Once the nurse educator and clinical nurse manager gained a thorough understanding of the device, they developed nursing procedures and protocols that were an integral part of the training program and ongoing practice. Administrative discussion and approval of nursing actions to be taken in the event of device malfunction occurred at this time.

Concomitant with course materials preparation, thought was given to development of resource materials to be maintained on the unit. Our reference was developed before training induction and was distributed to the target audience in advance of course attendance. The VAD Nursing Procedure Manual content includes (1) Nursing Care Plan (complete systems approach), (2) preparation for admission, (3) admission procedure, (4) device and console operation, (5) alarms, emergencies, and special circumstances, (6) documentation required, (7) patient transport procedure, (8) patient monitoring requirements, (9) laboratory test schedules, (10) dressing change procedure, and (11) key personnel identification, including phone and pager numbers. This manual functions as the training manual and remains on the unit at all times.

Once the training elements had been defined, another consideration was who would be trained? It was our decision to train only a core group of nurses before program

VAD Workshop Objectives and Class Schedule

On completion of the workshop, the participant will:

1. Describe the device and its components.
2. Identify the indications for implantation.
3. Compare the indications for the various mechanical assist devices utilized (i.e., IABP vs. Novacor).
4. State the physiological goals of the implant.
5. Differentiate the modes of operation and describe how each one operates.
6. Identify the operational components of optimum timing.
7. Identify the cause of alarm conditions and relate the steps to be taken by the nurse in such an event.
8. Identify the necessary backup equipment.
9. Discuss the nursing care plan for the patient and significant others.
10. Demonstrate nursing actions for specific emergency procedures.
11. State the required nursing documentation.
12. Perform correctly in the laboratory simulation.

Class schedule

8:00-8:30	Introduction to program
8:30-9:00	Description of device
9:00-10:30	Console components Modes of operation
10:30-11:15	Unit preparation for admission Admission procedure
11:15-12:00	Lunch
12:00-1:00	Physiological determinants of timing Assessing for optimal timing
1:00-2:00	Nursing care plan
2:00-2:30	Special circumstances Alarms and emergency action
2:30-4:00	Laboratory—mock circulation loop Demonstration Return demonstration

Fig. 24-1. Sample VAD workshop objectives and class schedule (specific to each device).

implementation rather than the entire staff. It was believed that it would be important to develop expertise and comfort with repeated exposure to the equipment and patient care needs. With this experience, early established policies and procedures could then be refined and utilization of a small working group of nurses could facilitate this process. Our initial core group consisted of 15 nurses. The negative side to this decision was that careful work scheduling of this small group had to occur to provide continuous patient care.

As the program has developed, we have studied and adjusted our practices to a point of relative stability. All of the staff have been trained to provide a continuum of acute through chronic care.

COURSE CONTENT

The training program for nurses has also been changed and revised over time (Fig. 24-1). In its current format the program begins with an explanation of the Artificial Heart Program development and institutional goals. The process for acquisition of both governmental and institutional approval for participation in clinical trials is discussed, as are related documentation requirements. Both institutional candidate selection process and patient consent procedure are reviewed. Indications and device selection, if more than one is to be used in a given center, must be included. Current statistics for our institution and worldwide experience are reviewed. This information is gained from internal sources and newsletters published by the manufacturers.

The operative procedure is explained, aided by slides. Nurses are urged to view an implant from the OR domes when possible, and are also welcome in the OR in small numbers during implantation.

A complete description of VAD physics, mechanics, and the complementary console is necessary. This portion of the course may be very time intensive, depending on device complexity and the nurses' prior level of understanding of mechanical assist devices. The entire console and control panel are reviewed, with focus on those components important for nursing management. Several of the devices also incorporate physiological monitors necessary for device function or patient transport, which must also be reviewed. A thorough understanding of the waveforms generated by the device is necessary. VAD effectiveness is assessed, and mode and setting adjustments are based on this information. We emphasize the relationship of the assist device to physiological outcome for increased understanding.

Procedures for admission of the patient to the Cardiothoracic ICU are outlined. Admission practices are identical to those already in place for other types of cardiothoracic surgical patients, with the added considerations of console placement and VAD monitoring.

Ongoing patient care practices are taught, using the complete Nursing Care Plan as the framework. Each major organ system is reviewed with respect to VAD function,

Clinical Competency Checklist

1. Demonstrated proper procedure for dressing change of mediansternotomy, cable exit site.
   Date:
   Initials:

2. Demonstrated competent nursing care for (fill in device name) recipient, 1 day of care during which nurse was responsible for all direct care, documentation, implementation of the nursing care plan.
   Date:
   Initials:

3. On completion of the patient care day, the nurse will have 2 days assigned for machine responsibility. These days are observed by the engineer:

   a. Correct monitoring of (fill in device name)
   Date:
   Initials:
   Date:
   Initials:

   b. Correct timing of (fill in device name)
   Date:
   Initials:
   Date:
   Initials:

   c. Correct assessment of waveforms
   Date:
   Initials:
   Date:
   Initials:

   d. Correct documentation of flowsheet
   Date:
   Initials:
   Date:
   Initials:

   e. Review of emergency procedures with engineer
   Date:
   Initials:
   Date:
   Initials:

Fig. 24-2. Clinical Competency Checklist. These are specific to each device. One list is completed for each nurse on each device for which he/she has been trained, and is kept on file in the unit.

assessment, and possible side effects. Infection control is emphasized, with particular attention paid to the specialized sterile dressing change technique we have implemented for VAD patients. Emphasis is placed on early mobilization (passive or active), pulmonary care, desired early extubation, and nutritional support. Also reviewed are the particular psychosocial needs of the VAD implanted patients and their families, privacy concerns, and news media considerations.

Transportation of VAD implanted patients is an additional area for training. To ensure patient safety during transport, procedures are reviewed in detail. Before developing these procedures, some transportation "dry runs" using all the equipment (bed, console, IV poles, personnel) should be made to ensure that elevators and travel pathways will accommodate the equipment and necessary personnel.

One of the most important training session components consists of device and console hands-on practice. The VAD is placed in the artificial heart laboratory mock circulation loop, and a functional console is attached. The class participants are able to observe VAD and console function, assess waveforms, make timing and mode adjustments, and observe the outcomes of those adjustments. They are given time to practice, and are required to give a return demonstration of previously identified activities, particularly waveform assessment, timing, alarm recognition, and emergency procedures.

On completion of this 1 day training session, clinical competency must be ensured and maintained. Under the observation of the clinical educator, clinical nurse manager, or designee, the nurse must demonstrate delivery of competent nursing care and documentation for a patient on the type of VAD for which training occurred. The nurse must also demonstrate proper procedure for mediansternotomy dressing change and VAD cannula(e) exit site(s). On completion of the patient care day, the nurse must also complete 2 days during which he or she assumes responsibility for the console, under the artificial heart engineer's direction. They must demonstrate competency in various areas on this day (Fig. 24-2). Only after the nurse has demonstrated competency will he/she be assigned autonomously to the patient.

Thereafter, on an annual basis nurses are assigned times for return to the artificial heart laboratory for review of principles and practice on the mock circulation system. Repeat competency testing is also done at this time and includes a written test and a skills demonstration. Sometimes extended time periods occur between clinical implants. Therefore the clinical educator and engineers organize periodic inservices to review the device, console, and priority care components.

It is our practice to conduct separate training classes for each of the devices that we use. Although there are some commonalities between the devices in principle, they are not interchangeable, and the differences are not insignificant. It is important that the nurses are well versed in the principles, function, waveform generation and assessment, alarms, and emergency procedures for each device. Classes are conducted on a repetitive cycle each year, and there are usually several weeks or months between classes for any given nurse to prevent training overload and allow time for assimilation of information and competency demonstration.

In some of these patients, a prolonged length of implantation necessitates their recovery in the step-down unit. Separate training classes are conducted for this nursing staff because nursing diagnoses and care goals differ.

LESSONS LEARNED

VAD program development at the University of Pittsburgh Medical Center has been an ongoing process that even today results in expansion and change. As the program has grown, it has been necessary to adapt and change our practices to meet the needs that increased experience and consumption of resources dictate. Continuous evaluation of patient care practices, division of workload, training, the environment, and available resources is necessary. It is then necessary to adapt, change, and improve practices based on this information.

CONCLUSION

Involvement in the implementation of VAD usage at UPMC has proven to be an exciting and rewarding experience. Ongoing changes and advances in the field of mechanical cardiac assistance present a continuing challenge for nurses. The continuing commitment to provision of quality nursing care necessitates a high level of nursing involvement in ventricular assist device programs. Nursing practices in this area should not stagnate, but should be constantly reviewed, questioned, and altered with the goal of a more positive patient outcome, and taught to all nurses involved in this exciting area of practice.

ACKNOWLEDGMENT

Thanks are extended to John Pristas and Dr. Keith Stein for their input and review. The authors wish also to voice their continued appreciation for the support and dedication of the Cardiothoracic ICU nursing staff at Presbyterian University Hospital and University of Pittsburgh Medical Center, and their important contribution to the success of the program.

REFERENCES

1. Walsh TR, Guttendorf J, Dummer S et al: The value of protective isolation procedures in cardiac allograft patients, *Ann Thorac Surg* 47:539, 1989.
2. Pristas JM, Borovets HS, Kormos RL et al: Biomedical engineering management of Novacor left ventricular assist system (LVAS) patients, *Perfusion* 5:181, 1990.

PART FOUR

ETHICAL AND PSYCHOSOCIAL ISSUES

CHAPTER 25

Ethical issues associated with a ventricular assist device program

Jay Katz and Susan J. Quaal

INTRODUCTION

Spectacular advances in the technology and application of cardiovascular ventricular assist devices (VADs) raise many professional, humane, economic, and moral questions about when, how, and with whom they should be used. These questions cannot be easily resolved; they require careful, sustained thought and debate.

We would like to comment on some of the ethical issues these questions pose in the spirit of opening up these complex issues to examination by healthcare providers, patients, and the public at large. At the same time, we shall force ourselves to provide answers. However, our answers should not be taken as final. We present them as challenges for devising better answers and raising better questions about issues that we may have overlooked or insufficiently considered for the real world in which decisions have to be made.

We come to this collaborative inquiry from different disciplines. One of us is a cardiovascular clinical specialist (S.J.Q.), with considerable practical clinical experience. The other is a physician (J.K.) with considerable theoretical training in biomedical ethics. We thought that a pooling of our respective expertise would permit us not to stray too far from the real problems that confront the participants whenever the employment of VADs is contemplated.

PROBLEMS

Heart failure afflicts approximately 4,000,000 patients in the United States and causes 400,000 deaths per year. A study conducted by the Working Groups on Mechanical Circulatory Support of the National Heart, Lung and Blood Institute predicted that 17,000 to 35,000 patients could annually benefit from some form of circulatory support.[1] If these devices were made available, a considerable number of patients' lives could be prolonged, even to the extent of living comfortably and productively. However, determining who will benefit and who will not is beset by much uncertainty and, for those who may benefit, more expensive devices could be used that may not be readily made available for many reasons.

Cost is a major factor that could limit device use. Providing 30,000 patients per year with the most advanced devices would add $3.1 billion per year to the $8.8 billion already expended on patients suffering from heart failure during their last 6 months of life.[2] Currently the Thoratec external pulsative VAD costs approximately $51,000 to $83,000 ($40,000 to $70,000 per console and $11,000 to $13,000 per device).[3] Less expensive devices, such as the centrifugal cardiac assist system, which costs approximately $11,500 ($150 per disposable pump head and $11,000 per console) are also available.[3] Centrifugal assist devices, however, have limitations. They can be employed only for a limited period of time and their success, beyond prolonging life for a short period of time, depends on the heart's ability to be restored to reasonably normal functioning or on the immediate availability of a heart for transplantation. Moreover a centrifugal VAD implantation necessitates activity restriction to prevent cannula dislodgement. Immobilization can lead to complications such as deep vein thrombosis and pneumonia. On the other hand, patients placed on an implantable VAD, such as the Thermedics Heart Mate, Novacor, or a pneumatic VAD, can progress to ambulation.

Thus choices have to be made in individual cases that are also dependent on, and often determined by, monetary considerations. We shall return shortly to the problems of cost that arise in individual encounters between a physician and his or her patient. First, however, a number of secondary problems spawned by the expense of these devices must be identified. Some of the devices, because of their cost, may not be purchased in adequate quantities by hospitals performing cardiac catheterization, angioplasty, or coronary bypass surgery. Thus, to the extent VADs are available, they have to be rationed and implanted in selected patients.

Two other problems of cost deserve mentioning. First, in addition to the centrifugal assist device, external pneumatic VAD, and implantable VAD, emergency resuscitative systems exist that are also expensive. Their cost is approximately $21,000 per unit ($20,000 for a console and $1000 for a disposable patient circuit).[3] Resuscitative systems support cardiac and/or pulmonary functions during heart or lung failure and provide an opportunity for temporary, but life-saving, resuscitation while buying time for further evaluation. They too are often not available in sufficient numbers. Second, effective use of cardiac mechanical assist devices requires trained personnel at the bedside. Hospitals may not employ a multidisciplinary VAD team that includes perfusionists and clinical engineers to monitor and regulate the VADs. Physicians and staff nurses often are inadequately trained, if at all, to attend to these devices in case of malfunction.

Beyond the ethical problems created by cost containment, there are those related to informed consent. About 1% of patients undergoing coronary bypass surgery may be unweanable from extracorporeal circulation.[4] At that critical moment, a patient's myocardial recovery or suitability for heart transplantation cannot be satisfactorily determined. Thus the surgeon is confronted with the decision of which device to implant, whether to implant any of them without the patient's consent, or to implant only with a relative's consent. The meaningfulness of proxy consent by a relative is beset by considerable doubt because of his or her distraught state and the unlikelihood of informing him or her adequately during the limited time available in such an emergency.

Of course a patient's informed consent could be obtained before surgery from all who undergo this procedure. However, doing so is alleged to be anxiety provoking and thus raises concerns about upsetting all patients, most of whom will not have to make this choice, for the sake of the few who will be confronted with such an emergency. Here another problem arises: giving patients the authority to ask for device removal, whether implanted with or without their consent, whenever they request it because they find life not worth living under these circumstances.

A final problem is that employment of centrifugal assist devices and resuscitation systems does not require an Investigational Device Exemption (IDE) because similar technology existed before 1976. However, the newer and more promising devices are subject to regulation, including Institutional Review Board (IRB) review. In light of the advances in VAD technology, one could now advance the argument that centrifugal and resuscitation systems have become "experimental" once again. Thus a new problem has arisen. Devices once exempt from regulation by the "grandfather clause" may have to be reclassified as experimental and subjected to the same review procedures as their newer sister technologies.

QUESTIONS

We now pose a number of questions. They are designed to identify and sharpen the ethical conflicts that confront all participants under these tragic circumstances. We frame them as best we can but, as we have already suggested, they may not be all the questions that need to be posed. Our questions are interrelated and in the next section, we shall answer them, but not necessarily in the order in which they are here presented.

1. In light of the considerable cost of some of these devices and the necessity to employ them only occasionally, but then for life-saving purposes, what are the responsibilities of hospitals and surgeons to ensure the devices adequate availability at centers that perform coronary bypass surgery and other invasive cardiac procedures?

2. Because some of these devices require constant skilled monitoring, what depth of staffing must be provided? Must surgeons and Intensive Care Unit (ICU) nurses be proficient in monitoring and maintaining these devices, particularly in hospitals that do not employ a VAD team of perfusionists and clinical engineers?

3. What information about the availability of these devices and the level of training of postimplant care givers must be provided to patients before they undergo invasive cardiac procedures or to those with poor ejection fractions?[2]

4. Because centrifugal and resuscitation systems are currently exempt from FDA regulations and the newer devices are not, should hospitals that perform cardiac surgery requiring insertion of cardiac assist devices promulgate regulations that subject all of them to IRB review?

5. Because myocardial pump failure will occur in approximately 1% of patients undergoing cardiac surgery, should consent for possible VAD implantation be obtained from all patients before surgery? If not from all patients, should at least those who are likely VAD candidates be fully informed and asked to give their consent?

6. In case of emergencies with patients who have not given their consent, should relatives be asked to give proxy consent?

7. In light of the uncertainties about who will or will not benefit from implantation (e.g., prospects of comfortable and significant prolongation of life and the likelihood of the availability of a heart transplant), what authority should be vested in the surgeon not to recommend or use the most optimal device because of its cost?

8. Because some third-party payers may not reimburse costs, should surgeons inform patients and their relatives in instances when no device, or a less expensive device, will be employed that the decision is based not on medical, but on economic, grounds?

9. Do patients have the right, once they awake from anesthesia or during their postoperative course, to ask that the device be removed, even though it may mean certain death?

10. Is it the professional responsibility of cardiac surgeons to alert Congress, state legislatures, and the public that patients may not receive optimal medical treatment because of fiscal constraints?

ANSWERS

The realities are these: (1) scarcity of expensive resources for all patients who could benefit from them and for those who may require them when complications arise during cardiac surgery, (2) death or marked quality of life impairment if these treatment modalities are not available, (3) absence of, or infringements on, patients' decision-making authority whenever obtaining informed consent is not deemed to be in their "best interest." Thus health care providers are confronted with making tragic choices whenever some form of unusually expensive treatment is unavailable that can at least preserve or sustain life for a period of time.

We would like to pursue our answers from two perspectives: (1) problems created for all participants by the general scarcity of these resources and (2) specific scarcity of resources when a patient is suddenly in need of them, secondary to acute heart failure.

The general scarcity of resources

At present patients who could benefit from cardiac mechanical assist devices may not receive any of them because of their expense. This problem is even more far reaching because, among the available devices, some are more expensive than others, and the more expensive assist devices may ensure a better quality of life and promise a greater chance for the prolongation of life than the less expensive ones. Moreover, even if available, third-party payers may not reimburse patients for the expenses incurred.

We believe that it is the responsibility of professional organizations to bring these problems to public attention. Such concerted action, joined by public interest groups, could lead, as it did for making hemodialysis and renal transplantation more generally available in 1972, to congressional action, which extended Medicare payments for these interventions under §299I of the 1972 Social Security Act Amendments.[5] In the meantime, and until support for these treatments becomes adequate, consideration has to be given to the selection of patients in need of these devices. Katz and Capron explored these issues for other scarce resources in their book *Catastrophic diseases—who decides what?*[6] They suggested that selection should "rely on medical criteria to narrow the initial field of persons down to a pool of those who can reasonably be said to be likely to benefit from treatment. From this pool, regular drawings could be held whenever additional treatment spaces become available. It would probably be necessary for the system, although national in scope, to be subdivided by region and locality. . . ."[6]

Here a more fundamental question arises. Should policies about which diseases to treat with these expensive devices be formulated that may or may not encompass some or all patients suffering from congestive heart failure? We can only flag this question and note that although a public commitment of $3.1 billion could meet the yearly cost for making the most advanced devices available to needy patients, the same amount of money could provide ambulatory care of a general nature for countless poor people.

In a recent article Victor L. Poirier[2] explored the question of "whether the financial investment for our society in applying this technology to an individual is a sound financial investment" from the perspective of ensuring that such an "investment [can be recouped during] a reasonable payback period [and in turn promise] an improvement in the financial structure of the economy?" His tentative analysis suggests that the initial yearly expenditure of $3.1 billion could be recouped by patients' earning potential during a 5-year survival period that would add their income to the gross national product. He also noted that, of course, "those individuals with a higher earning power [would have] to support those individuals with a lower earning power." Even if his analysis turns out to be correct, society would still have to bear the medical costs, which would add another .05% to healthcare expenditures.

Poirier, who is an economist, argues that "we can treat individuals with chronic heart failure as machines that have reached the end of their productive lives. Do we remove these individuals from the productive side of the equations, or do we invest in them to bring them back into a productive mode, generating income for the business (or society)? One way to answer this question is to use basic financial analysis techniques to determine the value of the investment and the payback period."[2]

Poirier's observations are important. They suggest that from an economic perspective, initial costs can perhaps be offset by a person's earning power after having been restored to productive life. He commendably also suggests that those with higher earning power can support those who do not possess sufficient economic resources to fully pay their way. Yet nagging questions remain. If his economic analysis turns out to be too optimistic, when, if ever, and by whose authority, should life be foreshortened for monetary considerations? In putting it this starkly, we do not wish to imply that tragic choices may not have to be made because our resources are not unlimited and therefore may have to be allocated for more important ends. We suggest only that the question be openly debated, if only because such choices should not be made on the basis of individual patients' wealth. In our view, this could violate a fundamental, albeit contested, constitutional principle: equal protection of all citizens, which, in theory, also proscribes discrimination on the basis of financial disparity.

The specific scarcity of resources

It is our impression that many hospitals that perform coronary bypass surgery or other cardiac operations have not formulated general policies (1) on the availability of cardiac assist devices and which kinds, in case of emergencies, or (2) for the depth of staffing, including trained ICU nurses, perfusionists, and clinical engineers. Such policies need to be formulated. We raise only in passing the question of whether such policies should be promulgated by an appropriate national professional organization to avoid unnecessary duplication of effort. If that were to happen, hospitals could then adopt or modify the policies according to their particular circumstances.

In the course of setting forth such policies, many other questions will emerge that require resolution, such as when in the absence of particular assist devices, must vulnerable patients (e.g., those with poor ejection fractions) be referred to other hospitals, or when must cardiac operations be delayed, if possible, because trained VAD teams are already overextended, caring for patients in need of these devices?

More generally we believe that even though centrifugal and resuscitation systems do not require an IDE, hospitals should ask their IRBs to formulate policies for their use that comport with the policies that have already been established for employment of the newer technologies. Both older and newer technologies expose patients to risks and benefits, and in light of the many available alternatives, more encompassing policies on their use need to be established. The policies will offer patients greater choice and avoid the danger of resorting to older devices because of the lack of "cumbersome" constraints on their employment.

Also, hospitals must establish policies on what patients need to be told before cardiac surgery regarding available resources and the possible necessity to implant a mechanical assist device during surgery. Major problems are at least threefold: (1) the hospital may not have available all the existing devices, including experimental ones, that are considered promising; (2) only 1% of patients undergoing coronary bypass surgery cannot be weaned from extracorporeal circulation after attempts have been made to remedy any problems that may arise during the operation by pharmacological means or intraaortic balloon/pumping, and then different devices, some more expensive than others, can be utilized; and (3) some devices are considered experimental and are therefore subject to federal regulations. The problems are intertwined but we shall treat them separately.

We recommend that all patients and their families be informed of the range of devices available. In turn, they must also be informed about facilities that are better equipped so that patients have a choice of where to go. However, this immediately raises the second problem. Because only 1% of patients require these devices, the majority of patients could be burdened with anxieties over complications that will never arise. This concern has often been raised, but it is supported only by anecdotal accounts. Thus it is not at all clear that patients will so react when confronted with situations when the risk for them is that minimal. Indeed the opposite concern can equally be raised; namely that patients will disregard the risk because it is so small. We believe that high-risk cardiac surgical patients and their families must be apprised of the potential need for a cardiac mechanical assist device not only, and perhaps not even primarily, because the small risk is a real one, but for other important reasons. Without this information, discussions cannot be meaningfully carried on about the devices that are or are not available at the hospital in case of emergencies and about preferences over using one of the more or less expensive devices. Two other questions deserve mention. Should patients, who during cardiac surgery appear to be unweanable from extracorporeal circulation, be given a choice about first resorting to intraaortic balloon pumping before implantation of external cardiac mechanical assist devices? Or should that decision be left to the discretion of the surgeon?

We appreciate that physicians generally do not inform patients of such rare eventualities in ordinary clinical practice. Instead, in case of an emergency, they do the best they can, relying perhaps on a family member's consent if it can be hurriedly obtained. We also appreciate that the law of informed consent is unclear on what constitutes nonnegligent professional conduct during these rare emergencies. One could argue that the potential risk of not being able to wean a patient from extracorporeal circulation following surgery must be explained under the general duty to disclose. One could argue that in these instances the life-threatening emergency exception applies, which permits surgeons to use their best judgment.

In deference to the widespread, though undocumented, belief that it is too burdensome to apprise all patients of risks from which most will be exempt, we suggest that reliance on surgeons' clinical judgment be entertained only if hospitals have all devices available and implantation will not be guided by considerations of cost but by what seems to be in the patient's best interest. However, in light of uncertainty of what constitutes best interest during an emergency situation, we also suggest that the surgeon be prepared to use a device that promises the greatest comfort and best chance of prolonging life.

Some of the newer cardiac assist devices are subject to regulations under the Medical Devices Act.[7] Some years ago Angela R. Holder[8] discussed a research project that had been submitted to an IRB, which was designed to investigate left-ventricle assist device safety and efficiency. The investigators "estimated that about 10% of patients on a bypass cannot be weaned easily; 8% respond to what is now considered standard therapy; and only the remaining 1% or 2% would be candidates for this device." Since it could not be predicted which patient might need it, the IRB was confronted with the question of "what form of consent would be appropriate and by whom should it be given." The IRB members who argued against obtaining informed consent pointed to an ambiguous exception to informed consent in the Medical Devices Act. This exception permits use of such a device whenever: "(1) a life-threatening situation involving the human subject of such testing necessitates [it], (2) it is not feasible to obtain informed consent from the subject, and (3) there is not sufficient time to obtain such consent from the subject's representative."[9] We have already noted the ambiguity contained in the phrase of what is "feasible," depending on whether it refers to consent *before* or *during* surgery.

According to Holder,[8] after having discussed and rejected options of no consent from any patient, consent from all patients, or consent from family members, the IRB ruled that "only those patients who were, as a matter of clinical judgment, more likely than most to need the device, [needed] to be approached before their operations. In the course of obtaining surgical consent, [only] patients in this group would be told that one of the risks of major cardiac surgery is death, which in a small percentage of cases could result from an inability to 'get them off the pump.' The patients would then be told that a new device might work in this situation. If the patient agreed [to pursue the matter further], three alternatives would be presented: (1) the right to refuse detailed discussion [and instead delegating a family member to make the decision], (2) the right to participate if need occurred, and (3) the right, preoperatively, to refuse [participation]."[8]

Although the IRB ruling was most thoughtful, we reject it on the following grounds. The persons involved in the research project are patients, some of whom, unless in the vulnerable group, would remain ignorant that they had been recruited for a research project until after the device had been implanted. Moreover since the experimental device is available and could save lives, all patients should be apprised of this alternative. Good medical practice and respect for persons requires such disclosures.

In the alternative we suggest that the device be used only with the high risk patients whose consent has been obtained. It would then take longer to complete the study, but it would eliminate the common danger in clinical research of confusing one's obligations to patients and their care with one's obligations to the research protocol and the advancement of science. In this process the patient can become objectified; he or she is no longer primarily a *person*-patient but an *object* of research.

We agree with the IRB's reasoning to not allow families solely to make this decision during an operation. It cogently observed that one cannot "always [assume] that family members have the patient's interest at heart; which [raises] other questions of a family member's right to refuse potentially life-saving therapy for a patient who would otherwise surely die."[8] Moreover in these emergency situations, family members can be too distraught to make considered choices. Should such situations arise, the preferable resolution is to rely on the surgeon's best judgment and his Hippocratic commitment that requires him or her to err on the side of prolongation of life.

Since patients can refuse implantation of cardiac assist devices, policies should be promulgated that give patients the right to ask for their removal if they find life intolerable. That choice probably should not be available to them immediately after surgery because one cannot be certain whether patients are reacting to postoperative discomfort, or have given the decision sufficient thought. Patients need to be talked with about such irreversible choices, but always with the understanding that the final choice is theirs to make.[9] To provide patients with this opportunity is particularly important because the surgeon's decision to implant a mechanical assist device may have been based on uncertainty about the patient's suitability for a heart transplant or about donor availability, which is in short supply. Those patients who do not qualify for heart transplantation should not be condemned to live out their remaining days or months on a device without hope, unless they prefer to do so.

We suggest finally that patients and their families be informed about decisions not to implant any device or not the most optimal one if that decision is based on economic and not on professional considerations. In the early days of hemodialysis, when dialysis was expensive and not covered by insurance, physicians often tried to shield patients from the painful truth that it was money that denied them access. Instead, patients were told that such treatment was medically contraindicated. This was wrong, both in the short and long run. Patients and their families were deprived of the opportunity to obtain necessary funds, and an aroused citizenry could not pressure its legislators to enact laws that would remedy the situation.

CONCLUSION: A FINAL REFLECTION

We have tried to provide answers to difficult questions. The answers we have given are shaped by our underlying convictions that medical decisions should be made jointly by patients and their physicians, and that this is possible only if doctors honestly disclose to patients what is at stake first. This is particularly true for the interventions that are the subject of this paper.

The astounding advances in medical technology that made cardiac mechanical assist devices possible confront doctors and patients with a vast array of therapeutic

options, each with its own known and unknown risks and benefits as well as consequences to quality of life. Thus it should be apparent that these decisions cannot be
made by physicians and hospital administrators alone. Nor, because the treatment
modalities are expensive, can these decisions be made solely by physicians and patients.
The public, through its legislators, must be included in the decision-making process.
Questions posed by these new technologies that will in time only become more sophisticated and even more expensive are awesome ones. Who shall benefit from them? Who
shall decide what constitutes benefit? Shall a person be denied life because he or she
has not enough money?

REFERENCES

1. The Working Group on Mechanical Circulatory Support of NHLBI. *Artificial heart and assist devices: directions, needs, costs, societal and ethical issues.* Bethesda, Md, 1985, National Heart Lung and Blood Institute.
2. Poirier VL: Can we afford circulatory support systems? *Trans Am Soc Artif Intern Organs* 32:540, 1991.
3. Smith RG, Cleavinger M: Current perspectives on the use of circulatory assist devices. *AACN's Clinical Issues in Critical Care Nursing* 2(3):488, 1991.
4. Miller CA, Pae WE, Pierce WS: Combined registry for the clinical use of mechanical ventricular assist devices: postcardiotomy cardioganic shock, *ASAIO Trans* 36:43, 1990.
5. Public Law No. 92-603, §299I, October 30, 1972.
6. Katz J, Capron AM: Catastrophic diseases—who decides what? New Brunswick, Canada Transaction Books, 1982. Reprint of 1975 ed., published by Russell Sage Foundation.
7. Medical Device Amendment of 1976, §21 USC, §321 et seq. Archara, A: Development of PMA Guidance for Ventricular Assist Devices and Total Artificial Heart. *IEEE Engineering in Medicine and Biology Magazine* 7:90, 1988.
8. Holder A: Consent to the use of an investigational assist device, *IRB* 1:6, March 1979.
9. Katz J: *The silent world of doctor and patient.* New York, 1984 The Free Press.

CHAPTER 26

Total artificial heart experience from the family's perspective

Una Loy Clark Farrer

INTRODUCTION

Before the onset of cardiomyopathy my husband, Dr. Barney Clark, had always been a very well and extremely active man. He had enjoyed a busy dental practice and was an avid golfer. In the spring of 1977 he retired from his dental practice and became involved in a small land development business. I believe he was happier at this time in his life than I had ever known him to be. However, in just 2 years he became plagued with an overwhelming fatigue, shortness of breath, and general weakness, which forced him to seek medical advice. It was in 1979 that he was diagnosed with cardiomyopathy myocarditis.

His cardiologist explained that cardiomyopathy myocarditis was a degenerative disease for which there was no known cure. We, as a family, faced and tried to accept the first major crisis in our lives, realizing that his life would slip from us a little each day and that there was nothing we could do to halt this process.

As I watched my husband decline from a healthy, robust man to a point where he was consuming approximately 39 pills a day to keep his heart muscle and other organs functioning, I realized that our most cherished dreams of our retirement years would be denied; I feared that he might become bitter. Then I began to recognize his personal strength and courage, and was in awe of how accepting he was of his illness, with a kind of quiet resolution. He never manifested any sign of bitterness, even when he was denied a heart transplant because they were not transplanting patients over the age of 50 at that time and Dr. Clark was 59.

During his 3 year illness we more or less learned to "cope" with the heartache and desperation of our situation, realizing our helplessness to alter things, yet having the comforting stability of being in our home, surrounded by friends, and able to gain strength from each other as a family. As a couple and family, we cherished every day and shared a closeness we had never known before.

CONFRONTING THE ISSUE OF A POSSIBLE ARTIFICIAL HEART IMPLANT

In October 1981 Dr. Clark's cardiologist informed us we had exhausted all of the then "proven" drugs that could stimulate his weakening heart muscle and referred us to another cardiologist in Salt Lake City who would try an experimental drug called "amrinone," hoping this might prove beneficial. However, the drug, when administered, was not tolerated by his system and the effort had to be aborted. Dr. Clark tried very hard to hide his great disappointment by saying, "Well, honey, we tried anyway, didn't we!" The cardiologist, realizing that we had no alternative, suggested that Dr. Clark be evaluated for a total artificial heart implant at the University of Utah. In response to this proposal, my husband fully realized its serious implications and must have read the fear in my eyes. He took my hand in his and said, "Thank you doctor. We'd be pleased to see the surgeon at the University of Utah."

Dr. Clark, who was now greatly debilitated, and I made our way to the University of Utah Medical Center 2 days later and listened intently as we were shown the total artificial heart (TAH) and were given a detailed account of how it had performed in the animal model. The team had learned all they could from the animal model and were seeking a human volunteer who could comply with the rigid requirements of the University of Utah's Institutional Review Board and the Food and Drug Administration (FDA). We were also informed that to be a recipient of the TAH, the volunteer and his spouse must be interrogated and approved by a special panel. This panel needed to agree unanimously that the TAH recipient must:

1. Fully understand the surgical and experimental procedures to which he or she must submit.
2. Be very near death.
3. Be mentally capable of handling stress and be able to be confined within a 6 foot radius of the heart drive unit.
4. Live near the medical center the rest of his or her life.
5. Have the complete support of his or her entire family.
6. Sign a 12 page consent form for the surgery and experimentation that set forth, in the bleakest manner, the complications that may occur as a result. This consent form was to be signed twice—24 hours apart—in order that the volunteer could, at any time within those 24 hours, withdraw from the experiment.

The next day we visited the Artificial Heart Animal Laboratory at the University of Utah. We observed two animals implanted with the TAH as they fed and walked on a treadmill; they appeared normal in every respect, except for the drivelines coming from their sides, tethering them to the TAH drive unit. We also visited the Mock Circulation Testing Laboratory where numerous TAHs had been pumping for many months, undergoing durability testing. I was impressed with Dr. Clark's enormous interest and reluctance to leave, and because of this was not greatly surprised when he announced that it would give him a "great deal of satisfaction if he could receive the TAH and perhaps make a contribution to medical science."

Returning to our home in Seattle 2 days later, we decided we would not discuss the possibility of volunteering for the TAH implant with anyone except our physician and our children. We also determined to be careful not to ask their advice because we did not want them to feel any responsibility for our decision or its outcome.

During the next 6 weeks as Dr. Clark's condition worsened rapidly, we prayed diligently, searched our souls, examined our motives, beliefs, our strengths and weaknesses. One evening, after a particularly difficult day, Dr. Clark requested that I share with him my innermost feelings about the artificial heart. He said "I cannot help but feel I have been a burden to you for many months, and perhaps, in fairness to you, I should just let nature take its course and allow you to continue on with your life." He said that he knew his decision would affect me as much as it would him and he had a real need to know exactly how I felt. As I choked back the tears, I quickly assured him that he had never been a burden to me, that he *was my life,* and that I would support him whatever his decision might be.

THE INSIGHT INTO OUR MAKING THE DECISION TO VOLUNTEER FOR TAH IMPLANT

We believed that God's most precious gift to us was the gift of life and the innate intelligence He endowed us with that we might gain knowledge and progress in all things. We also believed that man's desire to preserve and prolong life (as long as there was quality of life) was a manifestation of our gratitude for this gift and was also a form of progression. Therefore we had no problem with the moral/ethical aspect of the TAH. We were at peace that what we were considering was *not* contrary to God's plan and that conviction did a great deal to fortify us in our decision making process and in the entire experience.

Dr. Clark, having had medical training himself, was well aware of his critical physical condition and had long since faced reality regarding his mortality. He was very much aware of the experimental nature of the implantation and did not expect any great personal miracle. He was simply faced with two alternatives. He could let his disease run its course to a relatively painless demise or he could elect to volunteer for the TAH, hoping, at best perhaps, to be able to breathe without struggling, to enjoy a good book, to take meals at the table with his family, to move comfortably about his home, and most important of all, to continue to share interactions with his children, grandchildren, and friends. He knew that by volunteering he would be submitting to a totally unpredictable future. There had been no promises made to him.

The facts that were paramount in making his decision were (1) he believed that he owed a debt to those who had undergone the clinical trials with the drugs that had prolonged his life for the past 3 years, (2) he knew there were rigid requirements to be a candidate and not everyone could meet those requirements, and (3) he believed strongly that the TAH could offer prolonged life to some of the thousands suffering from heart disease, but that it must be implanted in a human being in order to evaluate this possibility, and that *regardless of his personal outcome,* much could be learned to benefit the medical world and future heart patients. He confided in me, "I would be somewhat less than satisfied with myself as a human being, knowing all this, if I did not volunteer. I would like my life and perhaps my death to count for something." The children and I could not argue with his reasoning, and we determined to be totally united behind his decision, whatever it might be.

THE TAH IMPLANT EXPERIENCE

By Thanksgiving Dr. Clark's condition was such that I suggested we forgo our usual family dinner, but he said he was particularly anxious to spend Thanksgiving with all of us. He made the effort to fully dress and had his sons bring him downstairs to the dining room where he sat at the head of the table and took charge as he always had done. He blessed the food and then, in a simple prayer, asked the Lord to bless us as a family, with strength, with courage, and with a strong desire to remain close to each other and to support each other. When he finished there was not a dry eye at our table; we realized that this might be our last Thanksgiving together.

Because of their father's total exhaustion, our sons assisted him back to bed immediately after dinner. Later that evening as we retired, he asked me to please contact the University of Utah TAH team in the morning and tell them that he had decided to volunteer for the TAH. I have often recalled the feeling that swept over me as he shared his decision. I did not feel the fear and anxiety I thought I might—only a sweet calmness and assurance that I had not felt in many months, and could only interpret that to mean that the Lord had guided us to the right decision and that He would sustain us.

Neither of us slept that night. We realized we were saying goodbye to the life we had always known, to the circle of friends we were so comfortable with, and to having our children and grandchildren nearby. We were taking a path no one had ever walked before and we knew not where it would lead us.

Dr. Clark refused air ambulance transport to the University of Utah. We traveled instead by common carrier. I did not understand how he could tolerate the flight as ill as he was, but thought he was trying desperately to keep things as normal as possible. When we landed in Salt Lake City, however, it was immediately apparent that things were not normal. Two security officers immediately boarded the plane. One stood directly opposite our seats and one instructed the passengers to deplane as rapidly as possible. Dr. Clark was taken off the rear of the plane and put aboard a hospital helicopter; I was escorted through the terminal to my brother, who took me to the medical center.

Immediately on our arrival at the medical center we learned that news of Dr. Clark's hospital admission had been "leaked" to the press and the medical center was besieged with reporters. I was advised that I should remain in the ICU wing for the next several days because it was important that I not be confronted by the press at this time. Only then did I realize that we had never considered or prepared for the effect our decision would have on the media and the people throughout the world. As I look back now, I wonder how we could have been so naive, so completely oblivious to the intense interest the implant operation would create.

I suddenly began feeling the strain of Dr. Clark's long illness, the stress of our decision making, the fear of being interviewed by the selection panel and the secrecy and urgency of our arrival. At this time I noticed a group of people walking toward me; one nice-looking lady seemed to be in charge as she put her arms around me, welcomed me, and introduced herself as my social worker. Although her arms around me were like those of a long lost friend and her warmth was like a shot of adrenalin, little did I know at that time just how much I would learn to depend on her and what a moral strength she would be to me during the next 4 months. She introduced me to the other team members, who, each in turn, welcomed me. I had not expected such warmth, and it was most comforting.

Until very late that evening, and all the next day, I visited with TAH team members, even sharing lunch and dinner with one or two of them, and I was very much impressed by their friendliness and interest in me and my family.

The next morning, it was obvious that Dr. Clark's condition had deteriorated considerably and I was concerned that he would be too ill to be interviewed by the selection panel and would not be approved for TAH implant. That evening I expressed my concern to the social worker, who took me totally by surprise when she said, "Oh, didn't you know? Both you and Dr. Clark have already been interviewed; that is why you have been visiting with so many members of the heart team." Dr. Clark had been unanimously approved for the TAH implant, which was scheduled for December 2, 1981.

Despite his critical condition, Dr. Clark never lost his sense of humor. When he was asked if he was going to sign the required second consent form, he replied, "Of course, but I'll bet if I said *no* there would be a lot of long faces around here."

Because it was feared that Dr. Clark would not live until the scheduled surgery on December 2, he was taken to surgery at approximately 11:00 pm on December 1, 1981, and some 10 hours later, we were allowed to visit him in the ICU. I feared my legs would not support me as we neared his room, and although we were not prepared to see him as we did, with tubes emerging from everywhere, the respirator's "clicking" sound, and the artificial heart driver emitting the burst of compressed air as it drove the heart, I could not help but notice the beautiful pinkness of his skin, which before the surgery had been grey and lifeless looking; thank God for this wonderful blessing. He was awake, took my hand, and placed it on his chest, so that I could feel the artificial heart beating, and looked up at me questioningly. I know not why, but my response was, "Yes dear, you have an artificial heart, but I hope this does not mean that you do not love us anymore." He made a brave attempt to smile, but could not because he was intubated.

I knew he was happy to be alive and to know that so far, he and the heart team had done well.

THE POSTOPERATIVE EXPERIENCE

As we lived the 112 days following the implant, it was like living on a roller coaster. One day our hopes and expectations would soar, and the next we would experience disappointment and even despair. In spite of all the complications, Dr. Clark endured; I think the seizures were the hardest and most challenging for him and the family. For over 2 weeks, he was in and out of reality. Visits by psychologists were a part of the scheduled routine. They would ask him such things as "What is your name?" "What day of the week is it?" "Do you know where you are?" and "Who is the President of the United States?" Even though I realized they were just doing what was required of them, it was upsetting because I felt it was demeaning to Dr. Clark. He was a very proud, intelligent, and decisive man, and I felt he had good reason to be confused at times. Aside from the results of the seizures, his days *and nights* were filled with endless procedures and I wondered how he could separate night from day, let alone be cognizant of what day of the week it was. Except for those weeks following the seizures, Dr. Clark was very much in control of his mental faculties and indicated many times to all of us his desire to proceed with the experiment.

I was privileged to be close to my husband throughout the 112 day ordeal. I was provided with housing in a hospital room very close to the ICU and knew from moment to moment what was happening. Our children, on the other hand, were 900 miles away, besieged by the press, who, in most cases, because of their direct contact at the hospital, actually knew more than the family did. It was either through the press calling or what the children viewed on television that kept them informed as to their father's status. They were unprepared and uninformed regarding how to handle the intense interest of the public and the press. They could not have a meal without being interrupted with telephone calls. The only times they saw their father were when he was in crisis. These visits were not comforting, and the children would return to Seattle with a heaviness of heart.

When Dr. Clark was moved out of the ICU, it was a triumph for him. From his spacious hospital room, he could enjoy the sunsets and the wonderful view out over the Salt Lake Valley. It was there we enjoyed our 39th wedding anniversary with a huge wedding cake made by the hospital chef and shared with as many of the patients as it would serve. This was a very special time for us. When I asked what he would like as an anniversary gift, he expressed the desire for a clock with big black numbers to be hung directly on the wall in front of him so that he could see it at any time. He said, "Nights are long and I want to pace myself mentally by it." He seemed to feel better knowing what time it was during the night and how much longer it was until morning.

On March 1, 1982, Dr. Clark gave his only interview on public television. It was in the evening after a difficult day and he was tired. I wondered why that particular day was chosen, but felt there must be a valid reason. I have read one reporter's criticism of this interview:

"From the public's perspective, that interview was one of the most striking and controversial aspects of Dr. Clark's case. It was the only time the public saw him with his artificial heart, and to most, he came off looking like a zombie. Dr. Clark looked like he was staring off into space, unable to look at his interviewer."

I was present at that interview. Dr. Clark was not a "zombie"; he was a very ill man, struggling to sit up and communicate to the public how he felt, and he was not looking at his interviewer because he had been instructed to "look directly at the camera," and that was exactly what he was doing. I believe the interview afforded an opportunity for the world to know how he felt about the entire experience. "All in all," he said, "it has been a pleasure to be able to help people." That statement personified his attitude, the reason he volunteered for the artificial heart, and why he was able to survive those 112 days as he did. I am hopeful that the general public was kinder and more accepting of Dr. Clark's special circumstances than the reporter was.

On the morning of the 112th day, I entered Dr. Clark's hospital room and thought he was sleeping. I walked over to the heart driver unit to check the dials and knew immediately there was a very serious problem. I immediately alerted the nurses' station, who in turn, alerted the cardiologist. At 10:05 that evening, Dr. Clark was declared "brain dead" and the heart driver was turned off. I knew then he was gone. As I stood there by him, I was never more proud of him, nor had I ever loved him more. Although my heart was aching and I knew life would never be the same again without him, I could not wish him back.

A REFLECTION ON THE ISSUES 10 YEARS LATER

After Dr. Clark's death we struggled, as all families do when they lose a loved one, to adjust to life without him. We were comforted and at peace in the knowledge that he was at last at rest and that though his days with the artificial heart were "stormy" for the most part, he also had many good days and his desire and purpose to give the experiment "his best" and make a contribution to medical science had been accomplished. In our eyes it had been a "success." We also were comforted in the hope that the Artificial Heart Program would continue—that there would be approval for another volunteer, whom we hoped would have an easier time than Dr. Clark, and from whom much would be learned to eventually benefit mankind. However, as the months went by, the IRB failed to approve another candidate and the papers and magazines were filled with criticisms by portions of the medical community and others about the implantation. As a family, we grew weary and very disheartened. Each day it seemed, there would be another article such as "Dr. Clark's Voyage to Nowhere." "Was the implantation an extension of Dr. Clark's life or a prolongation of his death?" "Was Dr.

Clark a good candidate for the heart, or should they have chosen someone else?" "What about informed consent, had he been properly informed or not?" and "What about Quality of Life?" Each time an article would appear in the newspaper or other publication, reporters would call to ask how I felt about it. I could say only that I was sorry, that it was impossible for me to comment on other people's opinions, but I believed we had done our best and I was very much in favor of further artificial heart experimentation.

At this particular time in our lives we were very tender about Dr. Clark, the heart team, and the experiment and were vulnerable to the point that we took these criticisms very personally.

It was with relief that we learned of the proposed conference at Alta, Utah in October 1983, sponsored by the University of Utah Medical Center and the Texas Health Science Center at Houston. Thirty of the local participants and 15 extramural consultants were invited to attend to discuss the many troubling issues that arose before, during, and after the artificial heart implantation. Following the conference a book entitled "After Barney Clark" was written and published, not only for the medical community, but for the public. Margery Shaw, the editor of the book, sent a copy to my family. We were deeply appreciative of this kindness because when we read it, we realized the criticisms were not directed at us personally. We could put it all in perspective and know that it was just, proper, and responsible to discuss and try to overcome many of these problems before another person received an implant and the experimentation continued.

We had been hopeful that the conference would lessen the pressures felt by the IRB and those who had been most critical of the experiment and that the FDA would be more cooperative. However, as the IRB and FDA failed to move forward, the artificial heart program disintegrated into a state of "limbo." The Utah Heart Team broke up out of their frustration and their desire "to get on with it." Had we not realized the depth of the heart team's frustration (because we too were so frustrated) we may have felt this breakup a desertion of sorts, but knowing our own disappointment over the inertia, we could only have sympathy for the heart team. After all, they had been involved in the planning for this experiment months and years before we were involved and, no doubt, had more to lose than we did.

It was a blessing in my life, when I seemed to be the most discouraged, that the American Heart Association invited me to be a volunteer-ambassador for them. Although I was concerned regarding my ability to be effective for them, I felt I must do something to carry on Dr. Clark's legacy, and I accepted. For the next 4½ years I traveled throughout the United States and Canada sharing the total artificial heart experience and encouraging the fight against heart disease. This was a comforting and healing experience for me at a time when I desperately needed to know that I was doing something positive and was not deserting those thousands of people who had supported Dr. Clark, and our family, and who had hoped for so much.

Perhaps I can best explain the family's perspective of the artificial heart experience by responding to the criticisms that were so prevalent after Dr. Clark's demise.

My family and I are deeply proud of our dear Husband and Father. We know for a fact the reason he volunteered for the artificial heart implant—it was not that he was desperately grasping for anything that would give him a few more days of life; it was because he found himself in a position in which he could possibly make his life count for something in prolonging life with quality for those to come after him who were suffering from end-stage heart disease, and also to express by his actions, his gratitude for the many who had tried and proven the drugs that sustained his life for the 2½ years after the onset of his illness. He had long since accepted the fact he was going to die, and when he learned that he might be useful in the artificial heart experiment, he believed he could not be satisfied with himself if he did not offer himself for the trial. He was not on a "voyage to nowhere," but rather on a "voyage to somewhere" for those who came after him.

If, through the implantation, he could survive the surgery and live for even a few hours, it would prove the artificial heart could support life in a human. If he lived a week, a month, or nearly four months as he did, that would be even better. If we could learn an artificial heart did not change one's personality or any of the human emotions, that would be something. If they could learn whether or not an artificial heart was painful inside one's chest—they could not ask the animals—that would be something. If the patient could adjust readily to the noise of the drive system, to the somewhat exaggerated beating of the heart, to the clicking sound of the valves as they opened and shut, that would be something. The fact is, they simply did not know what might happen until the device was actually implanted in a human being and they could "observe" what would happen and could "ask the patient."

It took great courage for Dr. Clark to go back to surgery four times, not knowing if he would have to go back seven or eight times more, not knowing what agony and pain he may have been subjected to, and not knowing from one second to the next if that heart would stop through some mechanical failure, or through some physical response of the body. It took great courage, when he could simply have died a relatively painless death, to submit himself to having his own heart cut out and an artificial heart placed in his chest—to see what happened! Dr. Clark surely was not on a "voyage to nowhere." He took one step toward a therapeutic treatment to prolong life for those whose natural hearts could no longer do so.

I would say the implantation was "prolongation of Dr. Clark's life" not his death. When you are breathing, you can think, smell, feel, taste; all of these are proof you are "alive." When you see your loved ones, interact with them, enjoy seeing the sun rising in the morning—any of these things we take so for granted—you are "alive." Even if you cannot run a mile, walk a block, or get up out of a chair on your own, if you can talk, hear, enjoy television or a good book, you are "alive." Unless you are in constant and terrible pain, or comatose, or a mental vegetable with no hope of getting any better, being with restricted functioning usually is better than death. You do not "prolong death"; it does not come until it really happens and it is pretty sudden and final when it occurs.

From the standpoint of whether or not Dr. Clark was a suitable candidate physically for the implant, I cannot judge because I have no medical expertise. I know only that when we were referred to the cardiologist at the University of Utah Medical Center, he did not believe that Dr. Clark's condition met the protocol set up by the IRB. That protocol required that the candidate have "cardiomyopathy Class IV congestive heart failure for 8 weeks." Dr. Clark and I returned to our home in Seattle, where we considered the artificial heart more thoroughly. When we returned to Salt Lake City in November, he was reevaluated. His clinical findings fit the TAH protocol and he was diagnosed as a suitable candidate. If, after the surgery, it was learned his pulmonary system was somewhat less than ideal, that was regrettable. We did know, however, that as far as his attitude, willingness to cooperate, eagerness to do all that was necessary for them to "learn," and his mental stability were concerned, he was an excellent candidate for the artificial heart.

Many people have asked me, "Do you have any regrets?" For a long time after Dr. Clark's demise, I answered *no* to that question. Now, 10 years later, I find that I do have two regrets; one of them is that Dr. Clark did not receive the artificial heart sooner, before he had cardiomyopathy and Class IV congestive heart failure for 8 weeks, as was necessary in the IRB protocol. I would not only wish this for my dear husband, but for any candidate that may be implanted in the future. Although I realize guidelines are necessary when we are dealing with human experimentation, such as artificial heart implantation, I believe we become so involved in red tape and bureaucracy that we deny progression of a technology that is desperately needed in a society where there are more deaths each year from heart disease than from all other causes combined. I believe that the patient and the doctor should have more latitude in deciding when a patient is physically ready, and that one set of rules cannot apply to each individual patient. I believe that had Dr. Clark had the heart even 3 weeks earlier, he would have done better and been better able to accomplish his purpose, to make a contribution to medical science.

If there is one question I can answer unequivocably it is "Was Dr. Clark properly informed?" Yes, he was. We had a conference with the implant surgeons 6 weeks before the implant, during which we were shown an artificial heart, informed of the materials from which it was made, how it worked in the animals, and the results of their animal experimentation. We were given a consent form that we reviewed with them, and they gave us a copy to take home with us. We visited the Artificial Heart Animal Laboratory where we saw a calf with an artificial heart and also a calf just coming out of surgery after implantation. We saw the Mock Circulation Testing Laboratory where TAHs were tested for durability. We visited the laboratory where a technician was making a heart in a dust-free room. We studied the consent form in the privacy of our own home. We asked for spiritual guidance many times and searched our souls, examined our motives, beliefs, strengths, and weaknesses.

We were somewhat concerned with the "morality" of removing one's heart and replacing it with an artificial one, perhaps because there had always seemed to us to be some connection between the heart and the soul, and it was through our prayers that we resolved our concerns. Therefore we had no problem with the TAH moral aspect. We were at peace that what we were considering was not contrary to God's plan; that conviction did a great deal to fortify us in our decision making, as well as through the entire experience.

Many people questioned the quality of life one would experience with an artificial heart, and rightly so. "Quality of life" is a very flexible term, and it can be present in varying degrees to different people under varying circumstances and periods in their lives. Of course you could not compare a completely well person who could go and do about anything he chose to do with a person who was implanted with a TAH and was tethered to a 395 pound drive unit by a 6 foot tube that was emerging from his side. True, the person with the artificial heart would not have a quality of life as satisfying as the person with his own heart who was mobile; that does not mean that the person with the artificial heart did not have a quality of life that was better than a person who was in constant pain from some physical disorder. Many people would rather be somewhat restricted with an artificial heart than dead.

Dr. Clark did not have a reasonable quality of life before his implant, nor did he have a quality of life he enjoyed after the implant. We all knew, or should have known, that no experiment has total success the first time it is tried. What was hoped was that this might offer personal benefit to Dr. Clark. If it did not, at least a great deal would be learned that would benefit those who would come after, and that in the end, through their efforts, a quality of life that was truly enjoyable would be possible with an artificial heart. It was this hope that made Dr. Clark willing to continue in the experiment as long as God gave him life to do so.

One of the requirements Dr. Clark had to fulfill to be eligible for the artificial heart was the support of his entire family, and he had that. This requirement has been challenged. Although I would not refuse a candidate an artificial heart if he did not have a family, I do think it did make a tremendous difference to Dr. Clark. Our children were as supportive as they could possibly be. Even though they lived 900 miles away, they were with us as much as possible. Those of us who were at his side every day looked forward to the children's visits because of the way he responded when they were close. Dr. Clark's response at these times was "positive proof" that no part of the human anatomy, not even the heart, is responsible for man's moral and emotional nature, the seat of real life and vitality, nor is it man's moving force. It is man's soul, that intangible spirit, that makes us what we are. Dr. Clark's human response, his love for family and friends, and his desires for all that is good in life, were as truly manifested in him with his artificial heart as they ever were with his own natural heart beating healthy and well in his chest.

Spiritual guidance was also most important and comforting to us. The leadership in our church could not have been more attentive to our needs. There is another support system that I feel is very special. In circumstances where families have a loved one with a long stay in the hospital, a social worker such as I had was unbelievably comforting.

Even though my children and several of my extended family were with us as much as possible, there were times, because they were under stress also, that I had problems and fears that I believed would be unfair to discuss with them. Our social worker was there and available much of the time, and she had a special quality about her that gave me confidence in our relationship. I shared with her many things I wanted to spare others who loved Dr. Clark as I did. Our social worker was very much of a sounding board for me. I could express my fears and my anger, and shed tears with her without feeling that I was imposing on her in any way and without causing her distress. Also, she opened up her home to the family and served us several meals when our children visited from Seattle. Being able to be with the children in a home atmosphere relaxed us, helped us to turn our full attention to each other, and to regroup before they had to leave again.

There has also been a great deal of speculation regarding whether or not the experiment was considered "a success." I suppose the criteria for that would depend on how you define "success" and what one hoped to gain. I would have to say that we considered it a success because Dr. Clark did what he wanted to do. He lived through the surgery, was able to survive almost 4 months, during which time things were learned that would be beneficial to those who came after him. The thing that would enhance that success for us would be that the experiments continue until a technology has been developed that would truly be a therapeutic treatment for heart disease.

I read that when the surgeon, Dr. DeVries was asked whether he considered the implant a success, he replied, "I had hoped to make Dr. Clark well enough to go home. But if Barney Clark had no regrets, then the procedure was a success." Dr. Jarvik said from the researcher's standpoint, it would have been impossible not to learn something. But, like Dr. DeVries, he felt that for the procedure to be called a success, "the patient must say it was worth it." I think they should feel it was a "success" because although Dr. Clark did not say it in those exact words, he did say on public television, "it has been a pleasure to help people." What could be closer?

Many times it has been my observation that almost everyone seems to have been more concerned that Dr. Clark receive personal gain than they were about what they could "learn" from the procedure. However, Dr. Clark and I felt that the main purpose was to "learn," hoping that Dr. Clark might gain something personally. In fact, I have been in awe of the fact that things turned out so much like Dr. Clark said they would as he counseled me when he made the decision to volunteer. He cautioned me about expecting any "personal benefit" for him and said words to this effect, "if I should live through the surgery and about 3 months after that, I think that would be the best we could hope for under the circumstances." We were totally committed.

About 3 years after Dr. Clark's death, I received a letter from one of the very special nurses who cared for him while he was in ICU. She wrote to inquire how I was doing and expressed the hope that things were allright with me. She said she wanted to share something with me, hoping it would further substantiate how courageous and dedicated Dr. Clark was to the TAH experiment. She then told me that one night she noticed there was a tear running down his cheek and he quickly brushed it away and acted embarrassed. The nurse just touched his hand and said: "It's pretty tough, isn't it Barney?" She said he looked at her and forced a smile, winked his eye, and said "You better believe it, kid!" She said sometimes she had a hard time dealing with all that went on during his hospitalization, had a great admiration for him, and just wanted me to know how much she appreciated him for the fine person he was. I was very pleased she took time to write me and was very happy she had comforted him that night, but I also regretted that it had not been me there instead of her. I wish that Dr. Clark and I had forgotten our "commitment" just one time, broken down the barrier we had built to keep our courage up with each other, and just cried together.

My family and I are emotionally attached to the heart team, which to me means everyone we associated with so closely in those 112 difficult, challenging, yet somehow very special days. Never, do I believe, did a group of people respond more conscientiously with individual effort to make an experiment successful, and never have I been a part of anything where I have seen the people of the world respond with such enthusiasm, such hope and caring. I feel we were all blessed to have been a part of a special medical breakthrough.

As we learn of the many new devices available today and the real potential for a totally implantable TAH to reach its genesis, we are encouraged to hope that this decade represents the beginning of something positive about the development of the artificial heart and the hope we all shared 10 years ago.

ACKNOWLEDGMENT

The author wishes to acknowledge those individuals who provided extraordinary support throughout the TAH experience and/or assisted with the preparation of this chapter.

Willem J. Kolff, MD
William C. DeVries, MD
Lyle D. Joyce, MD
Mrs. Peggy Miller
Don Olsen, DVM
Ross Wooley, PhD
Robert Jarvik, MD
Linda Gianelli, RN
Susan Quaal, PhD, RN
Marjery Shaw, MD, JD
Helen Key, RN

CHAPTER 27

Spiritual support for patients requiring ventricular assist devices

Timothy A. Thorstenson

INTRODUCTION

It is an overwhelmingly confrontative experience to face the actuality, or even the possibility, of having one's life supported by a ventricular assist device (VAD). Whether used as a bridge to transplantation or in a temporary effort to allow the heart time to regain its own energy in hopes of extending life, both patient and loved ones are confronted by everything ordered in their lives changing dramatically and by a potential threat of limited life and even death. VAD support is a pervasive and multidimensional experience of terror and hope that generates a profoundly human struggle.

Coming to terms with one's own mortality and place in life inaugurates a search for meaning and reevaluation of one's values and belief system. Therefore life supported by a VAD provokes a deeply spiritual experience, one that needs to be processed and shaped to move through shock and confusion to the integration that promises acceptance and serenity. It can be a sacred journey of self-discovery and spiritual renewal that moves through an exploration of meanings, attitudes, and beliefs in a process that reconciles the patient to his or her world. With appropriate intervention and guidance, the experience of the VAD patient can be life giving to the spirit, as well as the body.

ALIENATING AND ISOLATING ASPECTS OF THE VAD EXPERIENCE

No matter how positively or optimistically VAD support is framed by the healthcare professional, the invasive nature of this procedure is viewed as intrusive by the patient. VAD implantation is in fact a profound intrusion, which recipients experience existentially as alienating and isolating. Patients become alienated from their former healthy existence and lose autonomy. It is as if everything that has provided order and meaning in life has been interrupted, causing disorientation and fear. The patients' abilities to interact with their environment on their own terms and to have a significant role in shaping their own destinies has been interrupted. Dependency on VAD technology

342

forces separation from spiritual ground; the patient, therefore, is challenged to reclaim that reference point.

FINDING MEANING AND ACCEPTANCE IN THE FACE OF ALIENATION

Finding meaning and acceptance in the face of alienation begins by exploring how the VAD experience came to be. The VAD patient does not initially focus on religious questions and ask, "Where is the Divine in all of this?" but rather struggles to make sense of the experience, unconsciously asking, "Where am I in this?" In so doing, the patient comes to grips with the critical reality of being implanted with a VAD. A shift of focus occurs from an attempt to interpret the Divine in life to an attempt to comprehend the changing nature of life itself and of the patient's place in it. He or she is forced to contemplate why a VAD is required, alongside the age-old question, "Why me?"

The question is not simply, "Why did this happen to me?" but "Why do I need a VAD?" and "What is existence for me, now that I have a VAD?" Posing such questions forces a patient to confront realities, relating to life with a VAD, straight on. In a powerful manner, such confrontation becomes the initial "leap of faith." Patients begin to move through the shock and denial about their changing and painful realities to a level of affirming life in the face of its limits. As Martin Buber (philosopher/theologian) stated, "Only (s)he who believes in the world can deal with it."[1]

Confronting the reality of requiring VAD support is not only a leap of faith, but also a leap into faithfulness because it assumes redemption, that healing can come out of this brokenness of life. Recovery is made possible by accepting the need and potential for adaptation. The patient is encouraged to come to terms with the realities of life in this high-tech world, rather than to rationalize or minimize its impact by looking to the Divine to somehow intervene and change reality. The patient begins the process of becoming fully human, rather than having life diminished.

OVERCOMING ALIENATION

The process of becoming "fully human" necessitates spiritual exploration and the revaluing of what gives life its meaning. The VAD patient is unwittingly forced to explore the eschatological tension between what is and what can be. He or she lives now in a "between" time, for what is yet to come in life is clearly different from what has come before, and remains, as yet, undefined and unknown. To accept and come to terms with such a major life transition and the personal violation of such technological intrusion is to literally "turn around" to that which is spiritually grounding. The crucial spiritual issue in the face of the experience of alienation is to find connection both with the world and with that which transcends the world. The experience of relatedness is fundamental, and "being" must be conceived relationally.

In practical terms, the patient requires the nurture and care of family and professional staff to process and reflect on the intrusion and dialogue with other perspectives. In so doing the patient develops a sense of security and hopefulness. Realistic assurance is critical so that the patient feels the autonomy and integrity of being treated as one who can handle reality, as well as the anticipation and hope of positive change. False reassurance and "smoothing over" of painful realities diminishes autonomy and blunts hope. Well-intentioned messages from caregivers denying the reality of the patient's experience and the potential for death create distance in the relationship and work against the process of acceptance and integration. Messages of false hope tend to unconsciously encourage the patient to suppress feelings, increasing stress and isolation.

It is through the honest and caring contact of caregivers that the patient begins the process, perhaps for the first time, of defining a spiritual ground and shaping a relationship with the transcendent power of life. When life itself is threatened, the honest care of other people is often experienced as "humbling" by patients, and invites reflection on their "place" in the world. Many patients describe this as a moment of "grace"— an active encounter with a benevolent life source and a confession/profession that there is Something beyond the self to mediate the pain of the present moment. This is the "turning around" or "turning back" to what gives life its meaning and focus. It is a process of acceptance and affirmation of life and of a transcendant power that underlies it, where alienation and despair are replaced by reconciliation and hope.

FACILITATING HOPE

The role of the caregiver in this process cannot be minimized. More important than simply having people be with the patient is *how* people are with the patient. In general, love and care are healing dynamics and are to be provided abundantly, but access to the patient needs to be carefully monitored.

Family members tend to go through a "parallel process" with the patient and only come to terms with the implantation and all its ramifications over time. To expect them to initially provide the care necessary for the patient's process of acceptance is unrealistic. Family members and loved ones need to be "grounded," as does the patient, before they can become truly effective caregivers. Family members need to be with the patient, just as the patient needs to have them present. The caregiver needs to work with the whole family to facilitate the process described above; the primary nurse in particular needs to monitor who provides the facilitation. Again, because of our own fear of mortality and alienation and our efforts to "have" and somehow make secure our being, the human tendency in a caregiver is to minimize the impact of technology and meet it with well-intended but ineffective efforts to provide reassurance and optimism, which may only increase the sense of alienation in the patient. At issue for the caregiver, as for the patient and family, is the natural and self-protective defense mechanism of denial. Denial generally serves a most important purpose. As Ernst Becker made so clear, without denial the human person would "see things too clearly" and be "driven insane at the terror of life."[2] Whereas denial in the patient needs to be honored until the patient is ready to move past it, denial in the caregiver can be destructive.

The spiritual task of the caregiver is the same as that of the patient and family, to acknowledge and come to terms with the limits of life and yet affirm the joy and meaning of life in the face of such limits. The caregiver can then express compassion and empathy authentically, as one who "walks with" the patient and family through their experience. One might say this is the spiritual task of becoming fully human. We, who are confronted daily by death and the limitations of life, must come to a deep level of acceptance in order to maintain our effectiveness as caregivers. For the patient, who may normally be sheltered from such realities, it may be precisely at that point where one is dependent for life on a machine that one can finally embrace one's limits and mortality. It is a matter of sheer grace, a leap of faith into the unknown, not by "holding on" to denial, but by "letting go." Because of the experience of being loved and cared for, the patient can be open to the future with anticipation—and even hope—and allow for change and wonder and surprise.

THREE VOICES OF THE CAREGIVER

Douglas John Hall holds that a part of the process of moving from alienation to reconciliation and renewal is to ask not just "Why me?" and "Why is this?" but also to ask, "What is the purpose of life, of *my* life?"[3] It too is a question that cannot be fully embraced in isolation, or perhaps it can be fully experienced only in relationship. He suggests the caregiver become steward, priest, and poet, three helpful categories to frame the interventive process of acceptance.

CAREGIVER AS STEWARD AND PRIEST

To be a steward and a priest is to step into the reality of the patient and fully engage the experience. It is to acknowledge the tragic nature of life, to acknowledge that there *is* violence and negation that affects us all. The steward will insist not only on embracing one's finitude and place in life, but also will insist on accountability for the trusteeship of life and on responsibility for its unfolding. This creates a partnership with the patient both to reexamine lifestyle patterns, decisions, and expressions that may have contributed to bringing the patient to the experience of the present moment, as well as to revalue what can now foster reconciliation and provide meaning to life yet to be lived. The caregiver as steward participates *within* the experience and provides "caring leadership" to begin to order once again the chaos. With the use of empathic and compassionate expression, a relationship is formed with the patient and family that invites reflection and a "sorting through" of past experiences. The question the steward leads to is, "Now what?" Reflecting on what life has been and now is invites the question, "What is now to come?"

The priestly role of the caregiver is initially that of confessor. The relationship often becomes confessional in nature as the patient seeks understanding and self-acceptance. The key spiritual task in such self-acceptance is acknowledging one's contributions to the pain of life—in theological words, to one's "sin." To "live into the future" necessitates coming to terms with the past, literally reconciling oneself to one's self and accepting one's humanness. In such a process the priestly role moves from confessor to mediator, providing representation in a twofold movement: that of the patient before the Divine and that of the Divine before the patient. It is to stand with the patient empathically and to acknowledge the brokenness of the world, as well as the redemptive activity that comes in response to brokenness, to both acknowledge "sin" and its effects and to speak the mediating words of hope. To be both steward and priest is to prophetically engage the world by insisting both on coming to terms with reality and, through the power of the transcendant, on breaking through the pain of that reality in ways that are life enhancing and enriching.

CAREGIVER AS POET

An even greater task, perhaps, is that of the poet. The VAD patient has a deep spiritual need to give expression, which requires the presence of an interpreter, of one who can articulate expressions both of nature and of the Divine. Words spoken by the poet, on behalf of the patient, articulate what is already there at life's core—horror and angst, yes, but also and perhaps ultimately most important, gratitude and unspeakable joy for *all* being, for all life. The alienation of disease and of becoming slaves to technology entices us into silence. It is the poet's task to speak for those who cannot, facilitating integration and acceptance. Poetry helps the patient incorporate the strains of life into consciousness and facilitates expression of feeling, providing acceptance and security. This is done by imagining a future and remembering the goodness of the past. Without a past, there is no future, no sense of purpose, no awareness of anything significant. Only in retrospect, only in remembrance, do we discover and create a universe full of meaning. The task of the poet is to engage and express the meaning of the past, to transcend strict stimulus-response causality. Augustine called it the ability "to feel and to measure time."[4] It is a process of gathering together past and future into a present full of meaning by telling the stories and the dreams that shape our identities. It is in the court of memory, to again quote Augustine, where we "confront ourselves with ourselves."[4] He believed the image of God that brings healing to the soul resides in the capacity for self-knowledge and introspection, rather than in the capacity for abstract thought. To lack memory is to be soulless. Apart from our transcendent center of meaning, we are "torn piecemeal."[5] We lose ourselves in the multiplicity of things and fail to envision a future. We are limited in our ability to discern and distinguish. We become subject to the conflicting and random forces within and around us. We exist in a vegetative state of life without truly living, whether as slaves of oppressive systems or as patients on life-support systems. The poet's task truly is to work to keep body and soul together. Together, the caregiver as steward, priest, and poet enters into a relationship with the patient not to resolve the pain of the patient's existential experience but to help the patient live with the experience creatively and discover serenity while in the mix.

EMPOWERMENT

The journey toward acceptance and serenity, if not toward wholeness and recovery, is a spiritual process of empowerment. The immediacy of disease and of technological intervention such as the placing of a VAD produces complex emotional responses and tends to segment the body, mind, and spirit, giving rise to feelings of powerlessness. Research suggests that a key factor in healing illness and in coping effectively with a medical crisis is found in mobilizing diverse resources of power (i.e., in enhancing the patient's sense of personal empowerment, a largely spiritual process).[6]

There is growing evidence in the medical and social psychology literature that human beings do not live in the physical world alone, but in a world mediated for them by symbolic meanings provided by their culture and faith traditions. Symbols cue and prompt responses in the central nervous system and the endocrine system. Since humans respond to an environment understood in symbolic terms, their conceptions of health, illness, and crisis are shaped and affected by culture and faith as well. A patient's *perception* of reality or attitudes and beliefs about his or her environment and experience give rise to automatic, unconscious feelings and expressions and may either increase or decrease the sense of empowerment. The first century Roman philosopher Epictetus recognized this fact in this statement attributed to him: "[Humans] are disturbed not by things, but by the views which they take of things."[7] The Bible says of the person, ". . . as a person thinks in his heart, so he is."[8] One might say that it is not so much that the road is rocky, but that we expect the road to be smooth that causes us problems. Belief creates our individual context of reality. The attitudes we hold and the manner in which we "receive" reality shape the responses we make. Indeed the impact of "stress" in daily life changes according to how we give power to our environment to affect how we feel about ourselves. The fact that one person becomes "worried sick" in the face of a potentially stressful stimulus while another remains relatively unperturbed is indicative of the power the person attaches to the stimulus to cause threat. It is necessary for the person to reclaim the power, and by so doing, to change perceptions and attitudes, to develop the capacity for equanimity.

We are wise to take care, then, how we introduce the placing of a VAD, being mindful that the information we provide can generate a mind/body split that gives rise to anxiety and can be experienced as very stressful. Providing information about what staff may see as a helpful and hopeful medical option may cue emotional and physiological responses in the patient and family that may initially be strongly reactive and can become deleterious over time, unless attitudes and perceptions are processed and reframed. Just as symbols and learned interpretations can break down the spirit, so can symbolic constructs provide movement and healing. If a patient perceives the potential for a VAD as symbolic of rapid deterioration and of an increased likelihood of death (i.e., if the denial about the disease process is broken with little resilience in reserve) then feelings of fear and desperation may ensue. If a patient sees it as a hopeful safe-guard against the likelihood of death and as a "welcome" intervention that may provide security, then empowerment and hope may arise. We need then to first discern how a patient or family will receive the information. Too often, medical risks and options are discussed only briefly or not at all before surgery, and then according to the physician's or caregiver's busy schedule. Personnel skilled in perceiving and responding empathi-cally to the feelings of the patient will maximize the potential for such information to bring serenity rather than anxiety. In general, the more control the patient has over when the information is received and the more time a patient has to process feelings about the information, the greater will be the benefit of the information, in fact, low-ering the stress to the patient.

CASE STUDY I

A couple with whom we recently worked can serve as an example. Mr. K. is an end-stage class IV ischemic cardiomyopathy patient awaiting transplantation. He had slowly deteriorated over the past 14 months, experiencing corresponding periodic episodes of despair and hopelessness, seen psychologically as reactive depression, but which he was always able to "rise above" with self-talk as he improved physiologically. Information about the Novacor implantable VAD was provided to Mr. K. and his wife on his fourth readmission with congestive heart failure. Both patient and spouse had ordered their lives with a deterministic faith system in which life would end or continue according to the will of the Divine. It provided them a meaningful framework for "making sense" of their experience and shaped their perceptions and attitudes about their world. Indeed it provided them an effective grounding point as long as Mr. K. remained relatively stable and ambulatory. However, introduction of the Novacor was perceived as a poten-tial threat to the order they had established, creating both a conflict of faith (cognitive dissonance gave rise to anger and spiritual confusion) and emotional disorientation as they began to recognize the limits of their own resourcefulness and the power of such symbols to affect their feelings. They initially felt alienated from the world, distrustful of the medical system, and at odds with their deepest selves. Questions and statements about life's fairness, divine providence, and their own inability to make sense of things anymore suggested a state of anxiety and powerlessness. Their attitudes and perceptions gave rise to deep spiritual distress.

The process of restoring this couple to trust and acceptance (i.e., of helping them become "grounded" again) required reexploring (1) the meaning they had attached to the symbols of Mr. K.'s illness and potential intervention, (2) faith concepts that were causing dissonance, and (3) feelings of alienation. Mr. and Mrs. K. were experiencing the very human and normal response that comes when a life crisis forces immersion in multiple, overlapping, and at times, conflicting levels of meaning and existence.

To move through Mr. and Mrs. K.'s initial reaction required working to restore balance and power, a process that has two primary components. The first step in restoring trust and acceptance is to create a state of openness and mindfulness by eliciting the relaxation response. First described as an interventive process of empowerment by Benson in 1974,[9] relaxation is a physiological response that decreases the symptoms that are exacerbated by sympathetic nervous system arousal. The antithesis of the fight or flight response, relaxation is intended to counter the felt anxiety by decreasing heart rate, breathing rate, oxygen consumption, and blood pressure, all of which give rise to increased stress and worry unless countered. By learning a technique to elicit the relaxation response, the patient is empowered to break the cycle fueled by sympathetic nervous system arousal and can reduce stress-related symptoms. In time the relaxation response contributes to an opening of the mind and feelings of peace and well-being, and facilitates integration of the often compartmentalized facets of the physical body, rational mind, emotional psyche, and intuitive spirit.

This state of openness and mindfulness is critical because it facilitates attitudinal changes. The patient can then explore his or her attitudes and beliefs in a reflective manner, once again engaging reality in a way that sorts through all the messages and provides a sense of "involvement" in life's events that is experienced as empowering.

That reengagement of one's attitudes and beliefs is the second critical step necessary for restoring balance and accepting what the future brings. Healing involves more than just the physiological response elicited by behavioristic and psychotherapeutic techniques. To move toward recovery and wholeness also necessitates engaging the spiritual dimensions of life, the nonrational, the intuitive, the longing for transcendant experiences, and the exploration of moral values. Today more and more therapists and theorists are exploring spiritual issues, the meanings and values people attach to life, and their concepts of grace and transcendence. To open up and enable such deep-level self-exploration is to move into the realm of what is sacred and holy in life. It is a journey that is in itself empowering. The journey is facilitated simply by acknowledging with the patient what is painful and/or frightening, and then inviting reflection on what provides meaning and hope in the face of the pain. Far from lifting up a sentimental optimism that a sense of connection to something greater than the self will take away the pain of being human or will substitute for work that must be done on a psychological level, it is a movement *into* the pain and uncertainty of life, an exploration of what provides meaning in the face of limitation and brokenness. This process gives rise to true hope as patients come to terms with their limits and their "place" by reexploring, challenging, and often deepening their affirmations of faith.

For Mr. and Mrs. K. this process involved reexamining their beliefs about life and about the workings of the Divine in their lives. As they talked about their current experience in light of their values and beliefs, they discovered they could affirm new concepts that they had discovered in the face of their painful reality. Such a process was empowering for them and brought a "quieting of the spirit" and reduction in anxiety and stress.

THE PROCESS OF ADAPTATION

Placing a VAD electively is one thing; having it placed during a cardiac crisis or "waking up" from open heart surgery on a VAD, with the decision having been made by surgeons and family members (or other surrogate decision makers), is quite another. In such cases the patient's experience is compacted and may cause strong, emotional, and behavioral responses, giving rise to spiritual confusion and questioning.

Given such circumstances, we do well to see adaptation and recovery as processes rather than as isolated and independent stages or experiences. Rarely does a patient move directly through such typical responses as shock, anger, and withdrawal to acceptance without cycling back through them in an ebb and flow process. So-called adjustment disorders, primarily anxiety and depression, are normal responses to such a sudden life change as the onset of a critical illness or the placement of a VAD, and the patient adapts over time, paralleling physical recovery. Adaptation, however, is a road filled with curves and detours, and the need to adjust and make midcourse corrections is constant and demanding.

We cannot easily predict postoperative emotional or psychogenic morbidity, and we do well not to draw conclusions based on behavioral expressions alone. People come to terms with major life changes and medical crises only over time. The anxiety and depression exhibited, especially in the absence of a psychiatric history, are generally rooted in the spiritual issues of powerlessness and despair; they diminish as patients regain a sense of control, and as hope and trust emerge. Anxiety and depression are generally proportionately related to the severity of the medical situation. The VAD or total artificial heart patient who awakens with a machine in his or her chest is confronted not only by extreme risk but also by an uncertain and foreign future that may invoke the necessity for transplantation, a frightening prospect in itself, particularly if the patient had not been educated and oriented toward that prospect preoperatively. An appropriate degree of anxiety and/or depression is in fact considered a healthy response and a predictor of positive postoperative outcome. Such symptoms may reflect an ability to remain in emotional contact with a patient's reality without becoming overwhelmed or shutting down.

We have learned that adjustment to the rigors of such technological intervention requires a certain degree of resilience and resourcefulness, as well as adequate coping skills, which people possess in varying degrees. When patients deny feelings about such intrusion and their own existential crisis and when they consistently act out maladaptively, one can reasonably predict a difficult course with poorer adjustment, requiring greater intervention. The basic spiritual need at such a point is the establishment of security and confidence, generally requiring the consistent presence of nurturing care-givers, direct and honest medical information, and the emotional commitment of the medical authorities (primarily physicians). We can then begin the process of trust building and centering described above, minimizing adjustment disorders. Again, some expressions of noncompliance may actually reflect a healthy inner dialogue and a claiming of autonomy. When seen as a natural element in a greater process of facing mortality, we can "stand with" our patients and help them find their own level of acceptance, thereby fostering greater long-term integration.

CASE STUDY II

Because of the radical nature of such an intrusive crisis, adaptation tends to be a life-long process rather than a short-term, once-and-for-all experience, and the trauma of not playing a role in such a dramatic event, together with the confrontative experience about the nature and meaning of life, can continue to cause open-ended spiritual confusion. The following is a case in point.

Peter M. was a young man in his mid-twenties who underwent surgery for valve replacement 5 years ago and required a BiVAD when his heart could not regain its own rhythm. The bridging was successful and he was transplanted 2 days later. Peter has gone on to develop a successful career and father two children, living a full and rewarding life. Yet Peter recently sought me out to reflect again on his experience and its impact on him. He articulated the effects of not being a participant in his own life-or-death decision, of "being asleep on the job" and "having no say" during the "biggest event" of his life. He is, I suspect, representative of others like him when he details his spiritual journey and the confusion and mystery of which he is daily reminded. To unwittingly become "a product of the medical machine" suggests to Peter that his life and his destiny are not fully his own, generating strongly ambivalent feelings. He acknowledges both the benefit and the burden of being singled out, of being "special," and of what that says both about the actions of the Divine in this world (why Peter and not others?) and about his own responsibility in light of such an event (What now? What is the purpose of my life?). Peter reports that he has not felt "settled" since his implant and is continuing the deeply spiritual journey of "putting the puzzle pieces back together."

CONCLUSION

Perhaps the most profound spiritual need of the VAD patient is to rediscover or discover for the first time a sense of balance in life (i.e., learning to live creatively and gently with conflicting and opposing feelings). It means trusting the process enough to be able to affirm life even in the face of its pain and uncertainty, to openly explore what gives meaning while holding firm to what gives hope, to continue to ask the reflective and heartfelt questions while deepening the faith convictions that provide grounding, and to experience both anxiety and serenity as the pieces of the puzzle take new shapes. For Mr. and Mrs. K., for Peter M., and for others like them, it is a sacred journey of self-discovery and spiritual renewal. The word "spirit" is derived from the Latin word for breath. The Greek and Hebrew words for spirit also stem from roots with the same meaning. The ancient peoples tended to conceive of life itself as defined by the breath that came into them, literally the "power of life" and the spirit of the Divine. The scriptures of various traditions refer to spirit as that divine breath that flows through us to give us life.

That spiritual flow begins with getting in touch with one's spiritual needfulness and then moving through an exploration of meanings, attitudes, and beliefs to the development of acceptance and peace. It means facing the terror and the alienation and then engaging that which mediates them and brings hope. To focus on breathing and on the divine breath that gives life enables the facilitation of the relaxation response and the "openness" to go deeply inward. And that is a journey that invites the patient to affirm life as a flowing and healing energy that empowers acceptance, and brings with it the "experience of salvation."[9] As the great Sufi poet Kabir wrote: "Jump into experience while you are alive! What you call 'salvation' belongs to the time *before* death. . . . What is found now is found then. If you find nothing now, you will simply end up with an apartment in the City of Death. If you make love with the Divine now, in the next life you will have the face of satisfied desire."[10] The experience of being on a VAD needs to be breathed in fully, for to breathe is to be alive. And to acknowledge and take in the transcendant power of life is to become fully human and to develop spiritual well-being, the cornerstone of health.

REFERENCES

1. Buber M: *I and Thou,* New York, 1958, Scribner.
2. Becker E: *The Denial of Death,* New York, 1973, The Free Press.
3. Hall DJ: *The Stewardship of Life in the Kingdom of Death,* Grand Rapids, Mich, 1988, Eerdmann's.
4. Browning DS: *Religious thought and the modern psychologies: a critical conversation in the theology of culture.* Philadelphia, Pa, 1987, Fortress Press.
5. Augustine: *Confessions,* New York, 1952, Pocket Books.
6. Eileen MS et al: Spirituality in health and healing: a clinical program, *Holistic Nursing Practice* 3(3):35, 1989.
7. Albert EM, Denise TC, Peterfreund SD eds, *Great traditions in ethics,* ed 4, Belmont, Calif, 1980, Wadsworth.
8. Proverbs 23:7.
9. Benson H: *The relaxation response,* New York, 1975, William Morrow.
10. Bly R: *The Kabir Book,* Boston, 1975, Beacon Press.

PART FIVE

UNIQUE ASPECTS OF MECHANICAL ASSISTANCE

Organization and experience of a mobile team to support European cardiac centers

Marco Meli, Roland Odermatt, †Jean-Pierre Brugger, and
Charles Hahn

INTRODUCTION

The activity described in this paper took place between 1986 and 1990. We set up a 24-hour per day on-call Mobile Team (MT) that was able to mobilize with the Pierce-Donachy Ventricular Assist Device (VAD)[1] and the modified Thoratec Pneumatic Drive Console (PDC) into any cardiac transplantation center in Western and Central Europe. The team consisted of three people, usually of different specialities (physician, engineer, nurse), and remained on site at the patient's bedside until transplantation occurred.

In 1990 we revised our MT policy to a more collaborative role. Before accepting support of a VAD center, we first clearly defined the framework of our collaboration. This might even include a previous training program (theoretical courses, in vitro and in vivo experiments) for the subscribing VAD centers. Our MT has narrowed services to implant support and initial 24 to 48 hours of VAD patient management. Thereafter the local hospital clinical team assumes responsibility for patient care management, but the MT, of course, always remains available for telephone consulting 24 hours per day. In case of necessity a member of the MT might even return to the VAD center for some time.

Historical background

Since 1982 our group has been prepared to clinically use different mechanical circulatory support systems (MCSS). Our goal was to implement an already established system that could readily be applied for myocardial support after open-heart surgery. After a review of what was potentially available, we fixed our choice on three systems:

---

†Deceased

two pneumatically driven VADs and a nonocclusive roller pump.[2] The roller pump was intended for right heart assist, if necessary. The two VADs[3] and a method of biventricular assistance were evaluated through acute and short-term animal studies. In the meantime it was confirmed[4] that a VAD could be clinically applied to support the right heart. We finally chose the Pierce-Donachy VAD,[1] as commercialized by Thoratec, for the support of both ventricles (BiVAD) and trained ourselves through BiVAD in vivo experiments. We eventually used VAD for postsurgical recovery in three patients.[5,6]

During this evaluation phase, we observed that the PDC was heavy and bulky. Starting from the same basic elements, we decided to reassemble them in a more user-friendly manner. We also realized that the management of a patient on MCSS, even if uncomplicated, is better assumed by a team not directly involved with the daily clinical routine activities and possessing a good knowledge of patient-related and technical aspects. These "specialists" can be trained via recurring courses and can rapidly acquire needed experience.

Thus the idea germinated to offer the competencies of our team to other cardiac surgery centers. This gained momentum in 1985 for several reasons. Our group, which is otherwise pursuing development of an electromechanical total artificial heart and implantable assist device, established itself as a freestanding Cardiovascular Research Institute (IRCV), independent of an affiliation with a cardiac surgery center. At the beginning of the same year, the use of VAD or BiVAD[7,8] as bridge to cardiac transplantation took off in the United States.

Rationale

The rationale of our original approach did not appear at first, but occurred progressively during the course of this activity. However, we strongly believe that there are good reasons for this kind of mobile team.

For those centers experiencing low-volume heart transplantation or cardiac surgery, it can be more effective to call on the services of a specialized, equipped, and well-trained team than to independently set up their own program. This can be seen from two different points of view. Economically speaking, they can avoid the investment in permanent equipment and the expenses of the associated maintenance. Such an arrangement also eliminates the cost of initial team training and ongoing skill maintenance, which requires frequent hands-on experience. Furthermore, a single team with an increased number of applications accrues experience and clinical expertise, leading to an improvement in clinical results.

For those centers having an increased level of activity, we believe that an MT can be of support in assisting them with the start-up of their own program. Financing and team motivation are easier when good clinical results can be demonstrated. Furthermore, the success of in vivo and in vitro training, once some of the real clinical problems have already been experienced, is increased. Clinical application can then be considered as a starting point and not as a hypothetical goal. In this context the possibility of

PREIMPLANT FILL OUT FORM

Generalities

Last name.............................. Weight .... Date ....
First name .... Height.................................. Surgeon....................................
Date of birth........................... BSA (sq.m.)........................... Medical center ....

Diagnostic ....
....

Cardiovascular system

Mechanical circulatory support: No   Yes   Type   Duration
                                                IAPB
                                                ECMO
                                                Other

Hemodynamics   **Pharmacological treatment**

Date and time   Dopamine
MAP (sys/dias)   Dobutamine
CVP/RAP   Epinephrine
MPAP (sys/dias)   Nitroglycerin
PCWP/LAP   Lidocaine
CO/CI   Other
O_2 Sat (PA)

Infections   **Central nervous system**

Temperature   Alert
WBC   Obtunded
Localization   Comatose
Organism   Under anesthesia

Respiratory system   **Hepatic function**

Intubated (duration)   Liver palpation
Pao_2 SGOT
Fio_2 SGPT
O_2 Sat   Bilirubin
Tidal Volume   Proteins
Rate   Ammonemia
PEEP

Coagulation system   **Renal function**

PT   Date and time
PTT   Urine output last 8 h
Platelets   Diuretics
Plasma free Hb   Creatinine
FDP (if ECMO or IABP)   BUN

our institute proposing training courses to the clinical teams allows an advantageous synergy.

We also strongly believe that developers of new medical technologies are more efficient, from all points of view, if they have a strong direct contact with the end users (medical staff, patients). All the experience gained by our research group during clinical use of MCSS is an advantage for the future clinical introduction of our own devices. We also believe that acceptance of a total artificial heart by the public, patients, medical community, and persons in charge of health policy can be reached only by the clinical introduction of progressively more sophisticated and more aggressive MCSS. Stepping from the animal use of a total implantable artificial heart to its clinical application, without having established this general acceptance, will surely cause a rejection despite technical success. We think that temporary clinical applications of devices that, in their technological aspects, are progressively approaching the goals of a permanent system, promote the general idea of an artificial substitution of the involved organ.[9]

MATERIAL AND METHODS
Medical organization

VAD program organization consists of three aspects: (1) patient clinical profile, (2) clinical centers, and (3) medical team caring for the assisted patient. The patient waiting for heart transplantation represented the best clinical indication. In fact the relatively low degree of emergency and the evolution of the clinical deterioration provided us the necessary interval for our intervention (travel, telephone agreement, installation of equipment). VAD patient-selection criteria were established from the clinical information provided with the initial request for service. The clinical history, hemodynamic profile, and evaluation of the different organ functions, based on metabolic variables, permitted us to have a general evaluation of the patient's clinical profile. To improve data collection standardization we developed a preimplant form easy to complete during a telephone interview (see the box on p. 357).

The contraindications were age > 60 years, active infection, body surface area < 1.5 m^2 or > 2.2 m^2, evidence of preformed antibodies to human lymphocyte antigens, and use of continuous flow assistance for more than 6 hours before VAD implant.

We have decided to support any properly equipped cardiac center in Western and Central Europe. Geographical boundaries were dictated by flight times, which were established at less than 3 hours, to ensure a safe time limit for the implantation procedure. Each center was requested to have a well-developed heart transplantation program, with a high-level medical and nursing staff; other departments were requested to have adequate competencies and collaboration for supporting this program in its different clinical aspects (e.g., nephrology, immunology, infection, and hematology).

In our opinion the MT ought to have a multidisciplinary organization covering the three different aspects of a patient on MCSS: medical (patient selection, pre- and postoperative management), technical (maintenance and repair, logistical help), and nursing (prevention of infection and thromboembolism).

After implantation of the support system, three members of the MT assumed responsibility for monitoring both patient and the assistance system during the entire bridging period, in collaboration with medical and nursing staffs.

Technical organization

Regarding technical aspects, we organized our VAD MT equipment needs to be completely independent of any receiving hospital's equipment. The required organization comprised not only the MT and the transportable biomedical equipment, but also the in-house facilities and resources to manage the required support services. Furthermore an MT activation system and transportation strategy were necessary.

Transported equipment

Transported equipment consisted essentially of four components:

1. The PDC itself in four main parts (Fig. 28-1): (a) two electropneumatic command and control modules (drive modules), (b) intermediate stage with electrical connections, (c) bottom stage with compressors and vacuum pumps, and (d) a cart, two cylinders of compressed air, tie-down devices, and fittings completed the PDC. All the functional parts, mainly the two drive modules, are identical or equivalent to those of the original Thoratec PDC. We redesigned the housing to decrease weight and to facilitate the assembling, disassembling, and transportation of the components.
2. A two-track digital memory oscilloscope to visualize two pneumatic pressure waveforms, provided by the Thoratec PDC, which are mandatory to control ventricular function.[10] This allows early detection of inflow or outflow constriction or hemodynamic pathological conditions (tamponade).
3. A clinical set of three pumps and corresponding cannulae. Two pumps (biventricular assistance) were usually used for a bridge-to-transplant operation, the third being a spare pump. This disposable equipment was kept in stock in our facilities, after having been inspected and sterilized.
4. A kit comprising electrical and pneumatic plugs for the different European countries and some tools and spare parts for repair.

Facilities and background team

IRCV collaborator competency levels and research facilities allow building and testing of assist devices and the total artificial heart. In practice the IRCV can develop most prototype parts for in vitro and in vivo testing. These competencies and facilities were also used as a logistical basis for the MT activity. Each of our collaborators (15 to 20 persons, depending on the period) was to a certain extent involved in this work. PDC

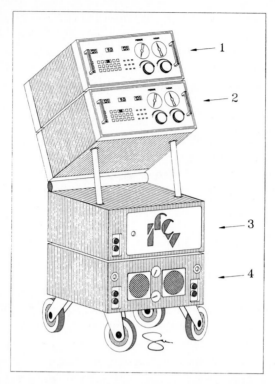

Fig. 28-1. Schematic of the transportable pneumatic drive console (PDC). *1* and *2*, the left and right drive modules; *3*, electrical connection and empty casing; *4*, compressors and vacuum pump assembly.

evolution can be summarized under three subcategories as follows.

Mechanical workshop. Conception of transportable PDCs. Routine maintenance and drive-unit pneumatic component customization is performed on receipt from the United States. After a three-component transportable PDC was developed and evaluated, four PDC units were constructed in the four-component version previously described. Based on input from Pierce and Thoratec consultants, we designed and fabricated a few accessories to facilitate cannulae implantation: (1) a dummy connector that de-airs the auricular cannula, (2) a cone that facilitates subcutaneous passage of the cannulae, and (3) a punch, making apical ventricular cannulation quicker and easier.

Electronics. These activities consisted of (1) conception and development of the transportable PDC electrical components, (2) inspection and repair of the drive module electrical components on receipt from the United States, (3) periodic inspection and maintenance of the electrical components (particularly the batteries), (4) installation and testing of new release software versions, (5) conception, realization, and testing of the external "ventricle full" detecting system. IRCV facilities were used to repackage, when necessary, and gas sterilize the ventricles, cannulae, and accessories shipped unsterile to Europe, as well as our in-house manufactured accessories.

In vitro and in vivo facilities. These facilities were used to train our MT and some external teams for clinical readiness. The PDCs were tested and evaluated in vitro after construction and after each repair or modification. A secretary assisted with all the administrative work, including (1) customs paperwork (temporary and permanent exportation of equipment), (2) scheduling flights, and (3) activity accounting.

Call system and transportation

During working hours the MT could be reached at the institute. After hours the MT was contacted through an answering telephone service and beeper system. Once the MT was notified of a potential VAD implant, a private flying company (usually from Sion) was contacted to prepare the plane and notify the pilot. Once the decision for VAD implant was finalized, the flight arrangements were continued. Equipment and MT were transported by car to the Sion airport. On occasion, because of weather conditions, departure had to be arranged from Geneva. Customs formalities, which can be cumbersome and time consuming in metropolitan airports like Geneva, were facilitated in Sion. VAD equipment was charged on the plane and secured for the flight. The receiving hospital was asked to send a vehicle to the destination airport for transportation of the MT and their equipment to the hospital, and if possible, to advise the local customs personnel and facilitate entry formalities. Again, if possible, small local airports were preferred to larger international airports where the transit time was always longer. When ground transportation was less than 3 hours, it was favored because of weather and financial advantages, or if air transport was unavailable.

Patient population

During the period from January 1986 through April 1990 the MT received 70 calls originating from 21 different cardiac surgery centers located in 6 European countries. Two cases were postcardiotomy failures and will not be considered in more detail in this review. We rejected 27 cases. Patients in 13 cases did not meet the protocol, in 11 cases the team was involved in another center, and in 3 cases the prosthetic ventricles were not delivered in time. In 3 cases the MT was on alert and equipment was charging on the plane in anticipation of potential implants for patients who were difficult to wean from emergency cardiac care (ECC) after cardiac surgery. Patients in 38 cases were accepted as being suitable for device implantation. In 3 instances the procedure did not take place (2 patients did not present an indication after a more accurate clinical evaluation and 1 patient died before our arrival). In 35 cases we proceeded to prosthetic ventricle implantation. There were 4 females and 31 males with an average age of 43 years (range 17 to 58).

The pathologic conditions responsible for terminal cardiac failure were (1) dilated cardiomyopathy (18), (2) acute myocardial infarction (7), and (3) ischemic cardiomy-

Table 28-1. Preimplant hemodynamics

Index/pressure	Parameter	Patients
CI (L/min/m²)	1.63 ± 0.34	24
RAP (mm Hg)	17.70 ± 6.40	27
MPAP (mm Hg)	40.12 ± 8.67	26
PCWP (mm Hg)	29.10 ± 7.31	21
MAP (mm Hg)	62.25 ± 14.44	31

CI, Cardiac index; RAP, Right atrial pressure; MPAP, Mean pulmonary artery pressure; PCWP, Pulmonary capillary wedge pressure; MAP, Mean arterial pressure.

opathy (5). The remaining 5 cases were respectively a large ventricular septal defect, a ventricular aneurysm, a donor-heart malfunction, a hypertrophic cardiomyopathy, and a postpartum cardiomyopathy.

In spite of maximal inotropic support and the use of the intraaortic balloon (13 patients) or extracorporeal membrane oxygenation (ECMO) (4 patients) the hemodynamic parameters indicated a very severe low output syndrome (Table 28-1). In 17 patients the implantation of the device was preceded by one or more cardiac arrests. Acute pulmonary edema was noted radiographically in 32 patients, and in 19, the pulmonary gas exchange was compromised to such an extent that mechanical ventilation was requested. The mean urinary output during the last 8 hours was 360 ± 353 ml. Five patients were anuric. Nineteen patients showed a certain degree of mental deterioration.

Patient management

VAD implantation was effected through a median sternotomy incision. There were 34 cases with biventricular support and 1 case with left support only. In 19 patients the procedure was effected without extracorporeal circulation (ECC). The sternum was always closed.

Implantation of left VAD occurred first. The inflow cannula was introduced through the interatrial groove in 19 patients,[11] the roof of the left atrium in 4 and the left ventricular apex in 2. The outflow cannula was sewn onto the ascending aorta by side-to-end anastomosis. After the connection of the prosthetic ventricle to the cannulae, it was run at low flow (2 L/min/m²) to avoid increasing the preload of a potentially impaired right ventricle.

For a right VAD, the inflow cannulae were always introduced through the right atrial appendage and the outflow cannula was connected to the pulmonary artery by side-to-end anastomosis. The cannulae were placed across the chest wall, below the costal margin and the prosthetic ventricle, and were positioned on the anterior abdominal wall.

Principle control mode was full to empty to ensure a maximal flow. The mean implantation time was 3 hours. We requested that the patient stay in an isolated intensive care room during the duration of assistance and that an accurate prevention of infection be accomplished as for transplant patients.

The anticoagulant regimen was based on a continuous low dose of intravenous heparin to maintain activated clotting time (ACT) between 150 and 180 sec. The treatment started when the chest drainage bleeding was less than 50 cc and the coagulation parameters were returned to normal values.

In the absence of preoperative infection, an antibiotic prophylaxis was accomplished for 48 hours with first generation cephalosporin. Only the cultured organisms were treated. The patient with only left VAD required inotropic assistance of the right ventricle with isoproterenol. Patients on BiVAD did not require inotropic agents but sometimes received vasoactive drugs to control the aortic pressure.

RESULTS
Patients

Mean response time between clinical team activation and arrival in the hospital operating room (OR) was about 3 hours. Support duration ranged from 1 to 66 days, with a total of 357 days and a mean support time of 10 days. Twenty-nine patients (83%) underwent heart transplantation in a period ranging from 19 hours to 43 days.

Six patients died on assistance because of uncontrolled bleeding (2), dislocation of the inlet left cannula followed by catastrophic bleeding (1), septicemia (2), and multiorgan failure(1). During assistance 21 patients were extubated, and 12 of 13 patients who presented a certain degree of nervous system obtundation before implantation recovered completely.

Of the 29 transplanted patients, 21 (72%) have been discharged from the hospital in good health. Hospital deaths were caused by right ventricular failure in two cases, graft failure in three cases, and in one case, acute rejection, multiorgan failure, and cerebral abscess. Two patients died after hospital discharge during the first year for chronic rejection. At present, 18 patients (62%) are alive and well, the follow-up ranging from 1 to 5 years.

Hemodynamic function

After the first 48 to 72 hours, characterized by hemodynamic instability (vasoplegia, bleeding, forced diuresis, and intra- and extravascular water shift), the system guaranteed a full circulatory support without any significant change in PDC setting and hemodynamic parameters for the duration of VAD assistance. These parameters are described in Table 28-2 for right and left VAD.

Our policy was to limit the flow through the pump during the first 12 hours to avoid reperfusion damage. After this critical period the pump flow was stabilized at 2.5 to 3 $L/min/m^2$ for the left VAD and at 2 to 2.5 $L/min/m^2$ for the right VAD. The left pump output was maintained 15% to 20% higher than the right pump output in patients who

Table 28-2. Drive unit and hemodynamic parameters during circulatory support with the Pierce-Donachy prosthetic ventricle

Phase	L V A D	R V A D
Filling		
Atrial pressure	10 to 15 mm Hg	5 to 10 mm Hg
Vacuum:		
Atrial cannula	−25 to −35 mm Hg	−15 to −25 mm Hg
Apical cannula	−0 to −10 mm Hg	
Ejection		
Systolic pressure	<120 mm Hg	<30 mm Hg
Ejection pressure	180 to 220 mm Hg	80 to 110 mm Hg
Ejection time	250 to 300 msec	350 to 450 msec

LVAD, left ventricular assist device; *RVAD*, right ventricular assist device.

did not present with significant ventricular arrhythmias, and 10% to 15% higher in patients with major ventricular arrhythmias. Five patients suffered sustained ventricular tachycardia, six experienced ventricular fibrillation, and one became asystolic.

In 30% of the cases, right pump flow was reduced after 4 to 5 days of assistance to accommodate partial right ventricle recovery and to reduce pulmonary artery peak systolic pressure. The level of reduction ranged from 30% to 50%.

Complications

In four cases (11%) the Hall effect switch broke. In one case we used the fixed rate control mode, closely monitoring pneumatic line pressure to evaluate complete VAD filling and emptying. In the remaining cases we replaced the system by an external switch. No embolic neurological events were reported. At explant most devices showed some fibrin deposits in the two seams between the polished valve ring and housing. Thrombi were found in the blood sac of one infected patient.

Among non-device–related complications, bleeding occurred most frequently (17 patients or 49%). Fourteen patients required a second exploration (40%) and two expired (6%). Bleeding was identified as due to surgery (5), coagulopathy (3), surgery and coagulopathy (8), and improper graft preclotting of the aortic cannulae (1). Two of the five surgical bleeding cases were related to dislocation of the left inlet cannula and could not be controlled in one patient. Of 35 patients, 11 (31%) had an infection during circulatory support, which in six of the patients already existed before implantation. In three cases the infection was located in the lung, in one case in the mediastinum, and in another case in the urinary tract. In the remaining cases, organisms were cultured in the bloodstream without specific localization (five septicemia, one septic shock). In another patient, positive cultures were identified on the skin around the transcutaneous passage without clinical effects.

In 11 patients, the creatinine level was greater than 2 mg/dl before implant. Renal function completely recovered in four patients on assistance (two cases with dialysis for 3 weeks and two cases with diuretics). Partial recovery occurred in three cases (one with dialysis and two with diuretics); renal function returned to normal, however, after transplantation. In four cases no recovery was reported on assistance. In three patients, renal function, which was normal before implantation, deteriorated immediately after VAD implantation. In two cases, there was no recovery.

DISCUSSION
Medical discussion

From a medical point of view the encountered problems can be grouped into two categories: general problems concerning hospital infrastructures and medical and nursing staff, and specific problems covering the clinical aspects of the patient on assistance.

General problems

Problems arose within three principle areas of the hospitals' infrastructure: (1) laboratory analyses (microbiology, coagulation, and hematology), (2) intensive care unit, and (3) team lodging condition.

Feasibility, reproducibility, and reliability of a number of laboratory analyses, especially for hemostasis and hemolysis, could not be guaranteed around the clock because of lack of personnel on some shifts, excessive workload, and equipment inadequacy. Laboratory equipment was not always sophisticated enough to perform necessary microbiological tests. The intensive care environment (surface, sterility, and equipment) has been the most serious constraint imposed. Excessive commuting distances between the MT's accommodations and the hospitals, excessive noise, exiguity of the rooms, and inadequate personal services posed problems at a few centers. When the bridging period was longer than 7 days these difficulties became more problematical. In most hospitals, intensive care nursing staffs were limited (one nurse for two or three patients), and their training was not always up to the standard of care required to competently care for a VAD patient. Many times nurses were not informed and trained for an MCSS, and no financial compensation was provided for this specialized work.

With the medical staff we encountered interpersonal and organizational problems such as an insufficient collaboration between the different departments concerning patient management. The lack of cooperation in establishing only one person to coordinate patient care, and sometimes a passive or negative attitude toward our team, created serious obstacles for our work.

Specific problems

A series of specific clinical problems characterized the course of the bridge-to-transplant procedure. In general proper VAD patient selection and timing of the heart transplantation are important for a successful procedure. Sepsis must be incorporated into the exclusion criteria. All patients in our series whose organ function did not recover in spite of hemodynamic stability suffered from sepsis. Clinical optimization of the bridged patients during VAD support is mandatory. During our earlier experience, support was considered as a real bridge where, for fear of device-related complications, patients underwent heart transplantation as soon as a suitable heart was available without regard to their clinical condition. With experience, we increased our knowledge of MCSS patient management, and the VAD was considered as a therapeutical intervention. Heart transplantation was performed only on clinically optimized patients. Our results reflect these different strategies. Survival rate after transplantation was 54% for our early group and 75% for the later group.

Extensive use of BiVAD (34 patients) was justified by a simplified postimplantation period regarding the hemodynamic management. In a few cases, BiVAD was a prophylactic decision to prevent right ventricular failure or major cardiac arrhythmias. Interatrial groove cannulation (29 patients) prevented cannulae crossing inside the pericardial cavity and also prevented the negative effects of the use of extracorporeal circulation in patients with a very poor peripheral perfusion. In very large patients (>2.2 m^2) left inlet cannula length and shape could not ensure a good placement and fixation in the left atrium. In small patients (<1.5 m^2) the support system did not guarantee physiological ranges of hemodynamic parameters; significant systodiastolic difference, low pumping rate compared to age, and high systolic peaks were the major constraints.[5]

No thromboembolic events have been documented. To prevent thromboembolism and minimize thrombus formation we have adopted a strict policy based on improvements made in artificial ventricle washout to avoid blood stagnation, preservation of an adequate intravascular blood volume, thus avoiding dehydration, and a strict anticoagulant regimen.

Concerning infections, a major problem of prosthetic hearts, three points should be stressed: (1) low incidence of mediastinitis (1 patient), (2) no infection from subcutaneous cannulae brought out through the chest wall, (3) very high risk represented by the presence of bacteria in the bloodstream with a high tropism for prosthetic material (*Pseudomonas* species, *Staphylococcus epidermidis*, or *Candida*). In two cases we had a subtotal occlusion of aortic and pulmonary cannulae by vegetation fixed to the Dacron graft.

During VAD assistance, we were impressed by the return of renal function in spite of a very compromised situation (creatinine > 2 mg/dl and anuria). Use of hemodialysis or ultrafiltration in 8 patients (23%) has extended renal recovery for up to 3 weeks without increasing morbidity.

Technical discussion

The discussion will be conducted from two points of view, one related to our side (material and organization) and the other related to the hospital infrastructure with which we had to interface.

Equipment. None of the PDC component failures experienced were life-threatening. However some of them were critical and would probably have been difficult to solve without the support of our excellent engineering team and ancillary personnel. We acquired the original Thoratec PDC in 1983; the first transportable prototype was subsequently designed. Thoratec has since released updated software and a new model of their PDC (Model II).[12] Some of the problems we encountered in the use of those earlier models were resolved with this hardware upgrade.

On delivery of the drive modules, three consistent problems recurred:

1. Unplugging of the electronic print boards. This was easy to isolate and correct, but reoccurred during subsequent system transports. We therefore added a mechanical fixation, thus ensuring immobilization.
2. Loosening of the pneumatic circuitry. We had to redo most of the electropneumatic valves and pneumatic circuitry components to ensure they were airtight.
3. The drive module front panels were arched because of the mechanical assembly. This led to an arching of the attached electronic print board. We remedied this problem by reassembling the mechanical structure of the modules correctly.

Problems appearing during use were:

1. Profound battery discharge (backup power supply of the electronics). This appeared because no "charge only" status was possible and no control of the charge was available without switching on the units. This was changed by Thoratec in the latest PDC versions, and we upgraded our older ones.
2. Drive modules accepting vacuum and pressure inputs from different sources connected in parallel through check-valves that eventually became sticky. The stronger source can then get lost in the others.
3. Current spike on start of the compressor/vacuum unit occasionally disconnecting from the main power 220 V circuit breaker. This was due to the presence of a transformer through which the pump and compressor motors were powered and the way they were connected. We were able to avoid this problem in the transportable PDCs.

The main electrical power source for the electronics was of course 220 V. The only redundancy was given by rechargeable batteries. Main pressure and vacuum sources were provided by compressors and vacuum pumps respectively. These were powered through 220 V only. In the beginning the first redundancy of these sources was the compressed air bottles, with generation of vacuum through a Venturi. A second redundancy was available through the wall pressure for the pressure source only.

Because it was inconvenient for us to travel with many compressed air bottles and it was not possible to refill them locally because of the the nonuniversal connections and related security regulations, we usually moved back and forth from the operating room (OR) to the intensive care unit (ICU) tethered to a long extension cord. In this way, we were able to conserve most of the compressed air in case of a main power failure. Furthermore the original Venturi efficiency was not adequate to obtain a satisfactory vacuum in some patient conditions. In the subsequent prototypes we exchanged the Venturi type for a much more efficient one and connected it so that the wall pressure could also generate vacuum. We then used wall pressure for pressure and vacuum sources with compressed air tanks as a backup. The vacuum in both cases was supplied by the new Venturi model.

The only problem we encountered with our modified transportable PDC was an anomalous heating of the compressor/vacuum pumps assembly after a few weeks of continuous functioning. This was due to the compactness of our construction and obstruction by dust of the filter, through which cooling air is circulating. We remedied this by systematically changing the filters after 1 week of continuous functioning or after each intervention.

The only technical VAD problems we encountered were related to the Hall effect switch detector. This switch is used to pump in the full to empty (volume) mode, which is the usual mode employed after the patient situation is stabilized. In four ventricles the switch ceased to function. We determined that the Hall element wiring was faulty in two ventricles. We were unable to locate the source of error in two VADs. We decided to build an external Hall sensor that can be attached to the ventricle housing and, through appropriate electronics, we can substitute the original switch signal.

Organization. From four to eight of our institute staff have been involved with MT activities. Three participated from the beginning in 1986 until 1990. In a few circumstances, we had two patients on BiVAD at the same time. Apart from the short vacation periods, the MT members were always on call and ready to respond 24 hours/day. This greatly intruded on their private lives and the institute's research activities, in which all the members were equally involved. At one time, we conceptualized forming a specialized professional service team devoted to the institute's VAD program. Many external circumstances did not allow us to realize this idea. In view of the decrease in bridge-to-transplant procedures, we believe this would not have been successful.

Infrastructures. Hospitals with which we interacted often were not specifically designed for cardiac surgery, but were modified from older structures. The main problems we had to face were transport distances between the OR and ICU, and inadequate power (electrical and air pressure) sources. Long distances between the OR and ICU made continuous connection to the main 220 V power supply difficult. Some of the elevators were so small that it was difficult to fit both the patient's bed and the PDC within the limited space. On occasion to succeed, we had to leave the patient on a narrow wheel stretcher and/or had to partially disassemble the PDC. This would not have been possible, of course, with the original model.

Europe is in the process of being unified, but electrical and pneumatic plugs are still not standardized. Electrical connections within the same country, the same hospital, or the same room are often incompatible. The emergency power supply was not always efficient, and it was sometimes tested without any advance notice. This was part of our motivation never to leave the patient in the care of an untrained person.

CONCLUSION

Clinical application of heterotopic VADs for temporary circulatory support has confirmed the hypothesis that prosthetic devices can provide adequate pump flow in a physiological range of hemodynamic parameters. Good vital organ function can be maintained without increasing patient morbidity.

No sophisticated control systems are needed to adjust pump flow to the patient's metabolic needs during the daily routine activities of the patient. Knowledge derived from these clinical applications has been useful for the development of our new implantable cardiac prostheses.

In fact the use of temporary support systems does not solve the problem of the scarcity of organ donors, and efforts should be accomplished in the development of permanent implantable devices as true alternatives to heart transplantation.

The (pneumatic) conception of existing systems is incompatible with long-term survival goals, quality of life, and the patients' security.

ACKNOWLEDGMENT

The experimental work necessary to prepare this activity was greatly supported by the "Fondation Centre de Recherches Médicales Carlos et Elsie de Reuter" (Geneva). We express our gratitude to the entire IRCV team for their continuing support during this period.

REFERENCES

1. Olsen EK, Pierce WS, Donachy JH et al: A two and one half year clinical experience with a mechanical left ventricular assist pump in the treatment of profound postoperative heart failure, *Int J Artif Organs* 4:197, 1979.
2. Richardson PD, Galletti PM, Trudell LA: Performance of the Rhone-Poulenc non-occlusive roller blood pump, *Proceedings 6th New England Bioeng Conf* 3, 1978.
3. Taguchi K, Murashita J, Fukunaga S et al: Preclinical studies on the use of a pulsatile paracorporeal assist device, *Hiroshima J Medical Sciences* 32:367, 1983.
4. Pennington DG, Codd JE, Merjavy JP et al: The expanded use of ventricular bypass sytems for severe cardiac failure and as a bridge to cardiac transplantation, *Heart Transplant* 3:170, 1984.
5. Lichtsteiner M, Meli M, Brugger JP et al: Pulsatile left ventricular assistance in an adolescent: the case for a pediatric-size ventricle, *ASAIO J* 8:186, 1985.
6. Brugger JP, Odermatt R, Meli M et al: Periodic failure and recovery pattern during cardiac assistance procedures, *ASAIO J* 8:182, 1985.
7. Hill JD, Farrar DJ, Hershon JJ et al: Use of a prosthetic ventricle as a bridge to cardiac transplantation for postinfarction cardiogenic shock, *N Engl J Med* 314:626, 1986.
8. Portner PM, Oyer PE, Pennington DG et al: Implantable electrical left ventricular assist system: bridge to transplantation and the future, *Ann Thorac Surg* 47:142, 1989.
9. Galletti PM: Artificial organs: learning to live with risk, *Technology Review, Massachusetts Institute of Technology,* 35, Nov/Dec 1988.
10. Pierce WS, Myers JL, Donachy JH et al: Approaches to the artificial heart, *Surgery* 90:137, 1981.
11. Carpentier A, Brugger JP, Berthier B et al: Heterotopic artificial heart as bridge to cardiac transplantation, *Lancet* 97, 1986 (letters to the editor).
12. The Thoratec Model II Dual Drive Console, Thoratec's *HEARTBEAT* 4.1:1, 1990.

CHAPTER 29

Cardiomyoplasty and skeletal muscle–powered mechanical assistance

Carolyne Desrosiers-Clarke and **Ray C.-J. Chiu**

INTRODUCTION

Although death from heart disease has been declining the last 20 years, the incidence of congestive heart failure continues to rise. When heart failure becomes unresponsive to maximal medical therapy, the only alternatives until now have been transplantation and the use of mechanical substitutes.

Over the years cardiac transplantation has provided outstanding results for patients with end-stage cardiac failure, yet donor organs are available to relatively few patients.[1] The artificial heart program continues to progress at a slow pace. However, complications arising from thromboembolism and infection seem to be major stumbling blocks.[2]

The concept of using skeletal muscle to assist the heart goes back many years. In 1959, Kantrowitz studied the use of the diaphragm as an auxiliary myocardium.[3,4] Since then a number of laboratories worldwide have examined the possibility of using skeletal muscle for cardiac assistance in either the direct or the indirect functional substitution approach. Both dynamic cardiomyoplasty and biomechanical cardiac assist have made considerable progress in recent years. At this point only dynamic cardiomyoplasty is being tested clinically.

Autogenous skeletal muscle cardiac assist has several advantages over other types of mechanical assistance for the failing heart. It does not provoke an immune response. There is also no need for donors and no requirement for awkward external power sources. In addition, autologous skeletal muscle is likely to preserve its potential for growth, which may make it suitable for the correction of complex congenital heart anomalies.

FATIGUE

Progress in the area of skeletal muscle cardiac assist could never have been made without first resolving the two major biological restrictions associated with this concept.

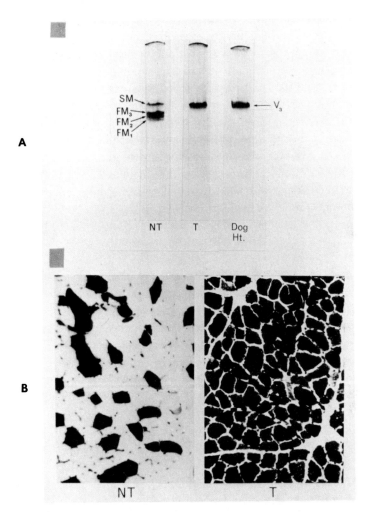

Fig. 29-1. **A,** Gel electrophoresis of myosin isoforms, showing that following transformation, the skeletal muscle myosin isoform becomes identical to that of the myocardium. **B,** Histochemistry (ATPase stain at pH 4.3), showing that mixed Type I (dark color) and Type II (light color) fiber muscle has been transformed into a virtually pure Type I fiber muscle, which is highly fatigue resistant. *NT,* nontransformed canine latissimus dorsi muscle; *T,* transformed canine latissimus dorsi muscle; *Ht,* canine heart muscle. (From Ianuzzo CD et al: Biochemical character of cardiac and transformed canine skeletal muscle. In Chiu RC-J, Bourgeois I, editors: *Transformed muscle for cardiac assist,* Mount Kisco, NY, 1990, Futura Publishing Co.)

The first problem is that skeletal muscle quickly fatigues when stimulated to contract simultaneously with the heart. Most skeletal muscles are composed of a mixture of type I fibers (slow twitch and fatigue resistant) and type II fibers (fast twitch and fatigue prone). Type II fibers are also highly anaerobic and their biochemical apparatus is geared for rapid, strong contractions rather than for sustained repetitive contractions.

The solution to the problem of skeletal muscle fatigue can be traced back to the work of Buller et al. in 1960.[5] Their cross-innervation experiments established the fact that the composition of fiber types in a fully developed skeletal muscle can be altered, introducing the concept of the "plasticity of muscles."

Subsequent studies by Salmons,[6] Pette,[7] and others led to the technique of transforming the skeletal muscle into a highly fatigue-resistant, purely type I fiber muscle using low-frequency electrical stimulation. Since then, extensive molecular and functional studies have been done to clarify and characterize the phenomenon of skeletal muscle transformation and its use in cardiac assist[8-12] (Fig. 29-1).

POWER OUTPUT

Another problem with using skeletal muscle for cardiac assist is related to the difference in the way the muscle responds to a single pulse of electrical stimulation. The heart, which is a syncytial tissue, contracts in an all-or-none fashion. Once the electrical current strength reaches the threshold level, the entire myocardium contracts with full force and in a sustained manner. In contrast the skeletal muscle, even following transformation, is composed of many individual motor units, and a single electrical impulse often depolarizes only a number of those motor units with only limited contractile force and duration.

Many investigators have attempted to find ways of generating greater power from skeletal muscle in response to electrical stimulation. Sponitz in the 1970s demonstrated that enough power can be generated from a skeletal muscle when burst stimuli were applied instead of a single electric pulse.[13] However, it was also recognized that the resulting tetanic contraction, although extremely powerful, produces rapid fatigue and subsequent loss of power within a short period of time.

In the late 1970s our laboratory proposed that a well-defined pulse train falling within a specific segment of the cardiac cycle may both augment the power output and at the same time prevent the rapid onset of fatigue in a skeletal muscle. In 1980 Drinkwater, reported on the first synchronizable burst stimulator.[14] It was determined that the sequential addition of stimulations in short pulse trains caused summation of twitches of the skeletal muscle. This augmented the force and duration of the muscle contraction without inducing fatigue.

Using this principle of summation our laboratory developed a stimulator that combines a component with R-wave sensitivity and its own delay and refractory period with a second component that functions as a pulse generator, able to multiply the simple pacer spike output from the first component into pulse trains of widely varying frequencies, pulse widths, pulse train durations, and morphologies.

ELECTRICAL STIMULATORS FOR SKELETAL MUSCLE CARDIAC ASSIST

The electrical stimulators for muscle-powered cardiac assist devices consist of a combination of features found in dual chamber pacemakers. They basically require output synchronized to sensed cardiac activity and a burst of pulses for skeletal muscle stimulation.

SP1005

The Cardiomyostimulator Pulse Train Generator (Medtronic, model SP1005) is an implantable stimulator that includes a sensing and a pacing channel. An electronic circuit synchronizes the stimulation of skeletal muscle contraction with the cardiac contraction after a programmed delay (4 to 250 msec). The system also determines the heart:muscle ratio (i.e., 1:1, 2:1, 3:1) depending on the mode selected and the heart rate. In atrioventricular block the system automatically acts as a cardiac pacemaker.

Pulse generator programming is achieved by radio-frequency telemetry. Battery life can be monitored by the same procedure, and pulse generator inhibition is possible by using an external magnet.[15]

The limitations of the Cardiomyostimulator became apparent following our laboratory's experience with the dual-chamber counterpulsator. The stimulator, which could be initially programmed to fire during cardiac diastole, became off phase and started to interfere with systolic unloading when the heart rate changed. It was then clear that a more versatile stimulator would be required because any augmentation of the aortic pressure during systole would be detrimental to the heart because it further increased the cardiac afterload.[16]

Prometheus

Biomechanical cardiac assistance by counterpulsation requires sustained muscle contraction during the period of the heart's diastole.[17] As a consequence stimulation of the skeletal muscle must be sustained for a period close to the duration of diastole using a burst of impulses. As heart systolic and diastolic times decrease with an increase in heart rate, the time of onset of muscle stimulation (time from QRS detection to onset of burst or synchronization delay) and the burst duration need to be adjusted when such variations in heart rate arise. This can be achieved by calculating the synchronization delay as a percentage of the previous cardiac cycle length. The burst duration should also adapt with the cardiac period. Muscle contraction would thus be inhibited when premature ventricular contractions occur. This requires accurate ventricular sensing, even during the muscle stimulation bursts.

A new, highly versatile microprocessor-based stimulator named "Prometheus" has recently been tested in our laboratory. The unit has a built-in microcomputer that is programmed through telemetry with software operated on an IBM-compatible personal computer. In our study,[18] software developed by Medtronic in collaboration with us for synchronized counterpulsation was programmed into the stimulator. It allows pulse burst stimulation of the muscle, synchronized to the cardiac R-wave. Timing for onset of delay of the pulse burst and its duration period is adjusted automatically by the stimulator, according to the varying R-R interval that occurs with heart rate changes. In addition, adjustment of the pulse voltage, frequency, and assist ratio can be easily made on the personal computer and sent via telemetry. A safety feature available with this pulse generator is an automatic shutdown of stimulation should sustained cardiac arrhythmias occur.

DYNAMIC CARDIOMYOPLASTY

Dynamic cardiomyoplasty is a relatively new surgical procedure in which a transformed, fatigue-resistant skeletal muscle is wrapped around the heart and electronically stimulated to contract in systole with the heart. This process increases the ventricular function of a failing heart.

The idea of using skeletal muscle to replace or repair a damaged myocardium can be traced back to the experiments of Leriche in 1933.[19] By 1966 Petrovsky of the USSR had reported on his experience using the diaphragm to repair cardiac aneurysms in 100 patients.[20] However, it was not until 1985 that the first clinical case of "dynamic cardiomyoplasty" was successfully performed by Carpentier and his associates[21] in Paris. They applied a latissimus dorsi muscle graft to the ventricular surface and stimulated it with a cardiac pacemaker to contract in synchrony with the heart. Experimental studies leading to the clinical application of dynamic cardiomyoplasty were carried out in our own laboratories and a number of others.[17,22,23]

Surgical technique

In our clinical series the surgical procedure for dynamic cardiomyoplasty is performed in two stages.[24,25] First the patient is placed in the right lateral decubitus position with the left arm elevated. A longitudinal incision extending from the axilla to the iliac crest over the lateral border of the latissimus dorsi muscle is made. The latissimus dorsi muscle is then dissected and freed from its insertions in the vertebrae, ribs, and iliac crest. The humeral tendon is also cut to prevent possible arm movements during electrostimulation of the muscle. The thoracodorsal neurovascular pedicle is preserved.

To stimulate the latissimus dorsi muscle, two intramuscular pacing electrodes (Medtronic SP5528, Medtronic, Minneapolis, Minn.) are implanted. These electrodes are woven into the muscle near the trifurcation of the thoracodorsal nerve for the negative electrode. Another electrode is woven 6 to 8 cm distally through the width of the muscle as the positive electrode. This configuration leaves the middle and distal portions, which will be wrapped around the heart, free of electrodes. It also provides for the preservation of the nerve and vascular branches, while providing a diffuse stimulation of the muscle flap.

Following the closure of this wound, the patient is turned to the supine position and a sternal splitting incision is made. Unless additional procedures are required, the cardiopulmonary bypass machine is left on standby and is rarely used. In anticipation of the need to supplement the cardiac wrap with a piece of pericardium, a reversed C-shaped pericardial flap is made in front of the right ventricle, which is hinged to the pericardium near the right phrenic nerve. The remaining pericardium is widely opened, and the left latissimus dorsi muscle is retrieved from the pleural cavity.

The muscle is then wrapped around the heart using the "no cardiac suture" technique.[26] Two stay sutures on the edge of the muscle flap are transfixed, one at the posterior pericardium near the left border of the pulmonary valve and the other in the posterior pericardium near the junction of the inferior vena cava and the right atrium. These sutures align the edge of the muscle to the posterior atrioventricular groove of the left ventricle. The remainder of the muscle is turned around the apex and approximated to the anterior and lateral borders of the heart with interrupted sutures.

In many patients with large hearts, the outflow tract of the right ventricle cannot be fully covered by the muscle graft, for which the previously developed pericardial flap is used to anchor the muscle edge, so that a 360-degree wrap can be accomplished (Fig. 29-2).

There are a number of variations of this wrapping technique. At present there is no definitive data in patients to establish the superiority of different fiber orientations used. In some patients partial rather than total wrap of the heart has been carried out, particularly to reinforce the left ventricle following venticular aneurysmectomy or resection of cardiac tumors.[21,27]

Long-term synchronization between the heart and the latissimus dorsi muscle is ensured by a sensing electrode placed in the epicardium or transvenously into the right ventricular endocardium. Both the sensing and stimulating electrodes are then connected to the Cardiomyostimulator, which in turn is placed in a subfascial pocket in the upper abdomen.

Postoperative management

Following 2 weeks of vascular delay (to allow the muscle flap to recover from ischemia associated with its mobilization), gradual working transformation of the muscle graft is carried out. Clinical and laboratory evaluations are then periodically performed according to established protocols.

Successful outcome of the cardiomyoplasty procedure in patients with poor ventricular function depends not only on the skills of the surgical team, but also on the availability of excellent anesthesia. It is important to avoid hypoxia because the left lung can be partially compressed by the graft and to prevent tachyarrhythmia when the heart

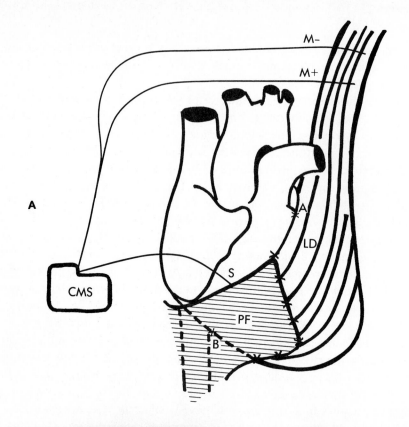

A

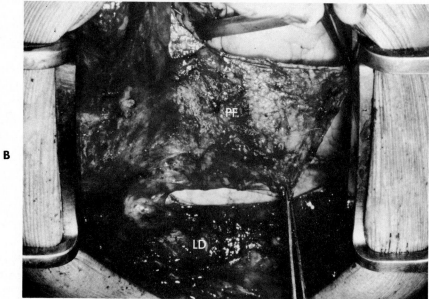

B

Fig. 29-2. For legend see opposite page.

is elevated to introduce the muscle flap behind the heart. Inotropes may be required during and immediately after the operation. Optimal medical support in collaboration with cardiologists is essential because the patients do not benefit from the dynamic cardiomyoplasty during vascular delay and the early phase of muscle transformation.

Clinical update

The most comprehensive data available have been compiled by Medtronic Inc. and reported by Grandjean.[28] The data were based on 78 patients who have been studied according to a specific protocol. Four of these cases had predominantly right heart failure, mostly in pediatric patients. Of the 74 patients operated on for left heart failure, 50% had ischemic cardiomyopathy and 34.6% had idiopathic cardiomyopathy. In this series, 55 patients, or 74%, received dynamic cardiomyoplasty with or without other concomitant operations. Most patients preoperatively were in functional class III or IV, with left ventricular ejection fraction ranging from 9% to 35% by radionucleotide scans. The average follow-up duration was 8.2 months, ranging from 0 to 32.8 months. The operative mortality was strongly related to the preoperative status of the patients. For those in preoperative New York Heart Association (NYHA) class IV, the early postoperative death rate was 33%, whereas for those in preoperative class III, the early death rate was less than half, 12%.

The most significant change noted in surviving patients, which was 60% overall and 81% in the subgroup of patients with class III functional status preoperative, is the improvement in NYHA functional classification. Of the 19 surviving patients with preoperative NYHA class IV, 50% attained class II status. In comparison, of the 20 surviving patients with preoperative class III status, 50% became class I, and 40% moved into class II. Altogether, 85% of the surviving patients improved in their NYHA functional class.

Today more than 150 patients have undergone the cardiomyoplasty procedure worldwide. Most of the hospital survivors have improved at least one NYHA functional class for heart failure; this improvement seems to be sustained for at least a couple of years.[28]

It is unclear at this point how cardiomyoplasty benefits these patients. In many, despite symptomatic improvement, hemodynamic changes have not been detected. Significant improvements in both hemodynamics and symptoms have been observed, however, in others.

Fig. 29-2. A, Schematic illustration of our surgical technique for dynamic cardiomyoplasty. *LD,* latissimus dorsi muscle; *PF,* pericardial flap; *CMS,* cardiomyostimulator; *S,* sensing electrode; *M−* and *M+*, negative and positive muscle stimulating electrodes. *A* and *B* are anchoring sutures in the posterior pericardium to fix the *LD* along the posterior atrioventricular groove. Anteriorly, the edge of the *LD* is anchored to the *PF* if the *LD* is not sufficiently large to encircle both ventricles. **B,** Operative picture just before sutures are placed to anchor *LD* to *PF.*

The mechanism of action of cardiomyoplasty will most likely be better understood in the near future as chronic heart failure animal models are developed with this procedure. At this time, there are no good chronic heart failure models in which cardiomyoplasty has been used. However, progress is being made in this area.

Dynamic cardiomyoplasty has moved rapidly from laboratory investigation to clinical trial. With improvements in the criteria for case selection and refinement of the surgical techniques, this operation can be carried out in patients with severe ventricular dysfunction with acceptable mortality. In surviving patients, gradual but significant functional improvements in quality of life have been observed. Further documentation of the functional improvements with concrete scientific data, such as maximum exercise capacity and oxygen consumption, are needed to understand the mechanism of improvement and to confirm the benefit of this operation.

MUSCLE-POWERED CARDIAC ASSIST DEVICES

The other application of skeletal muscle cardiac assist has been to use the skeletal muscle as a separate pump. In some cases the skeletal muscle is wrapped around the aorta. As the skeletal muscle contracts, it compresses the aorta. The skeletal muscle can also be wrapped around a mechanical device. As the skeletal muscle contracts, it causes fluid or blood to be pumped. In other cases, the skeletal muscle has been configured into a skeletal muscle ventricle and used directly as a blood pump.

Counterpulsation

The mechanism of counterpulsation to assist a failing heart was well-elucidated in the 1960s. The intraaortic balloon pump (IABP) has become the most extensively used form of circulatory assist. The physiological benefit of counterpulsation derives from the favorable balance between myocardial oxygen supply and demand through diastolic augmentation and systolic unloading.[29,30] The purpose of counterpulsation is to reduce systolic cardiac afterload and thus reduce the myocardial oxygen consumption. During

---

Fig. 29-3. A, Dual chamber counterpulsation device. In the blood pump, hydraulic fluid collapses Biomer membrane to eject 30 ml of blood during cardiac diastole, raising diastolic blood pressure. The blood pump consists of 10-mm Dacron graft (*a*), reduction plates (*b*), a flexible, thromboresistant Biomer membrane (*c*), a perforated inner casing (*d*), and 1-cm Neoprene tubing (*e*). Percutaneous Portacath (*f*) enables adjustment of resting volume and pressure in the hydraulic bulb (*g*). The 150-ml Biomer hydraulic bulb provides muscle stretch (*h*) during cardiac systole. **B,** Counterpulsation achieved with this device; *AP,* aortic pressure; *LVP,* left ventricular pressure. Arrow indicates diastolic augmentation. This device is activated at 2:1 ratio to the heart rate. (From Kochamba G, Desrosiers C, Dewar ML et al: *Ann Thorac Surg* 45:620, 1988.)

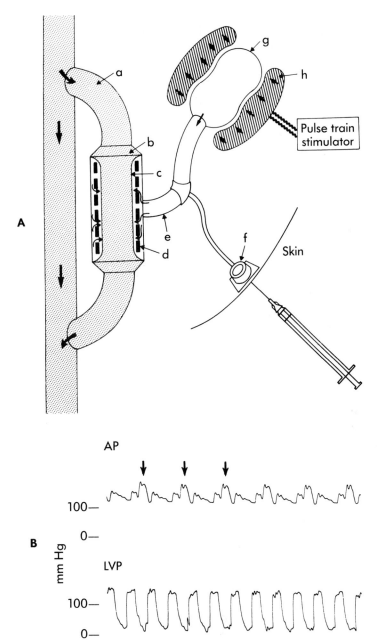

Fig. 29-3. For legend see opposite page.

diastole, the aortic pressure is augmented, which increases coronary blood flow and enhances myocardial oxygen supply. This is reflected *hemodynamically* in the increase in the diastolic pressure time product over the tension time index (DPTP/TTI) ratio. This results in greater myocardial recovery from ischemic insults, and consequently reduces the ventricular filling pressure and increases the cardiac output.

Counterpulsation does not require a device to generate unidirectional blood flow. It produces a back and forth displacement of a volume of blood approximating that of the stroke volume, timed precisely with the cardiac cycle to achieve the desired effects. Since it is not required to provide a unidirectional flow, there is no need for cardiac valves, which recent experiences have shown to be a frequent source of thromboembolism in various types of cardiac assist devices and artificial hearts.

IABP counterpulsation still remains one of the most effective modes of temporary cardiac assistance. However, blood biomaterial phase interaction, infection, and secondary thromboembolic complications limit the use of the IABP as a permanent or chronic mode of circulatory assistance.

Our laboratory therefore proceeded to study the following hypothesis: a skeletal muscle, stimulated with burst impulses and properly synchronized during cardiac diastole, should be able to produce an increase in the DPTP/TTI ratio comparable with those obtainable with the IABP.

Dual-chamber counterpulsator

Kochamba et al. in 1987 constructed a prototype "dual-chamber" counterpulsator (Fig. 29-3).[31] This rheologically superior implantable cardiac assist device consists of a blood pump with a Dacron graft at each end and is anastomosed end-to-side and parallel to the thoracic aorta, allowing continuous blood flow to minimize thrombus formation caused by stasis and turbulence. The blood pump is powered by a hydraulic bulb placed beneath the latissimus dorsi muscle, which is stimulated to contract during diastole using a synchronized burst electrical stimulator. This "dual-chamber" counterpulsator, which was totally implantable, proved to be hemodynamically effective, augmenting the DPTP/TTI ratio by approximately 50%.

A number of advantages associated with this configuration were also apparent. Because the hydraulic system can efficiently transmit the power, the blood chamber design may no longer be confirmed by the accessibility of the skeletal muscle to be used as the power source. In other words any suitable muscle can be used to generate power and the energy produced can be transmitted by the hydraulic system to where it can be employed for circulatory assist. This eliminates the extensive mobilization of the muscle and reduces interference to the collateral blood supply to the muscle. The advantage is to prevent the early postoperative ischemia of the muscular flap that had been noted by other investigators. As a result the strategy of "vascular delay" that was needed to address this problem can be eliminated, and the skeletal muscle–powered cardiac assist device can be immediately activated on implantation.

Aortomyoplasty

Another approach in biomechanical cardiac assist is the use of electrostimulated skeletal muscle in an extravascular position. Aortomyoplasty is a surgical procedure that consists of wrapping a latissimus dorsi pedicled graft around the aorta to compress it. The aim of dynamic aortomyoplasty is to create a new hemocompatible contractile chamber from the aorta. Studies have been carried out wrapping both the ascending and the descending aorta.

Dynamic aortomyoplasty was initially attempted by Kantrowitz in 1960. He was able to significantly augment diastolic pressure by wrapping a diaphragm muscle graft around the distal aorta and using an appropriately timed stimulation during diastole.[3,4] The disadvantages of this model include the risk of paraplegia caused by the interruption of the intercostal blood vessels.

More recently, Chachques et al. enlarged the native ascending aorta using an autologous pericardial patch to turn it into a ventricular chamber.[32] They then wrapped it with a latissimus dorsi muscle flap electrostimulated in a counterpulsation manner. The left ventricular afterload is thus more effectively decreased, and the counterpulsation is carried out at the vicinity of the coronary artery ostia.

The advantages of dynamic aortomyoplasty using the ascending aorta are (1) it avoids paraplegia due to spinal cord ischemia; and (2) it benefits from the larger diameter of the ascending aorta, which provides a larger volume of blood.[33] However, the creation of an iatrogenic aneurysm of the ascending aorta is of concern because the aorta may continue to dilate due to the effect of Laplace's law. Further chronic studies are needed to ensure its safety and its efficacy in cardiac assist.

Periaortic counterpulsation

To circumvent the problems of the blood biomaterial interface and to avoid the disadvantages of aortomyoplasty our laboratory is evaluating a method of periaortic balloon compression.[34] This model consists of fitting a segment of polyvinyl tubing snugly around the descending thoracic aorta. A 40 cc intraaortic balloon is slipped between the aortic wall and tubing, preserving the intercostal vessels. Significant diastolic augmentation and systolic unloading were observed, using both the IABP console and the skeletal muscle (latissimus dorsi) as a power source.

This avoids the potential complications that may arise from aortomyoplasty such as paraplegia or aneurysmal dilatation. Our approach also circumvents the thromboembolic risks of the blood biomaterial interface and may pave the way toward the development of a permanent implantable circulatory assist device.

Skeletal muscle ventricles

One of the methods of muscle-powered cardiac assist involves the construction of skeletal muscle ventricles (SMVs) or pouches that act as separate pumps connected to the circulation. SMVs have been constructed from a number of different muscles.[17] The latissimus dorsi seems to be ideal because it is a large, powerful, and nonessential muscle. After dissection, the muscle is wrapped in a spiral fashion around a conically shaped Teflon mandrel. Following an appropriate period of vascular delay for muscle recovery and for development of collateral blood vessels, the Teflon mandrel can be removed and the SMV can be connected to the circulation or to a mock circulation device for testing. A 6 week period of continuous electrical stimulation has been shown to transform practically all of the muscle fibers into the slow twitch, fatigue resistant type.

Macoviak and Bridges have now used SMVs to support the right-sided circulation.[35,36,37] In a series of acute studies, SMVs were capable of supporting the pulmonary circulation for many hours. Although SMVs supply enough power to replace the right ventricle, thromboembolic complications at low pressures encountered on the right side of the heart have hampered the development of a chronic model of right heart bypass.

Acker et al. tested SMV work output over several weeks with a totally implantable mock circulation device[38,39] and went on to develop the first model where the SMV pumped blood chronically in the circulation.[40] The SMVs were stimulated during diastole using an R-wave synchronous burst stimulator. Good diastolic augmentation was achieved in all animals, with one surviving 11 weeks. Unfortunately the animals suffered from continuous thromboembolic events originating from the SMVs, which caused multiple infarctions of the kidneys, resulting in renal failure.

A recent configuration using biological membrane (e.g., pericardium) as the lining for the SMV was successful in achieving good diastolic augmentation without such complications.[39] In a few long-term survivors, SMVs pumped blood effectively into the circulation for over 6 months. One dog continues to do well 16 months after connecting its SMV to the circulation.[41]

Right heart counterpulsation

Right ventricular (RV) failure is a complex entity capable of limiting overall cardiac performance.[42] It is commonly encountered in congenital heart disease and is being more frequently reported as the number of patients receiving cardiac assist increases, particularly in those with elevated pulmonary vascular resistance.[43] Therapeutic surgical intervention has ranged from pulmonary artery balloon counterpulsation to complete RV support with ventricular assist devices.[44-46] Because these modes of therapy all require continued tethering to external power sources, they are not ideal for chronic RV support. Most of the past work in the area of skeletal muscle–powered circulatory assist has focused on efforts to assist the systemic circulation with limited experience on the pulmonic side.

In our laboratory Li et al.[34] evaluated the feasibility and efficacy of pulmonary artery counterpulsation with skeletal muscle power in a pulmonary hypertension model. We did indeed find that effective PA counterpulsation can be obtained with a skeletal muscle power source. The degree of RV unloading correlated positively with the PA systolic pressures. Therefore skeletal muscle–powered PA counterpulsation can provide an alternative chronic implantable system for RV failure associated with pulmonary hypertension.

Patient management

The care of patients who receive skeletal muscle–powered cardiac assist would require a team effort, consisting of a cardiac surgeon, cardiologist, anesthesiologist, and critical care and cardiovascular nurses. In dynamic cardiomyoplasty patients the symptoms associated with severe heart failure will not be ameliorated immediately after operation, and intensive medical therapy aimed at stabilizing hemodynamics and combating arrhythmias will be needed. Since most of these patients may not require cardiopulmonary bypass, certain risks associated with extracorporeal circulation, such as postoperative hemorrhage, may occur less frequently. On the other hand, the presence of a large muscle mass in the left chest cavity can further compromise respiratory function in those with limited lung capacity, and thus require optimization of respiratory care.

Arrhythmia is common in patients who require cardiomyoplasty. Close monitoring and aggressive medical management of arrhythmias are important, not only in the perioperative period, but also throughout the patients' clinical course. Because of the many electrical leads and burst stimulators implanted, infection would be a particularly serious complication in such cases. The surgical dissection to free the latissimus dorsi muscle from its anatomical site creates a large skin flap in the back of the patient, and even with appropriate drainage of the subcutaneous space, seroma almost inevitably develops after this operation. Evacuation of the seroma is needed only when the collection is considerable. Tapping of the seroma should be undertaken only with the use of strict aseptic technique. The long-term monitoring of the burst stimulator function is similar to those required for ordinary pacemakers, and personnel familiar with programming these stimulators should be available.

Muscle-powered cardiac assist devices are still in the laboratory experimental stage. Therefore the clinical patient management issues cannot be fully foreseen at this time because the optimal devices and configurations for such assists to be applied to patients have not evolved. It is expected that the patient management protocols will be developed in parallel with progress in this field.

CONCLUSION

The ability to induce fatigue resistance in the skeletal muscle and the feasibility of modulating its power output with a modern electronic stimulator have ushered in the new approach of skeletal muscle–powered cardiac assist in recent years. Dynamic cardiomyoplasty is currently undergoing clinical trials, and muscle-powered assist devices continue to make progress in an increasing number of laboratories. If successful, a new approach will be added to the management of intractable heart failure in the future.

REFERENCES

1. Heck CF, Shumway SJ, Kaye MP: The Registry of the International Society for Heart Transplanation: Sixth Official Report—1989, *J Heart Transplant* 8:271, 1989.
2. Pae WE, Miller CA, Pierce WS: Combined registry for the clinical use of mechanical ventricular assist pumps and the total artificial heart: third official report—1988, *J Heart Transplant* 8:277, 1989.
3. Kantrowitz A, McKinnon W: The experimental use of the diaphragm as an auxiliary myocardium, Surg Forum 9:266, 1959.
4. Kantrowitz A: Functioning autogenous muscle used experimentally as an auxiliary ventricle, *Trans Am Soc Artif Intern Organs* 6:305, 1960.
5. Buller AJ, Eccles JC, Eccles RM: Interaction between motor neurons and muscles in respect to the characteristic speeds of their responses, *J Physiol* 150:417, 1960.
6. Salmons S, Sreter FA: Significance of impulse activity in the transformation of skeletal muscle type, *Nature* 263:30, 1976.
7. Pette D, Staudte HW, Vrbova G: Physiological and biochemical changes induced by long-term stimulation of fast muscle, *Naturwissenschaften* 59:469, 1972.
8. Ianuzzo CD, Hamilton N, O'Brien PJ et al: Biochemical transformation of canine skeletal muscle for use in cardiac assist devices, *J Appl Physiol* 68:1481, 1990.
9. Odim JNK, Li C, Desrosiers C et al: The remodelling of skeletal muscle for indefatigable hemodynamic work, *Can J Physiol Pharmacol* 69:230, 1991.
10. Kochamba G, Chiu RC-J: The physiologic characteristics of transformed skeletal muscle for cardiac assist, *ASAIO Trans* 10:404, 1987.
11. Brister S, Fradet G, Dewar M et al: Transforming skeletal muscle for myocardial assist: a feasibility study, *Can J Surg* 28:341, 1985.
12. Walsh GL, Dewar ML, Khalafalla AS et al: Characteristics of transformed fatigue resistant skeletal muscle for long-term cardiac assist by extra-aortic balloon counterpulsation, *Surg Forum* 37:205, 1986.
13. Sponitz HM, Merker C, Malm JR: Applied physiology of the canine rectus abdominis, *Trans Am Soc Artif Intern Organs* 20:747, 1974.
14. Drinkwater D, Chiu RC-J, Modry D et al: Cardiac assist and myocardial repair with synchronously stimulated skeletal muscle, *Surg Forum* 31:271, 1980.
15. Grandjean PA, Herpers L, Smits KF et al: Implantable electronics and leads for muscular cardiac assistance. In R C-J Chiu, editor: *Biomechanical cardiac assist: cardiomyoplasty and muscle powered devices,* Mount Kisco, NY, 1986, Futura Publishing Co.
16. Desrosiers C, Neilson I, Walsh G et al: Skeletal muscle-powered counterpulsator. In R C-J Chiu, IM Bourgeois, editors: *Transformed muscle for cardiac assist and repair,* Mount Kisco, NY, 1990, Futura Publishing Co.
17. Chiu RC-J, editor: *Biomechanical cardiac assist: cardiomyoplasty and muscle powered devices,* Mount Kisco, NY, 1986, Futura Publishing Co.
18. Li CM, Hill A, Colson M et al: Implantable rate-responsive counterpulsation assist system, *Ann Thorac Surg* 49:356, 1990.
19. Leriche R: Essai experimentale de traitement de certains infarctus du myocarde et de l'aneurysme du coeur par une graffe de muscle strie, *Bull Soc Nat Chir* 59:229, 1933.
20. Petrovsky BV: Surgical treatment of cardiac aneurysms. *J Cardiovasc Surg* 7:87, 1966.
21. Carpentier A, Chachques JC: Myocardial substitution with a stimulated skeletal muscle: first successful clinical case, *Lancet* 8440:1267, 1985.
22. Mannion JD, Stephenson LW: Potential uses of skeletal muscle for myocardial assistance, *Surg Clin North Am* 65:679, 1985.
23. Chiu RC-J, Bourgeois I, editors: *Transformed muscle for cardiac assist and repair,* Mount Kisco, NY, 1990, Futura Publishing Co.
24. Carpentier A, Chachques JC: Clinical cardiomyoplasty: method and outcome, *Semin Thorac Cardiovasc Surg* 3(2):136, 1991.
25. Chiu RC-J: Dynamic cardiomyoplasty: an overview, *Pace* 14:577, 1991.
26. Chachques JC, Grandjean PA, Carpentier A: Latissimus dorsi dynamic cardiomyoplasty, *Ann Thorac Surg* 47:600, 1989.

27. Magovern GJ, Heckler FR, Park SB: Paced skeletal muscle for dynamic cardiomyoplasty, *Ann Thorac Surg* 45:614, 1988.
28. Grandjean P, Austin L, Chan S et al: Dynamic cardiomyoplasty: clinical follow-up results, *J Card Surg* 6:80, 1991.
29. Weber KT, Janicki JS: Intraaortic balloon counterpulsation, *Ann Thorac Surg* 17:602, 1974.
30. Powell WJ, Daggett WM, Magro AE et al: Effects of intraaortic balloon counterpulsation on cardiac performance, oxygen consumption, and coronary blood flow in dogs, *Circ Res* 26:753, 1970.
31. Kochamba G, Desrosiers C, Dewar ML et al: The muscle powered dual-chamber counterpulsator: rheologically superior implantable cardiac assist device, *Ann Thorac Surg* 45:620, 1988.
32. Chachques JC, Grandjean PA, Fischer EL et al: Dynamic aortomyoplasty to assist left ventricular failure, *Ann Thorac Surg* 49:225, 1990.
33. Chachques JC, Grandjean PA, Carpentier A: Dynamic aortomyoplasty. In Carpentier A, Chachques JC, and Grandjean P, editors: *Cardiomyoplasty,* Mount Kisco, NY, 1991, Futura Publishing Co.
34. Li C, Odim J, Zibaitis A et al: Pulmonary artery counterpulsation with a skeletal muscle power source, *ASAIO Trans* 36:M382, 1990.
35. Bridges Jr CR, Hammond RL, Dimeo F et al: Functional right heart replacement with skeletal muscle ventricles, *Circ* 80(suppl. III):183, 1989.
36. Macoviak JA, Stinson EB, Starkey TD et al: Myoventriculoplasty and neoventricle myograft cardiac augmentation to establish pulmonary blood flow: preliminary observations and feasibility studies, *J Thorac Cardiovasc Surg* 93:212, 1987.
37. Bridges Jr CR, Woodford BA, Mora G et al: Use of skeletal muscle power to augment the pulmonary circulation, *Surg Forum* 41:267, 1990.
38. Acker MA, Hammond RL, Mannion JD et al: An autologous biologic pump motor, *J Thorac Cardiovasc Surg* 92:733, 1986.
39. Acker MA, Hammond RL, Mannion JD et al: Skeletal muscle as the potential power source for a cardiovascular pump: assessment in vivo, *Science* 236:324, 1987.
40. Acker MA, Anderson WA, Hammond RL et al: Skeletal muscle ventricles in circulation: one to eleven weeks' experience, *J Thorac Cardiovasc Surg* 94:163, 1987.
41. Pochettino A, Anderson DR, Hammond RL et al: Skeletal muscle ventricles: a promising treatment option for heart failure, *J Card Surg* 6(1) (suppl.):145, 1991.
42. Cohn JN, Guiha NH, Broder MI et al: Right ventricular infarction—clinical hemodynamic features, *Am J Cardiol* 33:209, 1974.
43. Sato N, Mohri H, Miura M et al: Right ventricular failure during clinical use of a left ventricular assist device, *Trans Am Soc Artif Intern Organs* 35:550, 1989.
44. Dembitsky WP, Daily PO, Raney AA et al: Temporary extracorporeal support of the right ventricle, *J Thorac Cardiovasc Surg* 91:518, 1986.
45. Flege Jr JB, Wright CB, Reisinger TJ: Successful balloon counterpulsation for right ventricular failure, *Ann Thorac Surg* 37:167, 1984.
46. Symbas PN, McKeown PP, Sentora AH et al: Pulmonary artery balloon counterpulsation for treatment of intraoperative right ventricular failure, *Ann Thorac Surg* 39:437, 1985.

Index

ISBN 0-8016-6442-X

90000>

9 780801 664427